DATE DUE

PRINCIPLES OF
SEATING
THE DISABLED

Editor

R. Mervyn Letts, M.D., M.Sc., FRCSC

Surgeon-in-Chief
Children's Hospital of Eastern Ontario
and
Professor of Orthopedic Surgery
University of Ottawa
Ottawa, Ontario, Canada

CRC Press
Boca Raton Ann Arbor Boston London

Library of Congress Cataloging-in-Publication Data

Principles of seating the disabled / editor, R. Mervyn Letts.
      p.   cm.
   Includes bibliographical references and index.
   ISBN 0-8493-6021-8
   1. Wheelchairs. 2. Physically handicapped. 3. Seating
(Furniture) I. Letts, R. Mervyn.
RD757.W4P75   1991
617.1′03—dc20   91-11940
                                              CIP

Direct all inquiries to CRC Press, Inc., 2000 Corporate Blvd., N.W., Boca Raton, Florida 33431.

© 1991 by CRC Press, Inc.

International Standard Book Number 0-8493-6021-8

Library of Congress Card Number 91-11940

Printed in the United States of America   1 2 3 4 5 6 7 8 9 0

PREFACE

A textbook on seating would have been almost unthinkable even a decade ago! In North America, specialized seating clinics were almost unheard of in the 1960s. The Ontario Crippled Children's Centre in Toronto, the Rehabilitation Centre for Children in Winnipeg, the University of Tennessee in Memphis, the Gillette Children's Hospital in Minneapolis, and the University of British Columbia in Vancouver were early pioneering centers in the struggle to address some of the difficult seating dilemmas and in the constant search to improve the materials and construction of the wheelchair to address the needs of handicapped users. The concept of fabricating the wheelchair to address the needs of the physically disabled gradually replaced the concept of trying to fit these individuals into so-called "standard off-the-shelf wheelchairs". The late 1970s and early 1980s saw centers of seating excellence spring up initially in numerous American and Canadian centers often associated with children's rehabilitation units and gradually, by the mid 1980s, many seating clinics were addressing the geriatric requirements.

Most textbooks addressing the seating issue have been devoted primarily to a few aspects of seating, i.e., looking at the problem from primarily engineering, therapy, or orthotic points of view. The purpose of this book is to try to amalgamate, in a multidisciplined manner, all the professional contributors to a good seating program. Emphasis has been given to the importance of prophylactic positioning in the wheelchair as a means of controlling and aborting deformities secondary to poor positioning in the wheelchair. The judicious melding of therapy, orthotics, rehabilitation engineering, physiatry, and orthopedic surgery has been stressed to ensure that the particular seating problem presented to the seating clinic can be properly addressed and corrected and hopefully, with good stable seating, prevented from recurring.

The recent technological advances in wheelchair design, communication devices, and neurosurgical techniques such as segmental stabilization of the spine and posterior rhizotomy have been discussed in terms of their contribution to the enhancement of the wheelchair user. Throughout the text the multidisciplined approach that has been so successful in most seating clinics has received perhaps excessive emphasis, but it is the key to a successful seating program. The more recent design of lightweight powered chairs, as well as the numerous varieties of sports wheelchairs, has added a new dimension for the physically handicapped, allowing much greater freedom and independence.

It is hoped that the reader will develop a different mind-set toward the needs of the physically handicapped during their wheelchair existence. The wheelchair person must be considered almost in the same light as an ambulatory individual who may have a particular problem with gait. In a similar vein, the seated person in a wheelchair who is developing pelvic obliquity, sacral sitting, or postural imbalance secondary to scoliosis demands the same approach to attain a stable sitting posture as does the ambulatory person with a dysfunctional abnormal gait.

It is hoped that this book will allow the various professional groups to appreciate the contributions of each others' professions in attaining the common goal of comfortable seating for the physically disabled and that all professions will respect the input and counsel from the wheelchair users themselves as well as their families and caregivers. If the text achieves only this last objective for most of the readership, it will, in my opinion, have succeeded!

R. Mervyn Letts
Ottawa, Ontario, Canada

THE EDITOR

R. Mervyn Letts, M.D., M.Sc., FRCSC, is Professor of Surgery, University of Ottawa, and Surgeon-in-Chief of the Children's Hospital of Eastern Ontario, Ottawa, Canada. Dr. Letts graduated in 1964 from the Faculty of Medicine, University of Manitoba, Winnipeg, with a BSc. (Med) degree in medical research and an M.D., with honors. Following an internship at St. Boniface General Hospital in Winnipeg and three years with the Royal Canadian Air Force and the United Nations in the Middle East, he obtained an MSc. in experimental surgery at Queen's University, Kingston, Ontario.

Dr. Letts is a member of the Canadian Orthopedic Association, the American Academy of Orthopedic Surgeons, and the Pediatric Orthopedic Society of North America. Following a year of postgraduate training at The Hospital for Sick Children in Toronto, he obtained his Fellowship in the Royal College of Physicians and Surgeons of Canada and his Fellowship in the American College of Surgeons. Dr. Letts is a Diplomat of the American Board of Orthopedic Surgery in the U.S.

Dr. Letts has a special interest in seating for the handicapped and was Clinic Chief of a pediatric seating clinic for 16 years. He has a particular interest in the biomechanics of seating and spinal deformity and hip dislocation and their influence on good sitting posture. He has numerous publications and presentations in the field of seating of the handicapped.

CONTRIBUTORS

Richard D. Beauchamp, M.D., FRCSC
Division of Orthopaedic Surgery
British Columbia Children's Hospital
 and Department of Orthopaedic Surgery
University of British Columbia
Vancouver, British Columbia, Canada

Jacques L. D'Astous, M.D., FRCSC
Myelomeningocoele Clinic Director
Children's Hospital of Eastern Ontario
 and Department of Surgery
University of Ottawa
Ottawa, Ontario, Canada

Eric Dehoux, M.D., FRCPC
Division of Rehabilitation Medicine
The Rehabilitation Centre
 and Department of Medicine
University of Ottawa
Ottawa, Ontario, Canada

Geoff Fernie, Ph.D., P.Eng.
Sunnybrook Medical Centre
Toronto, Ontario, Canada

Michael J. Forbes, P.Eng.
Special Devices Department
Rehabilitation Centre for Children
Winnipeg, Manitoba, Canada

Julie Huish, B.M.R. O.T.
Therapy Department
Rehabilitation Centre for Children
Winnipeg, Manitoba, Canada

Linda Kealey, B.Sc. P.T.
Myelomeningocoele Clinic
Children's Hospital of Eastern Ontario
 and Department of Physiotherapy
Ottawa Children's Treatment Center
Ottawa, Ontario, Canada

John E. Latter, M.D., FRCPC
Department of Rehabilitation Medicine
Children's Hospital of Eastern Ontario
 and Department of Medicine
University of Ottawa
Ottawa, Ontario, Canada

R. Mervyn Letts, M.D., M.Sc., FRCSC
Department of Surgery
University of Ottawa
 and Department of Orthopaedic Surgery
Children's Hospital of Eastern Ontario
Ottawa, Ontario, Canada

William G. Mackenzie, M.D., FRCSC
Muscle Diseases Clinic
Division of Orthopaedic Surgery
British Columbia Children's Hospital
 and Department of Orthopaedic Surgery
University of British Columbia
Vancouver, British Columbia, Canada

Barry Mason
Myelomeningocoele Clinic
Children's Hospital of Eastern Ontario
 and Spina Bifida Clinic
Ottawa Children's Treatment Center
Ottawa, Ontario, Canada

Richard A. F. Perry, OPAC, RTOrthop
Section of Orthopaedics
Health Sciences Centre
Winnipeg, Manitoba, Canada

Arthur Quanbury, M.A.Sc., P.Eng.
Department of Biomedical Engineering
Rehabilitation Centre for Children
 and School of Medical Rehabilitation
University of Manitoba
Winnipeg, Manitoba, Canada

Lori Roxborough, B.S.R. O.T./P.T.
Therapy Department
Sunny Hill Hospital for Children
Vancouver, British Columbia, Canada

Alison Kelly Stewart, O.T.(R), M.Ed.
Department of Occupational Therapy
Sunny Hill Hospital for Children
 and British Columbia Children's Hospital
Vancouver, British Columbia, Canada

Stephen Tredwell, M.D., FRCSC
Department of Orthopaedics
British Columbia Children's Hospital
 and Department of Orthopaedic Surgery
University of British Columbia
Vancouver, British Columbia, Canada

Erika von Kampen, P.T.
Therapy Department
Rehabilitation Centre for Children
Winnipeg, Manitoba, Canada

ACKNOWLEDGMENTS

It is a difficult task to document all the assistance received in the production of this text on seating, but I am indebted to numerous individuals for their suggestions, interest, and contributions to this endeavor. Many of the principles of seating, as well as my interest in this subject, were learned from and stimulated by Dr. Doug Hobson and Mr. Rhinhart Daher, two brilliant rehabilitation engineering specialists who have devoted their talents for many years to the field of seating, and by Dr. Robert Tucker, who taught me the principles of orthopedic rehabilitation. The staff of the Special Devices and Seating Clinic at the Rehabilitation Centre for Children in Winnipeg deserves a special thanks for assisting in my education in this field. To Kathy Mulder, Orthopedic Therapist, at the Children's Hospital in Winnipeg, to Inge Shaw and Erika von Kampen at the Rehabilitation Centre for Children in Winnipeg, and to Tam Yamishita at the St. Amant Centre in Winnipeg, a special acknowledgment for assisting in the solution in many of the problems discussed in the text. I am especially indebted to Dr. Gina Rempel and the nursing staff and physiotherapy staff of the St. Amant Centre in Winnipeg for testing many of the seating devices that were developed for severely handicapped children during my association with the seating team. The cooperation of my colleagues, Dr. Brian Black and Dr. Ron Monson, at the Winnipeg Children's Hospital, and Dr. Lou Lawton, Dr. Jay Jarvis, Dr. Bill McIntyre, Dr. Jacques D'Astous, Dr. Jim Wiley, Dr. Peggy Baxter, and Dr. Tim Carey, at the Children's Hospital of Eastern Ontario, in contributing cases and suggestions was greatly appreciated. To Ms. Pat Johnston and her library staff, a special thanks for their diligence and work in tracking down references and articles needed for the background research. Mr. Tony Cuillerier and his staff have provided excellent art work and photography, without which such a book simply could not be produced. The secretarial support of Ms. Maureen O'Neil and Ms. Sue Senn was instrumental in finally bringing the manuscripts to fruition. Their perseverance and cheerfulness in coping with revision after revision allowed the text to be completed by deadline. A sincere appreciation is extended to the coauthors for their excellent contributions recorded in the chapters of this text. The superb professional assistance of the editors at CRC Press, especially Ms. Carolyn C. Lea, is gratefully acknowledged. A special thanks to my family, wife Marilyn and sons, Ian, Eric, and Daron, for their tolerance in coping with revised chapters constantly lying about the house!

R. Mervyn Letts

This text is dedicated . . .
   to all the Seating Clinic personnel,
   to the parents and families,
      and, most importantly,
   to the wheelchair users,
      who are the primary focus of seating teams throughout the world.

TABLE OF CONTENTS

Chapter 1

GENERAL PRINCIPLES OF SEATING

R. Mervyn Letts

TABLE OF CONTENTS

I. GENERAL PRINCIPLES

l at least a third of our lives sitting. A smaller but ever-increasing
ion will spend all of their waking hours in the sitting position due
te because of congenital malformations, trauma, disease, or the
ntly, good, comfortable and functional seating is important to all

The days of simply manufacturing "a standard wheelchair" in small, medium, and large
sizes to which all the world could be fitted is fortunately gone forever. The varied modifications and accessories available for wheelchairs as well as the many varieties of specialized
mobility devices have greatly enhanced the approach to seating in the modern era.[1-6] However, in order to deliver the best possible seating chair to the handicapped population, a
team of knowledgeable individuals with various specialties and areas of expertise is required:[11,12,20,21]

1. Rehabilitation engineers to address the biomechanical problems and therapy, both
   physical and occupational, to ensure good function in the chair
2. Bioelectronic engineers and communication experts to ensure an adequate interface
   between the wheelchair and communication devices
3. A medical team which should include an orthopedic surgeon, to correct severe deformities and provide stable seating, a rehabilitation specialist to oversee the medical
   requirements of the handicapped sitter, and the individual's own physician — pediatrician, geriatrician, or family practitioner
4. Allied medical health professionals, including physical and occupational therapists, a
   clinic nurse, and an orthotist

All of these individuals and, indeed, the teachers, caregivers, and, most importantly, the
parents or family are intimately involved in the seating process[11,15,18,19] (Figure 1).

II. WHEELCHAIR GOALS

The wheelchair is much more than simply a device to deliver an individual from point
A to point B. It is essential for the education and, later, the employment of the wheelchair
person to ensure adequate interaction with the community. Fortunately, most handicapped
persons are able to function effectively from a wheelchair, and their mobility and independence can be ensured with good, comfortable, and functional seating.[24] Even those
individuals with a mental handicap and severe disability can often be managed much more
effectively with a good seating device in their own homes or group homes, avoiding the
necessity of institutionalization. A good seating program may also decrease the necessity
for extensive salvage surgery through the prevention of deformities occasioned by poor
seating in deformed positions.[5-8] The parents, family, and caregivers of the handicapped
sitter will also benefit from a good seating program since the delivery of care will be greatly
facilitated (Figure 2).

This entire book is basically devoted to a multidisciplinary approach to seating and, in
particular, to those situations that present difficult seating solutions for the treatment team.
It is the basic principles that are important and the goals that are essential rather than a
particular brand of wheelchair or this or that seating system. Just as there are many different
types of cars or computers, so, too, are there many varieties of seating devices to accomplish
the necessary goals of good stable sitting. The goals of a seating program are simple, but
often difficult to achieve without the combined efforts of the clinic group and the family.
The equipment, including the wheelchair and the wheelchair insert, if required, must be

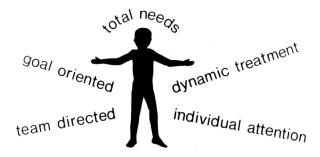

GENERAL APPROACH

FIGURE 1. A team approach to wheelchair prescription and design as well as the user's requirements is essential.

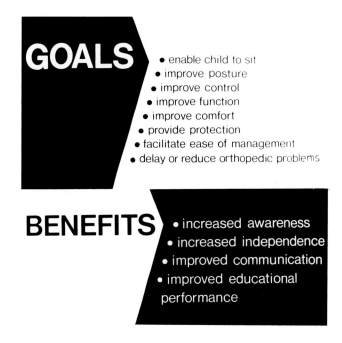

FIGURE 2. The goals and benefits of good wheelchair seating.

(1) comfortable, to enable the person to sit safely for 6 to 8 h at a time: (2) functional, to maximize the individual's potential learning and life experiences; (3) practical, to allow easy access to cars, toilets, the home, and the environment; (4) physiologic, to diminish the progress of deformity and dislocation and to prevent trauma; (5) mobile, to allow the person as much independence as possible; and (6) cosmetic, so onlookers will not be discouraged from offering care, transport, or other assistance to the physically disabled person using the device.[15-17]

III. BIOMECHANICS OF SEATING

Basic research into the factors that influence comfortable seating and stable posture in the sitting position has lagged behind the biomechanics research concerning spinal injuries and the upright spine.

AN   OBJECT   IS   IN   STATIC   EQUILIBRIUM   IF:

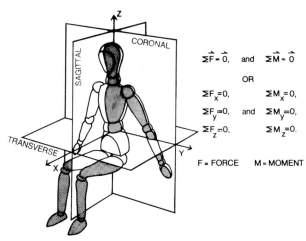

$$\sum \vec{F} = \vec{0}, \quad \text{and} \quad \sum \vec{M} = \vec{0}$$

OR

$$\sum F_x = 0, \qquad \sum M_x = 0,$$
$$\sum F_y = 0, \quad \text{and} \quad \sum M_y = 0,$$
$$\sum F_z = 0, \qquad \sum M_z = 0.$$

F = FORCE   M = MOMENT

FIGURE 3. Balanced or stable seating is achieved when there is a balance of forces and moments in all planes — sagittal, coronal, and transverse.

The physiological condition that has relegated an individual to a sitting existence frequently has an effect on trunk posture and pelvic stability. There are a number of factors that may alter the spinal biomechanics and result in poor seating. These include,

1.   Spasticity or paralysis, which will frequently predispose to spinal curvature with resultant imbalance of the upright torso in relation to the pelvic base
2.   Altered righting reflex, which may occur as a result of hypoxic brain injury *in utero* in the neonatal period secondary to intracranial bleeds or in later life, secondary to physical head trauma (The altered righting reflex will result in the individual not correcting a tendency to slump one way or the other.)
3.   Altered paraspinal muscle response, which occasionally occurs as a retained primitive reflex, the so-called Gallant reflex in which there is contraction of the paraspinal muscles on the side of the stimulus, resulting in a spinal curvature convex away from the point of the stimulus (This primitive type of reflex is often seen in profoundly retarded individuals.)
4.   Pelvic obliquity, which results in an inadequate seating base, resulting in obliquity of the spine and the development of a spinal curvature which may be part of the etiology of the obliquity or may be secondary to an attempt by the seated person to maintain their upper torso in a proper upright position
5.   Lower limb contractures, which may predispose to pelvic obliquity and make sitting very difficult and which have a direct impact on preventing a stable sitting position[24]

IV. WHAT IS STABLE OR BALANCED SEATING?

Stable or balanced seating is achieved if there is a balance of forces and moments in all planes. An object is in static equilibrium if the moments of forces in the transverse, sagittal, and coronal planes are equally balanced, as illustrated in Figure 3. If that is achieved, the head and neck will be vertical and the hips will be flexed to 100°, with the thighs abducted and shoulders slightly rounded. To achieve this, the arms need to be supported, as do the feet, and the back reclined slightly.[2-4] To achieve stable seating, there needs to be an appropriate mixture of support as well as freedom for the individual. Such a sitting

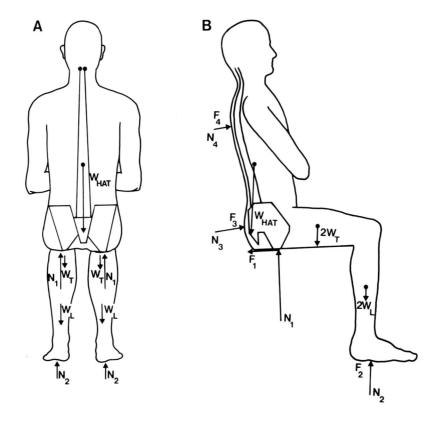

FIGURE 4. Forces exerted on a seated individual sitting in a chair with the feet supported. (A) In the sagittal plane; (B) in the coronal plane. WHAT = weight of head + arms + trunk; WT = weight of one thigh; WL = weight of one leg and foot; N = normal force; and F = resultant force.

posture must not only be balanced or stable, but also must be comfortable, functional, practical, corrective to some extent, and should facilitate the care of the individual as well as the mobility of the chair and its user (Figure 4).

V. SITTING POSTURE

The posture of a person sitting in a wheelchair is determined by both active and passive modalities. Active posture control consists of the maintenance of an adequate righting reflex, which, in turn, maintains an upright sitting posture by means of the musculature of the spine and activity of the upper extremities. A number of passive controls to maintain the posture exist within the torso, such as ligaments, bony interfaces, soft tissue stops such as menisci, discs, and, in some instances, mechanical features, such as a Harrington rod or other metal stabilizing device. Posture can also be controlled by external means such as braces or bolsters built into the wheelchair itself.[9,10,16,23]

VI. FORCES ACTING DURING SITTING

Poor sitting support for an individual prone to poor sitting stability will result in rapidly increasing deformities. A schematic diagram of forces acting on a person sitting on a chair with a backrest and foot support in the sagittal plane is illustrated in Figure 4. If such a person has a significant pelvic obliquity, the effect on medial-lateral sitting stability will be

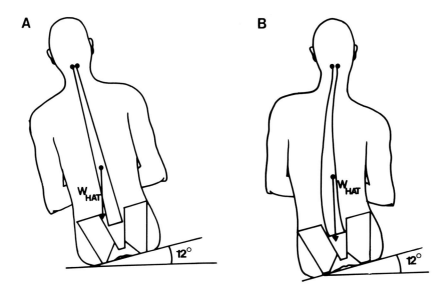

FIGURE 5. Effects of medio-lateral sitting instability as encountered with pelvic obliquity (A); (B) attempts to relocate center of gravity results in a long C-type curve.

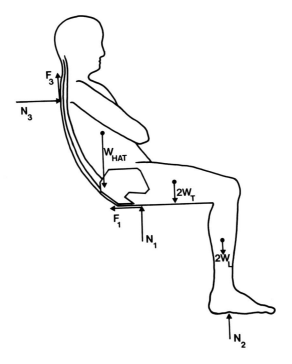

FIGURE 6. Sacral sitting due to hamstring tightness upsets the sagittal balance, leading to compensatory thoracic kyphosis.

a shift of the center of gravity of the head, arms, and trunk, with the result that at an angle of about 12°, a person with a straight back will fall sideways or, if he/she is able to counteract that tendency by attempting to shift the center of gravity back, a long C-type scoliosis will be induced (Figure 5). If tight hamstrings are present in such a sitter, sacral sitting will result, with a tendency to constantly slide out of the chair (Figure 6). In an attempt to

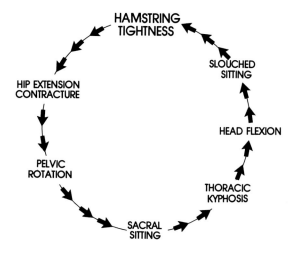

FIGURE 7. Vicious cycle of seating instability induced by hamstring tightness.

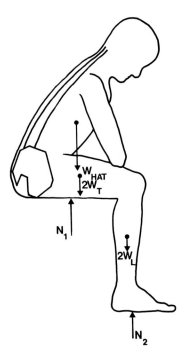

FIGURE 8. Paraspinal muscle weakness resulting in a falling forward in the chair and a postural kyphosis.

counteract this and to keep the head in a more forward functional position, the seated individual with tight hamstrings tends to develop a kyphosis as well (Figure 7). For those individuals with poor paraspinal muscle tone, there may be a tendency to increasing kyphosis and a falling forward, resulting in a defunctioning of the use of the arms, which are needed for support (Figure 8).

Just as it is important to correct deformity to ensure that the center of gravity is in a near-normal position in the upright ambulatory individual, so is it important to ensure in stable, comfortable sitting that there is a balance of forces around the pelvis and spine and

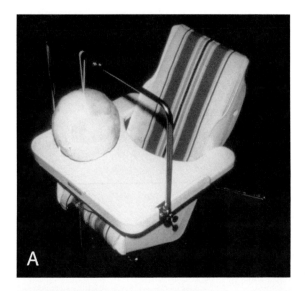

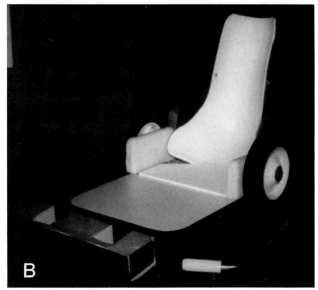

FIGURE 9. Examples of seating support for the handicapped young child. (A) Cozy Seat; (B) Castor Cart.

that the center of gravity of the seated individual is not displaced excessively to the point that other deformities must be developed in order to maintain the torso in an upright position. Such an individual may have to be assisted by good external support from the wheelchair itself or, in some instances, by corrective and preventative measures of a surgical nature in order to ensure comfortable sitting without excessive orthotic intervention.[6,13,17,21]

VII. TEMPORAL ASPECTS OF SEATING

A. BIRTH TO 18 MONTHS

The child with a severe disability is usually a late independent sitter and will require seating assistance, if only to allow the mother some freedom. A good, reliable seating device is required for the large child who is nonambulatory (Figure 9).

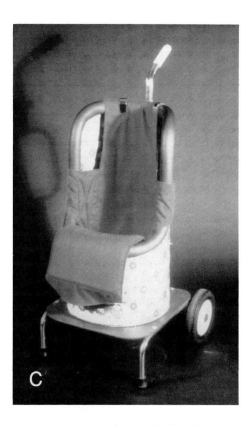

FIGURE 9 (continued). (C) Sleek Seat.

Cozy seat — At this young age, the Cozy Seat (Figure 9A) facilitates a normal flexed position which the child naturally wants to assume, i.e., the fetal position. It is comfortable for the child and provides a good, stable seat which can be transferred from one place to another.

CP floor seat — In the older child, i.e., over 1 year of age, the CP floor seat allows good abduction positioning and assists in changing the environment for the child as well as stretching the adductor muscles and keeping the hips nicely in joint.

GM car seat — the General Motors (GM) car seat is a very mobile and effective seating device for the child in the motor vehicle and is also used in the home in a manner similar to the Cozy Seat. In the younger age group, this form of seating is satisfactory.

B. 18 MONTHS TO 3 YEARS

Children in this age group have the added problems of developing deformities due to rapid growth and increasing weight, and will require a more aggressive approach to prevent deformities from occurring and recurring as well as to facilitate their care by their parents.

It is recommended that during the initial 18-month period any contractures of the adductor muscles that result in subluxation of the hip be released. It will not be necessary in all children, but in those where it is necessary, an aggressive approach must be taken if the hips are to be kept in joint. The same is true in the 18-month to 3-year-old age group, since, during this time, a soft tissue procedure is often effective in reducing or rectifying a deformity, whereas in a later age group, it may well require the addition of a bony procedure and a larger operation.

Modular insert — The child at this age is now too big for infant seating and requires, in most instances, a special approach to the wheelchair which may well include a modular insert. This consists of a specially designed insert on a tiny tot wheelchair base with appropriate bolstering and abduction seating with pommels or wing pads (Figure 10).

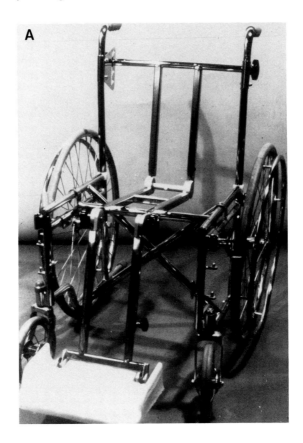

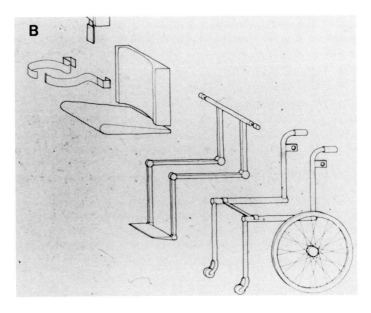

FIGURE 10.   Wheelchair base (A) to which insert can be added. (Reproduced with permission from Letts, M., Rang, M., and Tredwell, S., Seating the disabled, in *American Academy of Orthopaedic Surgeons: Atlas of Orthotics,* 2nd ed., C. V. Mosby, St. Louis, 1985.) (B) Construction of wheelchair base to accept seating insert.

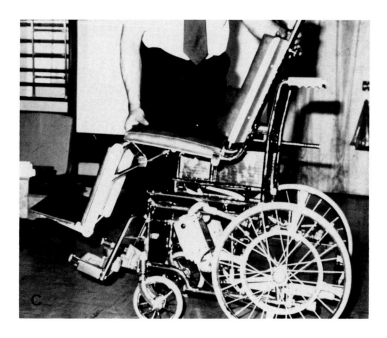

FIGURE 10 (continued). (C) Modular insert which is removable for ease of transport.

MODULAR WHEEL CHAIR

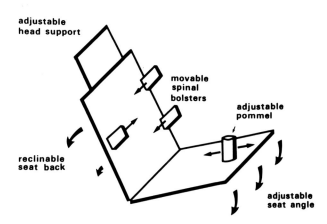

REMOVABLE INSERT

FIGURE 11. Bolstering may be sufficient to provide sitting stability
and defer the timing of an orthosis or surgery.

Bolstered wheelchair seating — In some instances, the child's trunk stability may be such that a spinal orthosis is not required and a modular insert with bolstering is all that is necessary to maintain a good sitting posture (Figure 11). Control of the pelvis at this age is essential.

Standing devices — Standing devices, although not strictly conventional seating, go hand in hand with the seating program (Figure 12). Standing devices such as an A-frame help keep the child's muscles stretched and are useful in the younger age group. Hamstring

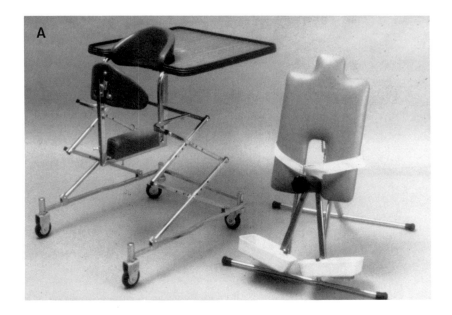

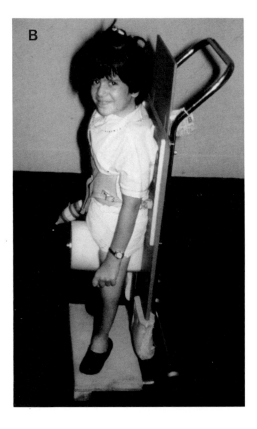

FIGURE 12.   Standing devices such as the pommel walker and prone stander (A) provide respite from the wheelchair and stimulate lower extremity function; (B) the standing frame allows controlled weight bearing through the adjustable pommel.

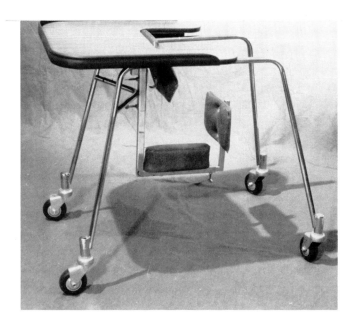

FIGURE 13. The pommel walker with a "seating" pommel allows an introduction to upright positioning. (Reproduced with permission from Letts, M., Rang, M., and Tredwell, S., Seating the disabled, in *American Academy of Orthopaedic Surgeons: Atlas of Orthotics,* 2nd ed., C. V. Mosby, St. Louis, 1985.)

lengthening and heel cord lengthening should be done at this age if the tendons are so tight that good seating is inhibited through pelvic tilt, marked knee flexion, or marked equinus.

Mobility devices — Mobility devices as well are really part of the seating program and many such units require specialized seating.[13,14] The pommel walker can be introduced at this age to stimulate the child and to allow a change from regular wheelchair sitting (Figure 13).

The pommel seat — Pommel seats allow good abduction for the child and are good postoperative prophylactic devices to prevent further contracture of the adductors (Figure 14).

C. 3 TO 6 YEARS OF AGE

In this age group, attention must be directed to both the hips and the spine since scoliosis often begins at this age. Vigilance must be exercised to prevent the hips from going out of joint, with resultant pelvic obliquity and scoliosis, the triad that is so notoriously difficult to rectify from both an orthopedic and seating point of view once it has occurred.

Modular wheelchair inserts — Wheelchair inserts must now incorporate bolstering to attempt good spinal alignment (Figure 15). Abduction seating is still desirable (Figure 16), and the addition of specialized trays to facilitate Bliss boards, school activities, etc. will be required (Figure 17).

Spinal orthoses — In some instances, it may be necessary to provide spinal bracing in the form of a polypropylene thoracolumbar spinal orthosis. This is not tolerated by all spastic cerebral palsy patients, but if the scoliosis is rapidly progressive, this approach together with the seating may be necessary (Figure 18).

Prone board — The prone board is another useful device that allows the child some time out of the wheelchair, with a further experience in upright positioning. A small number of children may ambulate during this period of time; however, generally speaking, if

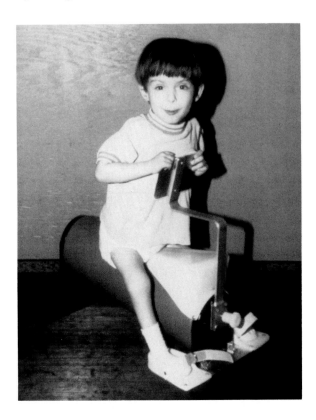

FIGURE 14.   The pommel seat provides abduction seating and is a "fun" type of seating device, providing short-term respite from the wheelchair. (Reproduced with permission from Letts, M., Rang, M., and Tredwell, S., Seating the disabled, in *American Academy of Orthopaedic Surgeons: Atlas of Orthotics,* 2nd ed., C. V. Mosby, St. Louis, 1985.)

ambulation has not commenced by 7 years of age in spite of no major contractures, the child will undoubtedly be a sitter.

D. 6 TO 12 YEARS OF AGE

Deformities that have persisted until this age become much more difficult to treat and usually require a bony procedure as well as a soft tissue operation. At this age, the team must weigh carefully the pros and cons of major surgery, although in some instances, with regard to a subluxated hip or markedly increasing scoliosis, surgery will be beneficial for future seating.

Wheelchair inserts — The wheelchair insert has to be constantly modified and changed as the child grows. The same objectives, good posture and spinal stability with level pelvis, must be achieved (Figure 19).

Foam-in-Place insert — In some instances, the older child will have major deformities that will not respond to typical orthoses or modular seating. In this regard, the Foam-in-Place insert is of great advantage and allows comfortable seating with some element of correction (Figure 20).

Mobility devices — At this age, the child may have achieved sufficient development to either propel the wheelchair on his own or to require a power device. Here again, careful assessment by the team is necessary and training with the control box is essential. Modifications to the joystick and positioning on the wheelchair may be necessary in order to

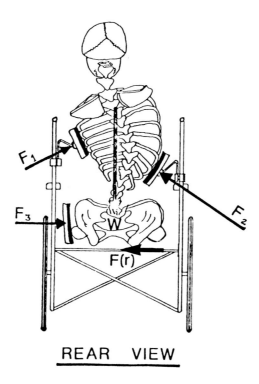

REAR VIEW

FIGURE 15. Three-point bolstering to provide postural stability. This seldom arrests curve progression, but may "buy some time" until more definitive treatment is necessary.

facilitate use (Figure 21A). This includes upper extremity and head control assessment. Since the upper extremities are important in seating, release of major contractures inhibiting function together with orthotic support of the head and neck (Figure 21B and C) should be part of the seating program.

Spinal orthoses — The spine at this age may become a major impediment to seating. Orthotic management of the spine in cerebral palsy is notoriously unsuccessful. It can be initially tried and may well slow the progression of the scoliosis, but if this is unsuccessful, serious consideration should be given to stabilizing the spine surgically if major seating problems are to be avoided in the future (Figure 22). Basically, this consists at this age of Harrington instrumentation or Luque rodding, which may well be sufficient to control the curve, although postoperative modular seating and orthoses are usually necessary.

E. 12 YEARS AND OVER

At this age, deformities are well established and the seating objectives will be primarily palliative, although good sitting posture is still important.

Modular wheelchair insert — The insert at this age should support the trunk in good upright sitting and be comfortable for the child. For the older child and adult, a seating "fitting" chair has been found to be useful by some seating teams.[11,17] This allows the wheelchair user as well as the professional staff to "try out" different bolsters, restraints, tilts, etc. before fabricating a definitive seating system (Figure 23).

Foam-in-Place inserts — The use of this type of seating modality will be more frequent in this age group, especially for those children with deformities so severe that the objective is for comfort only.

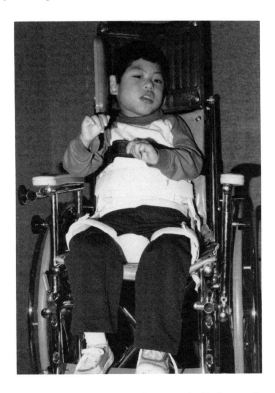

FIGURE 16. Abduction seating ensured with the use of a spinal-hip orthosis to control pelvic obliquity. (Reproduced with permission from Letts, M., Rang, M., and Tredwell, S., Seating the disabled, in *American Academy of Orthopaedic Surgeons: Atlas of Orthotics,* 2nd ed., C. V. Mosby, St. Louis, 1985.)

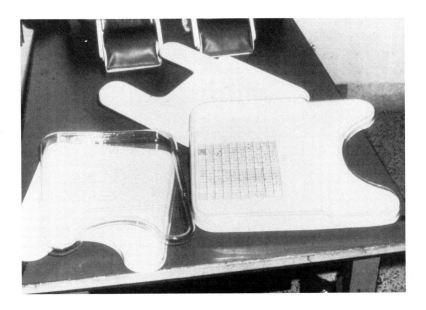

FIGURE 17. The wheelchair tray is part of the seating system, providing not only a work and play surface, but also serving as a trunk bolster and fulcrum for upper body support as well as a medium of communication through the Bliss board. (Reproduced with permission from Letts, M., Rang, M., and Tredwell, S., Seating the disabled, in *American Academy of Orthopaedic Surgeons: Atlas of Orthotics,* 2nd ed., C. V. Mosby, St. Louis, 1985.)

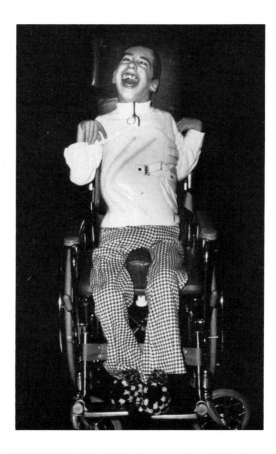

FIGURE 18. The additional support of a spinal orthosis may be necessary to augment the seating system in those with a mobile, collapsible type of scoliosis to provide sitting stability. (Reproduced with permission from Letts, M., Rang, M., and Tredwell, S., Seating the disabled, in *American Academy of Orthopaedic Surgeons: Atlas of Orthotics,* 2nd ed., C. V. Mosby, St. Louis, 1985.)

Spine — The spine can be a major impediment to good seating at this age (Figure 24). In selected individuals, stabilization of the long C-curve may be necessary with a combined anterior and posterior approach with good postoperative modular seating.

Powered chairs — The electric wheelchair and other powered devices such as the Pony™ or the Amigo™ provide considerable independence for the older child and adult. These often greatly facilitate schooling, education, and access to the work place.

The temporal approach to seating is an important concept and is often not appreciated by the seating team dealing only occasionally with pediatric seating needs. The above has been a summarization of the requirements faced by the seating team in the provision of stable seating systems from infancy to adulthood.

VIII. SUMMARY

Good, balanced seating requires adequate input and the participation of many disciplines if the major goals of stable sitting are to be achieved. The goals will often change at different ages, with some requiring more emphasis than others, but, in general, comfort, function, mobility, appearance, and reasonable cost are essential at any age. The team approach in a defined seating clinic will provide the best seating solutions for all of the varied requirements

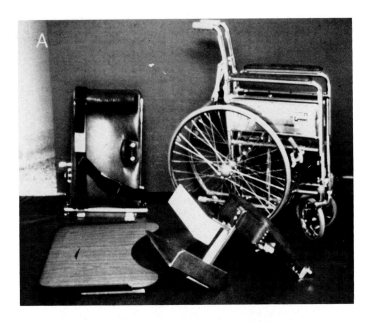

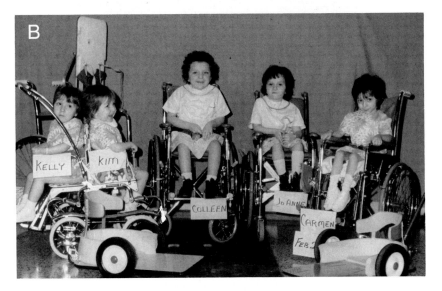

FIGURE 19.   Wheelchair inserts (A) require constant modification for growth in height and width. In cold climates, modification for heavy winter clothing is often necessary. (B) An example of the different seating requirements required at different ages for a family with five girls with an unusual familial form of muscular dystrophy.

of the seated population. The seating team must be constantly predicting and visualizing the child's future seating needs with the goal of achieving and maintaining a stable seating posture by the time skeletal maturity is attained.

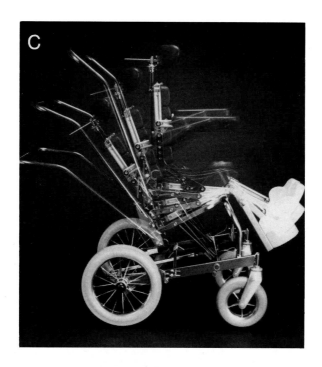

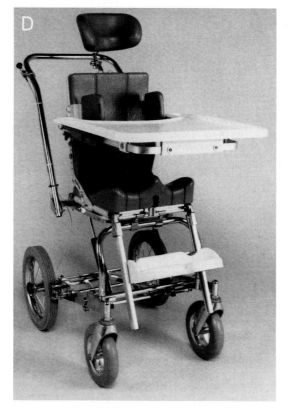

FIGURE 19 (continued). (C and D) Otto Bock modular seating systems with reclining bases.

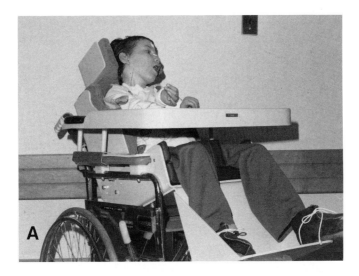

FIGURE 20.   Foam-in-Place seating provides total contact torso support, is comfortable, and maintains upright seating posture for severely handicapped wheelchair users.

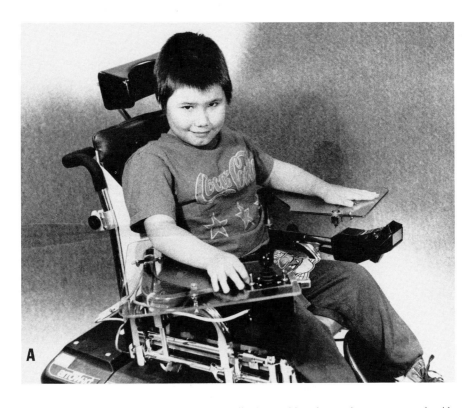

FIGURE 21.   Powered wheelchair (A) with centralized control box that can be swung out to the side.

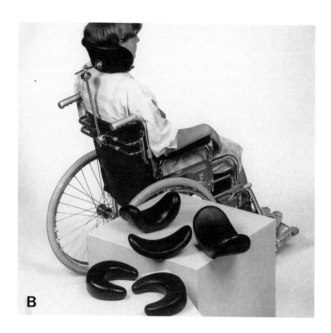

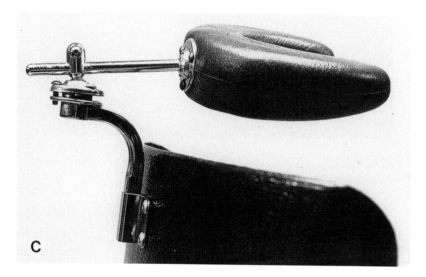

FIGURE 21 (continued). (B) Head support system anatomically contoured to give optimal support with comfort; (C) adjustable head and neckrest with two independent ball joints to give optimal support with comfort (Otto Bock Orthopedic Ltd., Winnipeg, Manitoba, Canada).

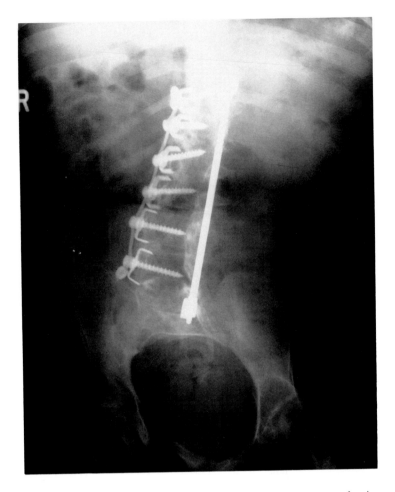

FIGURE 22.   Anterior and posterior stabilization may be necessary to control major scoliosis to facilitate stable seating.

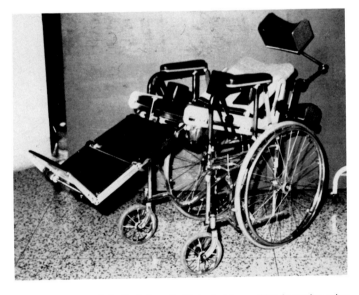

FIGURE 23.   A "fitting" chair to facilitate decision making in seating prior to permanent construction of an insert or seating system.

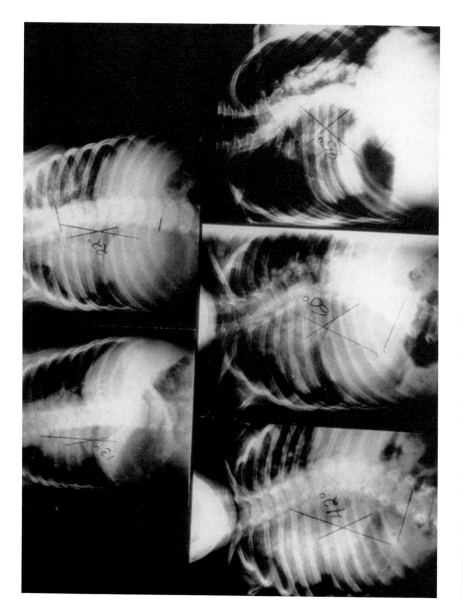

FIGURE 24. Progressive increase in spinal curvature in a child with cerebral palsy from age 2 years at 13° Cobb to age 18 years at 85° Cobb. In retrospect, this curvature should have been corrected and stabilized at age 13 years when the curve measured 42° Cobb, rather than trying to build the insert around the increasing deformity caused by the scoliosis.

REFERENCES

1. **Allison, B. J.,** Current uses of mobility aids, *Clin. Orthop.,* 148, 62, 1980.
2. **Adams, M. A. and Hutton, W. C.,** The effect of posture on the lumbar spine, *J. Bone Jt. Surg. Br. Vol.,* 67, 625, 1985.
3. **Anderson, G. B. J., Murphy, R. W., Ortengren, O. R., and Nachemson, A. L.,** The influence of back rest inclination and lumbar support on lumbar lordosis, *Spine,* 4, 52, 1979.
4. **Andersson, G. B. J., Ortengren, O. R., and Nachemson, A. L.,** Intra discal pressure, intra abdominal pressure and myeloelectric back muscle activity related to posture and loading, *Clin. Orthop.,* 129, 156, 1977.
5. **Behrman, A. L.,** Factors in functional assessment of wheelchair selection, in *Proc. Wheelchair IV,* Brubaker, C., Ed., RESNA Press, Washington, D.C., 1988, 17.
6. **Brubaker, C.,** Ergonometric considerations, in *Proc. Wheelchair IV,* Brubaker, C., Ed., RESNA Press, Washington, D.C., 1988, 37.
7. **Bull, M. J. and Stroup, K.,** New transportation solutions for children with special needs, in Proc. Seating the Disabled, Memphis, 1988.
8. **Chow, W. W. and Odell, E. I.,** Deformations and stresses in soft body tissues of a sitting person, *J. Biomech. Eng.,* 100, 79, 1978.
9. **Cooper, D.,** Biomechanics in postural control, in Proc. Seating the Disabled, University of British Columbia, Vancouver, 1990.
10. **Dolan, P., Adams, M. A., and Hitton, W. C.,** Commonly adopted postures and their effect on the lumbar spine, *Spine,* 13, 197, 1988.
11. **Fraser, B. A., Hensinger, R. N., and Philips, J. A.,** *Physical Management of Multiple Handicaps,* Brookes, Baltimore, 1990, 3.
12. **Graham, J. D.,** Experience with a special seating clinic, *J. Bone Jt. Surg. Br. Vol.,* 57, 1572, 1975.
13. **Hobson, D. A.,** Research and development considerations in engineering perspective, *Clin. Prosthet. Orthot.,* 10, 122, 1986.
14. **Kaye, J. C., Cairns, A., and Bennet, G. C.,** A mobility aid for paraplegic children, *J. Pediatr. Orthop.,* 5, 711, 1985.
15. **Letts, R. M.,** The special devices and seating clinic — a universal need, *Can. Orthot. Prosthet.,* 10, 19, 1978.
16. **Letts, M., Rang, M., and Tredwell, S.,** Seating the disabled, in *Atlas of Orthotics,* 2nd ed., C. V. Mosby, St. Louis, 1985, 440.
17. **Louis, D. S., Hensinger, R. N., Fraser, B. A., Philips, J. A., and Jacques, K.,** Surgical management of the severely handicapped individual, *J. Pediatr. Orthop.,* 9, 15, 1989.
18. **Nachemson, A. L.,** The lumbar spine: an orthopedic challenge, *Spine,* 1, 59, 1976.
19. **Scott-Taplin, C., Smith, M., McLaughlin, J., and Matthews, T.,** The wheelchair simulator: powered wheelchair assessment and training, *Can. J. Rehabil.,* 3, 1, 1989.
20. **Sussman, M.,** Setting up a seating clinic, in Proc. Seating the Disabled, University of British Columbia, Vancouver, 1990.
21. **Trefler, E., Ed.,** *Seating for Children with Cerebral Palsy: A Resource Manual,* University of Tennessee Center for Health Sciences, Memphis, 1984.
22. **Wilson, A. B. and McFarland, S. R.,** *Wheelchairs: A Prescription Guide,* Rehabilitation Press, Charlottesville, VA, 1986.
23. **Woollacott, M., Debu, B., and Mowatt, M.,** Neuromuscular control of posture in the infant and child: is vision dominant?, *J. Motor Behav.,* 19, 167, 1987.
24. **Zacharkow, D.,** *Posture: Sitting, Standing, Chair Design and Exercise,* Charles C Thomas, Springfield, IL, 1988.

Chapter 2

REHABILITATION ENGINEERING IN THE SEATING P

Michael J. Forbes

TABLE OF CONTENTS

E REHABILITATION ENGINEER

ing clinic to apply engineering principles and technology
a disabilities. Technology is opening more doors to the
to their seating. Rehabilitation engineers bring important
ing team. For example,

chanics, dynamics, and kinematics in relation to body me-

factors, human/machine interface design, and component

3.   Training ...   olving to manage consideration of trade-offs and alternatives
4.   An understanding of disabilities and conditions that cause them, and how these affect
     the patients' daily lives
5.   Design skills and knowledge of stress analysis, materials science, and mechanical
     design technology

Using these skills, the engineer must transform the therapeutic objectives into a successful
design. It is the engineer's role to translate the attributes of a seating system into drawings
and specifications that can be understood by the technicians responsible for making it. There
are trade-offs and alternatives inherent in any design. They need to be clearly communicated
to the rest of the team and discussed so that a workable design is produced. The engineer
is the team member who is best able to picture the finished seating device and to best describe
it to the patient and the rest of the seating team.[9,11]

II. ENGINEERING OBJECTIVES

Each seating system must address engineering objectives as well as therapeutic objectives. It is not always necessary to qualify these, but some measure of the expectations
placed on a seating system must be made. For example, an estimate of the length of time
the seating device will be used is needed in order to select materials and fabrication techniques
that will last for the duration of the seat usage.

A. MAXIMIZING THE FUNCTIONAL LIFE OF THE WHEELCHAIR INSERT
The useful life of a seating system directly affects the expenditures in materials and
labor required. It also may necessitate trade-offs in some other objectives. In order to increase
lifetime, more growth potential may be required or the fitting (patient) tolerances may need
to be relaxed. At this point, the therapeutic objectives impinge upon the engineering objectives and may limit the choices available. Specifically, if a close fit is required for therapeutic
reasons, the lifetime of the seating insert may be reduced.

B. OPTIMIZING THE COST OF SEAT PRODUCTION
Since the engineering decisions contribute to the final cost, the reduction of cost to a
reasonable level becomes an engineering objective. As well as the expected lifetime of the
insert, costs are affected by cosmetics, fabrication methods, choice of materials, complexity
of the design, and ease of modifications to accommodate change or growth. The target is
to produce a pleasing design that meets the therapeutic objectives for the least possible cost.

C. DEVELOPING PRACTICAL ENGINEERING DESIGN CONSIDERATIONS
There are certain properties that a well-made seating system must attain. It must fit into
the mobility base securely. If it will be removed regularly, removal must be easy and reliable,

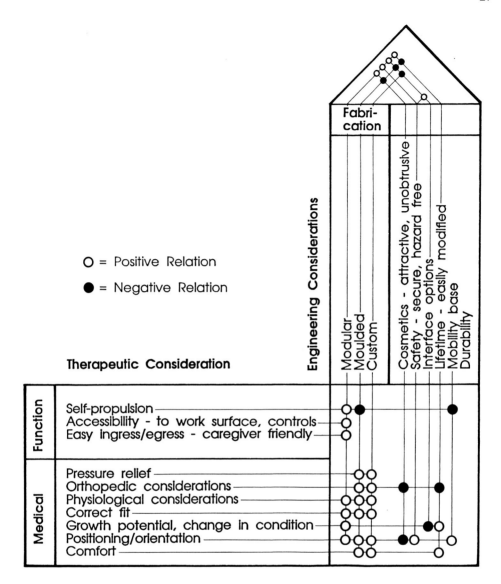

FIGURE 1. House of quality, showing relationship between therapeutic considerations and engineering considerations.

i.e., each time the seat is installed into the base, it must sit at the same orientation. The seat must provide the occupant with a safe environment. It cannot present any sources of injury at the least and, wherever possible, needs to limit the liability of injury. It must be easily cleaned and the materials used should not promote fungus growth.

The seating system should be compatible with the mobility base with which it is matched. A lightweight wheelchair for an active user is not an appropriate base for a complex insert supporting a multihandicapped patient. Similarly, a mobility base intended for a multiply handicapped individual would be mismatched with merely a seat and back cushion. Since the mobility base must be user appropriate, it is an integral part of the system and should be carefully selected to meet the user's needs and activity level.

D. ENHANCING THERAPEUTIC AND ENGINEERING OBJECTIVES

Figure 1 shows a "house of quality" which describes the relationship between therapeutic and engineering considerations. The therapeutic considerations are listed on the ground floor of the house, and the engineering considerations are listed on the second story. By comparing the two, we can learn which ones affect the others negatively and where trade-offs will be required. The roof shows a comparison of the engineering considerations. For instance, we find a ''●'' in the box that leads to both the custom-fabricated option and interface option. This indicates that the choice of a custom-made insert may complicate the interface requirements.

E. PROVIDING A COMFORTABLE SEATING SYSTEM

The major factors affecting seating comfort are relief of pain and freedom from irritation. Pain may be due to seating pressures or orthopedic and positioning problems. Relief of pressure can be achieved by good positioning and the right choice of a seating system. There are several seat cushions available which are designed to relieve pressure. The most common are fluid-filled and gel cushions. Fluid-filled cushions are actually a sealed reservoir of fluid. Because the pressure in a fluid system is equal throughout, these cushions will exert the same pressure at all points. With air-filled cushions, the pressure can be varied to suit the patient. Gel cushions have characteristics of both foam cushions and fluid-filled cushions. Custom foam cushions are often fabricated to relieve sensitive areas of pressure entirely by removing the foam from under those areas.

Freedom from irritation is a more difficult problem to address. Frequently, the source of the discomfort is unknown or the patient is unable to express it. If a patient can move independently within the seat, often he/she can reposition himself/herself periodically and avoid discomfort. Seating materials such as fabric coverings and open-cell foams that can store moisture often increase comfort. Synthetic materials are currently very common. However, people often develop sensitivities to these materials. Sometimes a change of covering materials is all that is required to restore comfort.

III. ENSURING DURABILITY OF MATERIALS USED FOR SEATING

The durability of a seating system applies to its ability to withstand the stresses of daily use and to satisfy the required lifetime objective. Failure to accomplish this may result from fracture of a major component or failure of a minor accessory such as a belt. Such failures are usually due to three causes: underestimating the loads, improper material selection, or improper construction methods.

The loads placed on a seating system by a handicapped person can often be two to three times their body weight. This is particularly true of clients who subject their equipment to impact loading. Seating materials often fail by fatigue failure through cyclic loading. This is aggravated with plastic components which also tend to creep under normal loads. Often, caregivers are the source of considerable abuse of the seats. A correct estimate of the load is required to properly specify the materials and construction, and affects all subsequent design decisions.[5]

Seating materials fail because they are placed in working situations beyond their capacity. Foams that are subjected to deflections beyond 65%, even locally, will tire and lose their support. Velcro™ is a very convenient closure, but is often the first component to fail. For belts that are to be used many times a day, buckles will last longer. Plastic seating modules frequently require reinforcing at areas of high stress.

Proper construction methods can increase the durability of a seating system. The components need sufficient support and must be interfaced into the mobility base in a way that reduces the stresses on them. Accessories such as belts, trunk bolsters, and headrests can often cause problems, the most common being failure at the point of attachment because of poor methods or the wrong fasteners. Large washers should always be used to attach belts

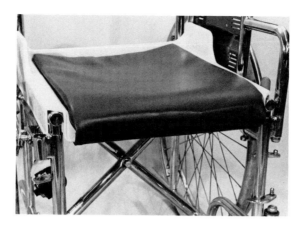

FIGURE 2.   Transfer seat of molded plastic allowing support loads
to be distributed along the entire seat length.

and plastic parts. The areas of joints should be large so as to distribute loads over a sufficient surface and avoid localized stresses.

A. CHOICE OF SEATING MATERIALS

For material selection, three parts of a seating system need to be considered: the interface hardware, the seat support elements, and the upholstery. The interface hardware connecting the seating system to the mobility base or supports it in free standing. The term "hardware" suggests metals and usually these components are steel or aluminum because of the high stress involved and the need for compact parts. Plastic or wood is used when the stresses can be distributed over large areas. For example, some plastic seat support elements are molded to conform to a wheelchair. In this case, the support loads are distributed along the entire seat length[10] (Figure 2).

Plastics such as acrylonitrile-butadiene-styrene (ABS) or polyethylene have the advantages of easy formability, easy cleaning, good appearance, and inexpensiveness. The disadvantages of plastics are their low stress levels, discoloration, odor in some cases, and allergic sensitivity. Thermoplastics are easier to form than thermosetting plastics and can be reshaped with heat to permit modifications. The most common shaping techniques are vacuum forming and hand bending, using a strip heater.[8,9] The insert back shown was hand formed after heating ABS on a strip heater (Figure 3).

One property of plastics which affects their performance is their tendency to creep.[1] A safety factor of four is required to protect against premature failure due to creep. Fasteners should be self-holding so that they will not loosen after the material creeps out from under them.

Metals, mostly steel and aluminum, are used primarily for the interface hardware that supports the insert in the mobility base. There is a wide range of commercially available hardware for seat interfacing. The majority are chrome-plated mild steel, although stainless steel and aluminum parts are available. Plated steel offers the most economical material with a good-quality finish. Stainless steel provides superior parts with high stress tolerance and an enduring finish. Aluminum is usually chosen for its light weight, formability, and finish (Figure 4).

Very often, wood is selected for both the seat support elements and the interface system. Wood is easily constructed into custom shapes, and wood-working techniques are understood by most technicians. It is difficult to predict the strength of wood because it varies greatly in performance.[2] Wooden parts are hard to keep clean and will soak up spills unless they are well protected.

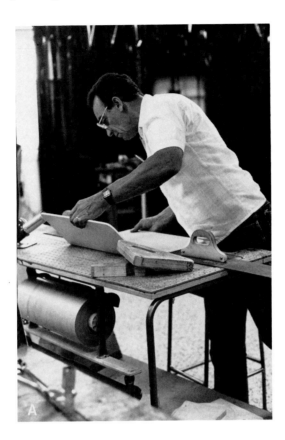

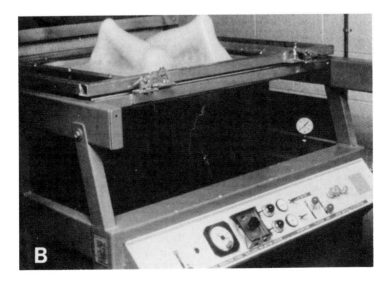

FIGURE 3.   (A) An ABS insert back being hand shaped after heating; (B) vacuum-forming machine allows rapid shape forming of thermoplastics, facilitating seat fabrication.

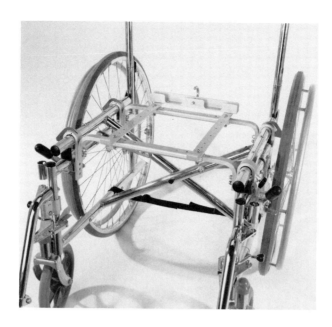

FIGURE 4. Otto Bock interface hardware using three metals — aluminum, plated steel, and stainless steel. (From Otto Bock Ltd., Winnipeg, Manitoba, Canada. With permission.)

The upholstery is made up of an elastic cushion material to accommodate the irregular anatomical shape and the protective covering. The cushion material of choice for most seating devices is flexible cellular foam. The factors that influence foam behavior are the types of foam, chemical composition, thickness, density, 25 and 65% indentation force deflection, and the support factor. The 25% indentation force deflection (IFD) is the force in pounds required to produce 25% indentation over an area of 50 in.[2] after 1 min at rest. Similarly, the 65% IFD is the force in pounds required to produce a 65% indentation over an area of 50 in.[2] after 1 min at rest. The support factor is the ratio of the 65% IFD to the 25% IFD. These deflections are specific to the original thickness of the foam test specimen and are good indicators of the hardness of the foam. Foams used in seating have 25% IFD values between 25 and 47 lb and 65% IFD values between 39 and 104 lb. For the purpose of special seating, foams should be selected so that their operating force deflections are between 25 and 65% IFD.[3]

The protective covering will be either a film material or a woven fabric. All film coverings are synthetic materials such as vinyl, but woven materials may be either natural or synthetic. The selection of covering materials depends on the conditions of use. Film coverings are preferred where incontinence and lack of cleanliness are experienced. They are extremely durable and long lasting. Woven fabric coverings provide a better exchange of air around the patient. They are preferred for patients who perspire excessively or live in humid climates. Woven fabrics offer a greater selection and so can more easily accommodate allergic sensitivities.

IV. FABRICATION TECHNIQUES

A. CUSTOM-MOLDED SEATING SYSTEMS

Custom-molded seating systems provide the user with a great deal more support than modular or plywood and foam seating systems. They accomplish this by close contact with the client's seating surfaces. To obtain this close contract and intimate shape, a cast or form

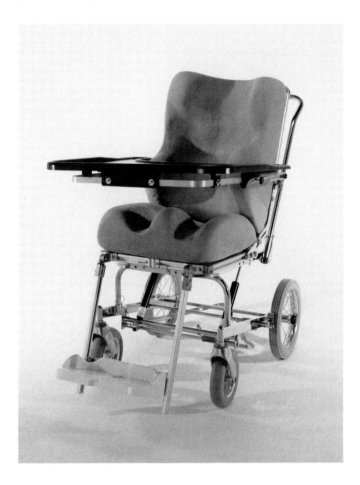

FIGURE 5.   Custom orthotic seating system provides custom-molded, total-contact support to maintain sitting stability in difficult sitting situations due to spasticity or deformity (From Otto Bock Orthopedic Ltd., Winnipeg, Manitoba, Canada. With permission.)

is made of the client. This approach is used for clients with severe seating difficulties such as orthopedic deformities and severe spasticity (Figure 5).

The client assessment for a custom-molded seating system will be much more detailed and time consuming than for a modular insert. Realistic expectations of what problems are correctable and what position is attainable are required. Custom molding is time consuming and expensive, and not compatible with a trial-and-error approach. A clear picture of the final seating system will help to prevent costly mistakes. The use of a multiadjustable ''fitting'' chair also facilitates assessment.[7]

There are two methods of casting clients for a custom-molded insert. The first involves an intermediate medium such as plaster wrap or a vacuum consolidation bean bag to obtain a reverse impression of the patient's shape. Once the reverse impression is made, it is used to form a seat cushion or shell which is a very close fit to the client. The final seat may be made from thermoplastic,[4] flexible foam,[5,6] or a rigid foam.[7]

The second method is a direct approach which does not use an intermediate medium. The client is positioned directly into the material from which the final seat cushions are to be made. This material may be either a mixture of styrene beads and slow-curing epoxy adhesive[8] or flexible polyurethane foam.[9] The pressure of the patient against the medium

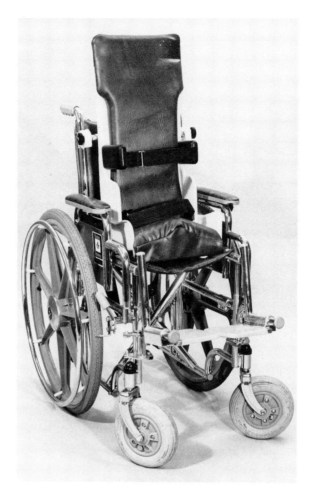

FIGURE 6. Modular wheelchair insert produced from vacuum-formed plastic and covered with cushions.

forces it to conform to his/her shape. In a short time, the material cures and maintains its shape.

B. MODULAR SEATING SYSTEMS

The principle of modular seating is to have on hand a series of prefabricated seating components from which a customized seating system could be made. The components have the features most commonly required and are produced in a range of sizes. By selecting and assembling the components with the shape and size needed, a seat can be readily constructed to suit a client with moderate requirements[10,11] (Figure 6).

Most modular seating components are made from vacuum-formed plastic and covered with cushions. They offer a great deal of flexibility in assembly and allowance for growth. Additional supports such as trunk and hip bolsters are available and can be used when required. Different types of headrests are available which can be attached with adjustable hardware. Since these seating systems are most frequently used as wheelchair inserts, hardware to interface into a wheelchair is usually available.

C. PLYWOOD AND FOAM SEATING

The first seating for the handicapped was made from plywood and foam. The seats were handcrafted onto plywood bases. Many hours of skilled and intensive labor were required.

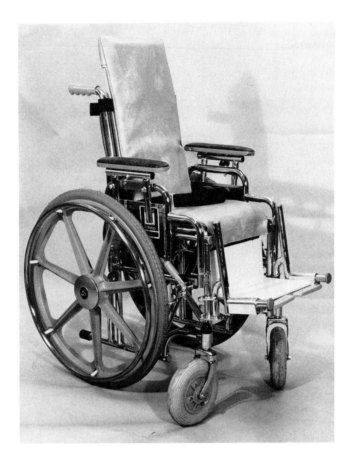

FIGURE 7.   Plywood and foam seating still has application for those individuals who have not been successfully seated with prefabricated inserts.

Most often, the seating was successful. The years of handcrafted plywood and foam seating systems were a learning period. The knowledge gained has been transferred to different construction methods.

There is a place for individually upholstered seating. No prefabricated system is suitable for every client and new ideas will need to be prototyped (Figure 7).

V. SUMMARY

The success of wheelchair seating is a meld between the needs of the wheelchair user, the type of insert prescribed, the therapeutic objectives, and, finally, the engineering design of the unit. Proper materials must be chosen and the engineering objectives must be in concert with the therapeutic requirements. Comfort, function, and cosmesis must be achieved, and it is the fabrication techniques and the use of appropriate materials that will enhance the achievement of these three major objectives. The engineer and technical staff must work closely with the seating team and user, and fully understand the needs of the potential user as well as the treatment objectives of other members of the seating team. Only in this multidisciplined environment will the optimum seating device emerge to satisfy the requirements of each wheelchair user!

ACKNOWLEDGMENTS

Many thanks to Gerri Weigle and Gay Kirby for their help in preparing this paper and to Rick Stevens and Ed Buyachek of Otto Bock Orthopedic Industries.

REFERENCES

1. **Carlson, J. M. and Winter, R.,** The "Gillette" Sitting Support Orthosis, *Orthot. Prosthet.,* 32(4), 34, 1978.
2. *Custom Orthotic Seating System,* Otto Bock Orthopedic Ltd., Winnipeg, Manitoba, Canada, 1990.
3. **Forbes, M. J. and King, M. W.,** Properties of foam and how they influence cushion selection, in Proc. Int. Symp. Adaptive Seating, University of Manitoba, Department of Continuing Education, September 1985.
4. **Forbes, M. J., von Kampen, E., and Iluk, G.,** Special seating at the Rehabilitation Centre for Children, paper presented at Int. Seating Symp., University of British Columbia, Department of Continuing Education, Vancouver, February 1986.
5. **Hobson, D. A.,** Foam-in-Place seating for the severely disabled, preliminary studies, in Proc. 5th Annu. Conf. on Systems and Devices for the Disabled, Houston, 1982.
6. **Hobson, D. A. et al.,** Bead seat insert seating system, in Proc. 6th Annu. Conf. of Rehabilitation Engineering, San Diego, 1983, 209.
7. *Optimum Seating and Positioning Aids,* Canadian Posture and Seating Centre, Kitchener, Ontario, Canada, 1986.
8. **O'Toole, J.,** Designing with plastics, in *Modern Plastics Encyclopedia,* McGraw-Hill, 1989.
9. **Schubert, P. B., Ed.,** *Machinery's Handbook,* 20th ed., Industrial Press, New York, 1975, 455.
10. **Silverman, M. and Silverman, O.,** The Contour-U Customould seating system, in Proc. 6th Annu. Conf. on Rehabilitation Engineering, San Diego, 1983, 194.
11. **Statt, B.,** A beginner's seating primer, *Phys. Ther. Forum,* 6(29), 1, 1987.

Chapter 3

THERAPY ASPECTS OF SEATING

Erika von Kampen

TABLE OF CONTENTS

I. INTRODUCTION

The therapist's role on the seating team is very important. As a team member, the occupational or physiotherapist is initially involved in the assessment, fitting, and follow-up of the seating requirements of each individual. This includes consultation and client/caregiver education and may necessitate home or school visits to assess special modifications in this environment.

For the nonambulatory population, the wheelchair or any wheeled mobility device has to fulfill a variety of functions. However, commercially available wheelchairs, strollers, etc. do not always provide the comfort and support a handicapped person requires for all daily activities due to the specialized needs of that individual. Therefore, being supplied with a good, comfortable, and functional seating system is essential. A thorough assessment and realistic goal setting must always precede the manufacturing of a seating system.[5-7] Although this is done within the context of the seating team, the approach outlined in this chapter reflects occupational and physiotherapy considerations.

II. ASSESSMENT

Given the medical diagnosis, the therapist gathers details regarding the client's specific disability. This includes history taking, observation, and testing. The present mode of sitting is observed, and the client and/or caregiver reports on the amount of time spent sitting daily (Figure 1).

The client is examined in a variety of positions: sitting, lying prone, etc. Orthopedic considerations at this point are skeletal abnormalities and joint contractures which would interfere with seating.[4,5]

Associated conditions such as seizure disorders, blindness, and deafness are recorded. It is important to find out if a mental handicap exists and to what degree cooperation from the client can be expected. Functional muscle testing is carried out, with emphasis on upper extremity function and head and trunk control. Skin sensation is assessed when necessary. Neurological observations are made regarding muscle tone and the presence of abnormal reflex activity.[2]

It is also important to note if other technical aids are going to be used by the client and if he/she is planning to wear orthoses when sitting. Transfers in and out of the wheelchair for all activities of daily living should be considered, observed, and discussed.

Consideration must be given to the client's mode of communication. It is important to know if the user of the seating system will require some form of accessible communication device.

To conclude the assessment, the following points must be discussed:

1. The client's lifestyle
2. Place where the client is living or going to live
3. Attendance at school or work
4. Wheelchair accessibility for routine daily activities
5. Transportation arrangements (car, bus, or handi-transit)
6. Environment in which the system is going to be used: variety of terrain (indoor, outdoor, gravel, snow, etc.) and climatic conditions (humidity and temperature)

The seating team together with the client and/or caregiver then decide on the type of base the seating system will require to meet the functional needs of the client (Figure 2). Generally speaking, three types of bases are considered:

1. A wheelchair which the client can wheel himself/herself

2. A stroller or a base with small wheels in which the client is pushed by an attending person
3. An electrically powered base

Before designing the system and setting goals, the team should also consider the following points:

1. Are pain and/or skin breakdown a problem?
2. Adjustments for growth should be provided when designing a system for children.
3. Safety — The system should be safe for the client to use and also allow the caregiver(s) to easily and quickly remove the user in case of emergency.
4. Cosmetics — The seating system should be as attractive as possible. The materials used should be durable and easy to clean. The seating system should also be as unobstructive as possible, placing emphasis on the person, not the device.

III. GOAL SETTING

In setting goals, the client's needs must be prioritized. Maximum function and maximum comfort are the ideal goals.

The therapist recommends the best functional position in which the client should be seated. Seating for a person with cerebral palsy should be tone reducing, reflex inhibiting, and supportive to facilitate maximum function and development.[1,2]

When seating head-injured clients, the system should be readily adjustable for the rapidly changing seating and positioning needs of a head-injured person.[3]

In the older population, comfortable support is the main goal. Facilitating and maintaining upright posture and easy transfers are also important.[3]

IV. FITTING

At the fitting appointment, it is the therapist's responsibility to ensure that the seating system fits comfortably and meets the prescribed criteria.

The therapist should check the padding of the seat, seat length, back height, seatback angle, belt lengths, foot supports, and other supports. He/she also ensures that the pelvis is positioned as level as possible, the trunk and head are in the midline, and the arms are well supported on armrests or on a wheelchair tray (Figure 3).

The client is observed in the new seating system (Figure 4). If changes and/or modifications are necessary, they are carried out and the client is observed again. The seating device and its use are explained to the user and/or caregiver(s). The user's opinion is requested to ascertain whether the device meets expectations. Instructions are given regarding the length of time to sit and the importance of good positioning in the system. Practical advice is given on taking the system apart (if applicable) and on maintenance and cleaning (Figure 5).

Alternate seating and positioning should be discussed at this point, as it is not advisable for anyone to remain in one position for too long. This is especially important for children, as change of position as well as the seating device facilitates physical and social development and allows them to interact at the same level with their peers.

Providing a person with a special seating device is only part of the overall management of his/her needs. Occupational and physical therapy continue, along with the monitoring of the client's seating and positioning devices.

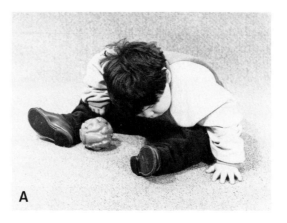

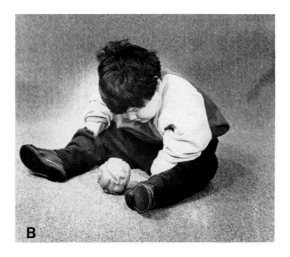

FIGURE 1.   Example of sitting assessment. (A) Child needs hands to be able to maintain a seated position; (B) poor sitting balance in spite of wanting to play with the ball.

V. FOLLOW-UP

Regular follow-up visits are necessary for the users of a special seating system. These take place at a team meeting or seating clinic every 6 to 9 months. The therapist must check the same items as at the fitting appointment. Necessary changes and repairs should be promptly instituted. The client and his/her caregiver(s) are asked how the system works for them and what adaptations they would like to have made. Reported time spent in the seating device gives a good indication regarding the comfort of the seat. Functional abilities are reevaluated and supports are added, replaced, taken away, or left in place as abilities change.

Seating goals must be reemphasized by the team to achieve maximum function with minimum restraints. The user is encouraged to keep in touch with the seating team and to ask for adaptations and repairs if and when they become necessary.

VI. CONCLUSION

As stated previously, a seating system is only part of the overall management of a handicapped person. Therapy is an ongoing process of which seating is only one aspect.

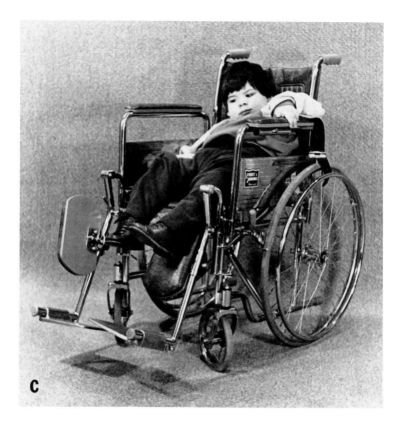

FIGURE 1 (continued).   (C) Stable sitting in an unadapted standard wheelchair is impossible.

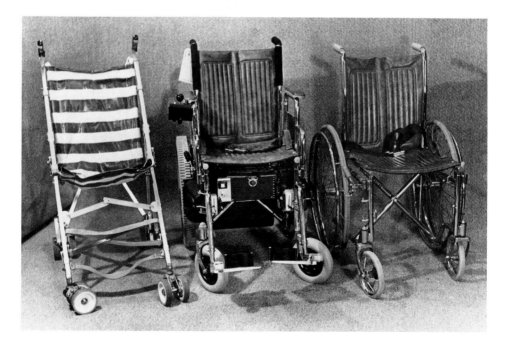

FIGURE 2.   Three commonly used bases for seating systems (from left to right): stroller, power wheelchair, and manual wheelchair.

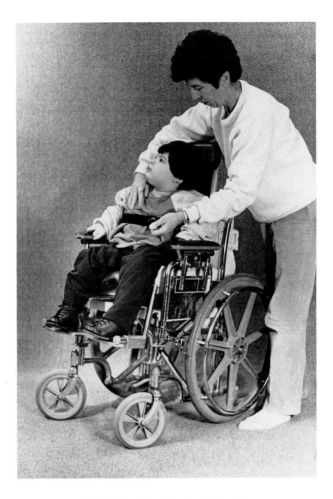

FIGURE 3.   Checking the belt length.

The therapist is available to carry out therapeutic measures and also to educate and encourage the client. Seating goals must be reevaluated periodically, and active cooperation between team members and client must be fostered at all times.

The therapist should be knowledgeable in new technological developments and, along with the other team members, take an active part in problem solving. With combined efforts and respect for the client as the most important team member, an acceptable, functional, and practical seating system will be designed, delivered, and used successfully.

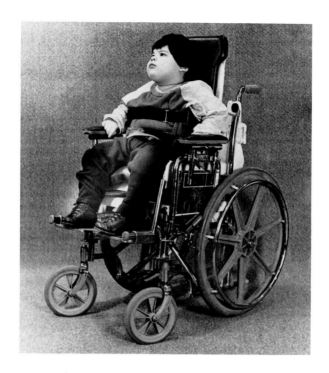

FIGURE 4. Trunk bolster positioning is ensured; foot placement is adjusted and body symmetry is observed.

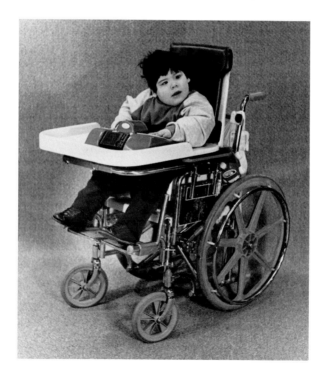

FIGURE 5. Addition of a tray improves shoulder and head control and encourages hand use and facilitates fine motor coordination.

REFERENCES

1. **Carlso, J. M., Lonstein, J., Beck, K. O., and Wilkie, D. C.,** Seating for children and young adults with cerebral palsy, *Clin. Prosthet. Orthot.,* 2, 176, 1987.
2. **Bergen, A. F. and Colangelo, C.,** *Positioning and Client with C.N.S. Deficits: The Wheelchair and Other adapted Equipment,* Valhalla Rehabilitation Publications, Valhalla, NY, 1985.
3. **Henderson, B. (Compiler),** *Seating in Review: Current Trends for the Disabled,* Otto Bock Orthopedic Industry of Canada, Winnipeg, Manitoba, Canada, 1985.
4. **Snow, C. J., Ed.,** *Proc. Int. Symp. Adaptive Seating,* Division of Physical Therapy and Department of Continuing Education, University of Manitoba, Canada, 1985.
5. **Trefler, E., Ed. and (Compiler),** *Seating for Children with Cerebral Palsy: A Resource Manual,* University of Tennessee Center for the Health Sciences, Rehabilitation Engineering Program, Memphis, 1984.
6. **Trefler, E., Tooms, R. E., and Hobson, D. A.,** Seating for cerebral palsied children, *Inter-Clin. Inf. Bull. Univ. Tenn. Cent. Health Sci. Rehabil. Eng. Cent.,* 17, 1, 1978.
7. **Trefler, E. et al.,** A modular seating system for cerebral palsied children, *Dev. Med. Child Neurol.,* 20, 199, 1978.
8. **Ward, D. E.,** *Positioning the Handicapped Child for Function: A Guide to Evaluate and Prescribe Equipment for the Child with Central Nervous System Dysfunction,* 2nd ed. rev., Phoenix Press, St.Louis, 1984.

Chapter 4

INFANT SEATING

R. Mervyn Letts

TABLE OF CONTENTS

I. INFANT SEATING NEEDS

Infants with disabilities do not require any seating assistance until 6 to 8 months of age and some, because of delayed development and small stature, may not require such assistance until 10 to 12 months of age. During the initial phases of their development, such infants are treated as any small baby and usually can be managed by the parents quite well without any special assistive devices. However, once the child attains the age of 6 to 8 months, at which time normal sitting stability usually develops in most children, a seating device or sitting support may be indicated (1) to assist the infant in sitting upright and relating to the environment; (2) to provide stimulation for further intellectual and motor development; (3) to facilitate support for the hips and lower extremities; and (4) to provide respite for the family or caregivers. Infants most in need of such support will usually be suffering from muscle hypotonia secondary to such diseases as spinal muscular atrophy or increasing spasticity secondary to cerebral palsy. Many other disease entities may necessitate a specialized seating approach to the infant, such as the extreme bone fragility seen in osteogenesis imperfecta or in patients with multiple congenital amputations or contractures secondary to arthrogryposis.[4]

II. COMMERCIALLY AVAILABLE INFANT SEATS

For most infants under 8 months of age, commercially available seating devices can probably be obtained on the market that will be quite functional and cost effective. These include the standard infant transport seat (Figure 1) and the Tumbleform™ seat (Figure 2).

III. MODIFIED INFANT SEATS

Most infant seats can be modified if necessary to provide trunk support, either with bolsters or with the addition of a tray (Figure 3). Headrest support can also be added. Custom-designed seating devices for infants such as the Cozy Seat can be useful, not only for supportive seating for these children, but also to facilitate feeding. A built-in reclining feature in most of these seats allows the child to be positioned appropriately for feeding, which is especially helpful for the feeding disabilities that frequently accompany many of the disease processes that result in poor sitting posture[2,3] (Figure 4).

IV. SPECIALIZED SEATING IN INFANCY

Future sitting stability is dependent on a stable pelvis and well-located and reduced hips. Acetabular development of the hip occurs most rapidly during infancy and is stimulated by the head of the femur being well seated within the acetabulum. This is an ideal opportunity for future problems, with dislocation of the hip to be avoided or aborted through the provision of abduction seating. No matter what type of device the child uses during his sitting activities, the hips should be positioned in abduction. A specialized seating device that takes this into consideration is the cerebral palsy floor seat which has abduction wings built into the seat and ensures that the child will sit with the legs abducted and, hence, the femoral head well seated in the acetabulum (Figure 5). In some infants who have significant spasticity to the point that abduction cannot be ensured, adductor tenotomies and iliopsoas recessions may be necessary to ensure good abduction of the hips. In this way, future subluxation of the hip and good development of the acetabulum may be ensured and the future sitting stability of the infant greatly enhanced.[5-9]

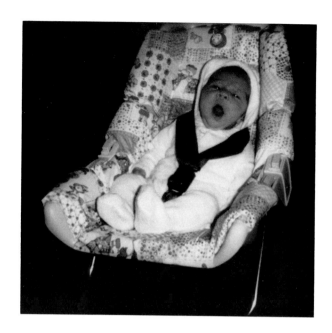

FIGURE 1.   Commercial infant seat.

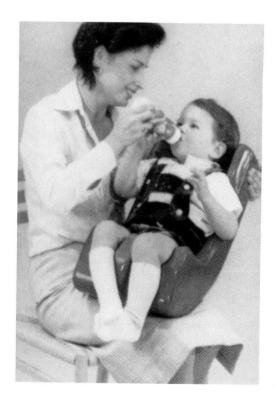

FIGURE 2.   Tumbleform™ infant seat.

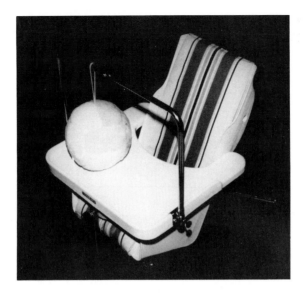

FIGURE 3.   Modified infant seat with tray and toy bar.

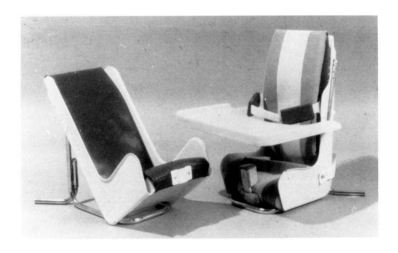

FIGURE 4.   Cozy Seats which are reclinable for feeding. (Reproduced with permission from Letts, M., Rang, M., and Tredwell, S., Seating the disabled, in *American Academy of Orthopaedic Surgeons: Atlas of Orthotics,* 2nd ed., C. V. Mosby, St. Louis, 1985.)

V. HIGHCHAIR SEATING

The infant who requires seating support will benefit from highchair modifications such as trunk bolsters, additional padding, and enhanced restraint belts (Figure 6). For infants difficult to feed or for very slow feeders such as spastic cerebral palsy children, the ability to recline the highchair seat a little is a welcome addition for the caregivers.

VI. MOBILITY DEVICES

During infancy, mobility is primarily related to the caregiver rather than the child. Children with good upper extremity function, such as in spina bifida, will be able to use a castor cart very effectively. The castor cart itself can be converted into a mini-stroller with

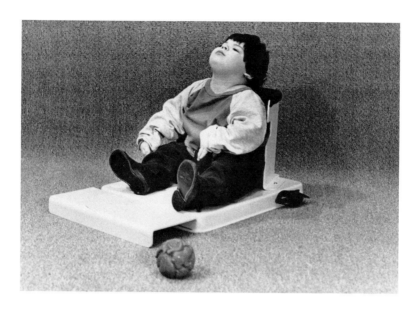

FIGURE 5.   Floor seat with molding constructed to keep legs abducted. (Reproduced with permission from Letts, M., Rang, M., and Tredwell, S., Seating the disabled, in *American Academy of Orthopaedic Surgeons: Atlas of Orthotics,* 2nd ed., C. V. Mosby, St. Louis, 1985.)

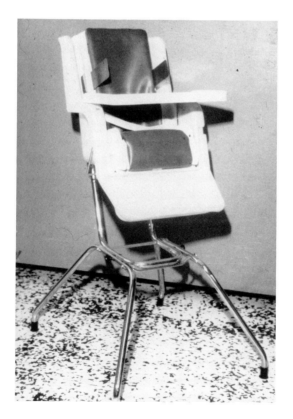

FIGURE 6.   Modified highchair for feeding infant with poor sitting stability. (Reproduced with permission from Letts, M., Rang, M., and Tredwell, S., Seating the disabled, in *American Academy of Orthopaedic Surgeons: Atlas of Orthotics,* 2nd ed., C. V. Mosby, St. Louis, 1985.)

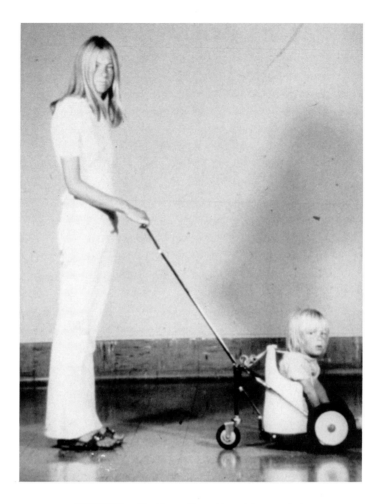

FIGURE 7.   The Castor Cart with push bar attached.

the addition of a push bar, and this facilitates the care and enhances the enjoyment for the child (Figure 7). For those children with more disability who require more supportive seating, the Pogan stroller can often be used as a base to fit a custom-made insert for the child (Figure 8). These inserts can also double as car seats for those infants who require a significant amount of support.

VII. INFANT CAR SEATS

For most handicapped children, the infant car seats available on the commercial market will be satisfactory and provide ample support during car rides. However, a small proportion of children with very severe disability may require more support, and it is these children who will also require more substantial sitting support in their strollers and highchairs. Inserts can often be constructed in such a manner that they can also be used as a very efficient car seat for the child. In some areas, this poses a potential legal problem for the seating team in that unless the seating device has been properly tested for its efficiency during a motor vehicle accident, there may be some question about appropriate authorization for such use. The Winnipeg modular insert was tested for its efficacy as a car seat by the National Research Council and was found to function as well as commercial devices manufactured exclusively for use as a car seat.[1] The standard General Motors (GM) car seat can be modified to provide

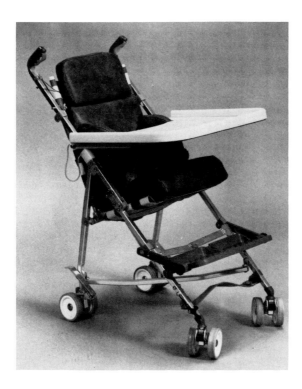

FIGURE 8.   Infant seating insert fitted to Pogan stroller base.

further support and functions very effectively for many handicapped children as a supportive car seat. Seating teams designing specialized infant car seats are advised to have them tested appropriately (Figure 9).

VIII. INFANT BATH AND TOILET SEATS

Infants under 6 to 8 months of age usually pose no difficulty for parents to bathe. However, between 12 and 24 months of age, very floppy infants are of a size such that handling may be very difficult and precarious in the bathtub arena. Polypropylene seats with restraint belts greatly facilitate the bathing process[5] (Figure 10). The bathtub frame (Figure 11), although designed for older children and adults, may also be useful from time to time for infants where showering plus sponge bathing is required. Modified commodes may also facilitate toileting in later infancy and provide some respite for the caregivers in coping with the training of these children (Figure 12).

IX. SUMMARY

Supportive seating will not be required for all handicapped infants, but in those with more severe disability, the seating team will be required to either modify the commercial infant seats or provide custom-made support in order to facilitate sitting as well as feeding and handling these severely compromised children.

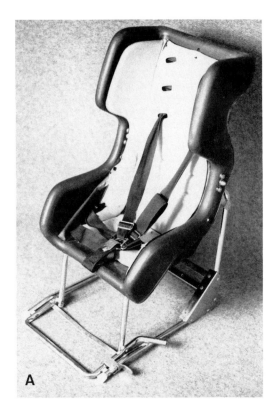

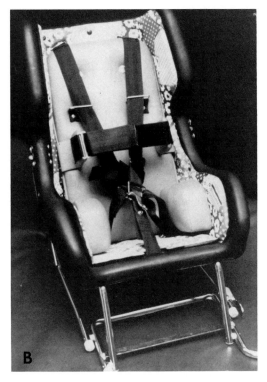

FIGURE 9.   Infant car seats. (A and B) Modified with foam inserts to facilitate seating support.

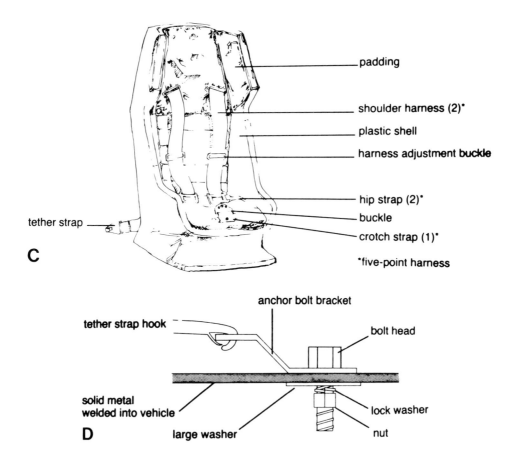

C

padding

shoulder harness (2)*

plastic shell

harness adjustment buckle

hip strap (2)*

buckle

crotch strap (1)*

*five-point harness

tether strap

D

anchor bolt bracket

tether strap hook

bolt head

solid metal
welded into vehicle

large washer

lock washer

nut

FIGURE 9 (continued). (C) Components of five-point harness; (D) anchor bolt assembly to vehicle to ensure solid fixation to the frame.

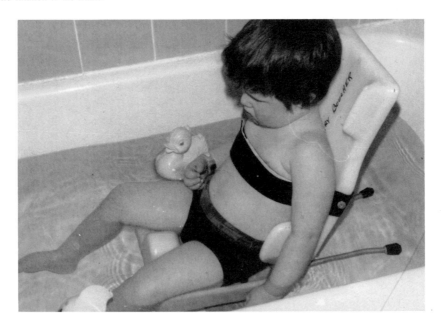

FIGURE 10. Polypropylene bath seat with reclining back and restraint belt. (Reproduced with permission from Letts, M., Rang, M., and Tredwell, S., Seating the disabled, in *American Academy of Orthopaedic Surgeons: Atlas of Orthotics,* 2nd ed., C. V. Mosby, St. Louis, 1985.)

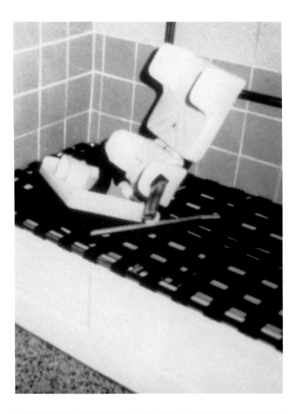

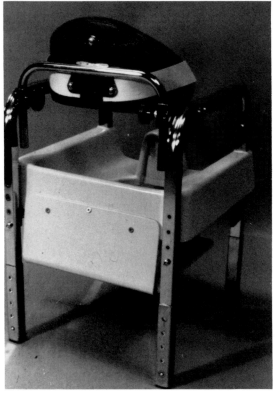

FIGURE 12.   Modified infant commode with back support and restraint belts.

REFERENCES

1. **Bull, M. J. and Stroup, K. B.,** Premature infants in car seats, *Pediatrics,* 75, 336, 1985.
2. **Carolson, J. M. and Winter, R.,** The "Gillette" sitting support orthosis, *Orthot. Prosthet.,* 32, 35, 1978.
3. **Dilger, N. J. and Ling, W.,** The influence of inclined wedge sitting on infant postural kyphosis, in Proc. Seating the Disabled, Memphis, February 26 to 28, 1987, 3:52.
4. **Letts, R. M.,** The special devices and seating clinic — a universal need, *Can. Orthot. Prosthet.* 10, 19, 1978.
5. **Letts, R. M., Rang, M., and Tredwell, S.,** Seating the disabled, in *Atlas of Orthotics,* 2nd ed., C. V. Mosby, St. Louis, 1985, 440.
6. **Motloch, W. M.,** Seating and positioning for the physically impaired, *Orthot. Prosthet.,* 31, 11, 1977.
7. **Rang, M., Douglas, G., Bennet, G. C., and Koreska, J.,** Seating for children with cerebral palsy, *J. Pediatr. Orthop.,* 1, 279, 1981.
8. **Tredwell, S.,** Shapeable matrix seating for the handicapped child, *J. Pediatr. Orthop.,* 2, 44, 1982.
9. **Trefler, E., Tooms, R. E., and Hobson, D. A.,** Seating for cerebral palsied children, *Int. Clin. Inf. Bull.,* 17, 1, 1978.

Chapter 5

JUVENILE SEATING

R. Mervyn Letts

TABLE OF CONTENTS

I. INTRODUCTION

There is probably no other age group in which seating is more important and, indeed, more difficult for the handicapped child with poor sitting stability than that from age 3 to 12 years. It is during these formative years that the child's social skills, peer group interaction, and overall self-worth becomes established. The seating team has a unique opportunity and, indeed, obligation to ensure that the child can interact with his environment and peer group in a manner that will allow psychological and motor development to the maximum of the child's potential. Children at this age also become quite heavy and can be a major burden and, indeed, medical liability to caregivers and family if they are unable to sit appropriately and constantly require lifting and carrying from one point to another. It is also during this age that deformities may become more fixed and interfere significantly with functional and comfortable seating.

II. PATTERNS OF DEFORMITY

Regardless of the etiology of the underlying sitting disability, three patterns of deformity are commonly seen: symmetrically slouched (Figure 1), asymmetrically slouched, and windswept. In this age group, such deformities may be controlled and prevented from becoming established and permanent to the point that future sitting during adolescence and adulthood will be severely compromised. No one seating solution may provide the appropriate seating need, and the involvement of the entire team with all specialties participating is essential. A combination of specialized seating and surgical correction of fixed deformity will be required for many of these patients. A brief analysis of some of the solutions to seating problems seen in this age group are outlined in Table 1.

III. GOALS OF JUVENILE SEATING

The major objective of seating in this age group is to allow the child full access to his environment by removing the necessity of the seated juvenile to spend most of the seating time concentrating on sitting posture, which defunctions both upper extremity activity and concentration on learning and intellectual matters. In order to accomplish this objective, the following goals should be accomplished regardless of the underlying disability that has necessitated a wheelchair existence for the child:

1. The head and neck should be vertical. If the head is too far back, the child will constantly be flexing the neck to bring it forward to see what is going on in the environs (Figures 2 and 3). If the head is too far forward and poorly controlled, the chin will lie on the chest.
2. The lumbar spine should be supported in some lordosis, but excessive lumbar bolstering should be avoided. Normal thoracic kyphosis should be maintained.
3. The hips should be flexed to 100°, which helps prevent the tendency to slide forward in the wheelchair (Figure 4).
4. The legs should be abducted to provide containment of the femoral heads in the acetabulae. This also assists in ensuring a straight pelvis, thus minimizing the development of pelvic obliquity with resultant asymmetric weight bearing (Figure 5).
5. The shoulders should be slightly rounded and do not need to be held back excessively. It is preferable to tilt the insert back 15 or 20° to minimize forward slouch rather than using chest and shoulder straps (Figure 6).
6. The arms should be supported to avoid fatigue and discomfort in the shoulders, which frequently occurs if they are allowed to hang free. A wheelchair tray is useful to provide arm support (Figure 7).

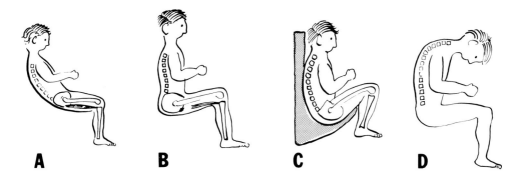

FIGURE 1. The symmetrically slouched child. (A) Hip extension contracture causes the child to slide forward. A pommel or tight lap belt is a poor answer. (B) Proximal hamstring lengthening allows the child to sit upright; (C) a wedged seat which permits excessive knee flexion is the best seating answer. (Reproduced with permission from Letts, M., Rang, M., and Tredwell, S., Seating the disabled, in *American Academy of Orthopaedic Surgeons: Atlas of Orthotics,* 2nd ed., C. V. Mosby, St. Louis, 1985.)

7. The feet should be supported. Foot supports decrease thigh pressure and control knee and hip flexion position (Figure 8). Contracture of the tendoachilles from a constant equinus position may also be avoided.
8. Freedom of motion must be ensured. Rigid support of all body parts is not practical or comfortable.

IV. TEMPORAL SEATING CONSIDERATIONS

In the juvenile age group, seating devices may be used for (1) short-term use, (2) medium-term use (3 to 6 h), or (3) long-term use. Seats intended for short-term use include, for example, car seats, in which the fit should be good and snug, but not necessarily structured for permanent or long-term use. Seats fabricated for medium-term use should fit more accurately, more like an orthosis, and provide support where required. Seating systems devised for long-term use should be safe and comfortable and provide a good means of transportation and good support for all-day use. This type of seat should also be well padded, with a reasonably loose fit to allow some movement. Tilting of the insert to redistribute the pressure widely will make prolonged sitting safer and more comfortable (Figure 9).

V. SEATING THE SYMMETRICALLY SLOUCHED CHILD

Controlling the symmetrically slouched child with modifications in the seating system itself may not be possible if the slouching is secondary to fixed contractures. As an example, contracture of the hamstrings often leads to the development of hip extension deformity, which, in turn, results in sacral sitting, pelvic rotation, and a tendency for the child to slip forward out of the chair. This may result in a fixed thoracic kyphosis as the child leans forward to counteract this tendency. Groin straps are frequently employed to control this problem; however, these are often a source of discomfort for the child and a source of aggravation for the caregivers. To correct this vicious cycle of tight hamstrings leading to symmetrically slouched sitting and further contracture of the hamstrings, surgical lengthening of the hamstrings is often required. Following the lengthening of the hamstring and the adductors, the child can often be seated much more comfortably and functionally with a 10 to 20° incline in the seat (see Figure 1). It should be emphasized that in a child with symmetric slouching, hamstring tightness often is undetected since hip flexion is usually examined with the knee flexed. It is best recorded by measuring the range of straight leg raising or the popliteal angle of Bleck (Figure 10).

TABLE 1
Trouble Shooting in Postural Seating

	Problem	Possible causes	Possible solutions
Pelvis	Posterior tilt (sacral sitting or sliding out of chair)	Hypotonia	Decrease seat length
		Tonic labyrinth prone (TLP) reflex (producing flexed posture)	Reduce seat wedge/roll height
		Limited active hip flexion (causing compensatory loss) of low lumbar curve)	Lumbar or sacral pad
			Change position of head in space and thereby influence TLP
		Tight hamstrings with seat too long or with too high a wedge in seat, footrests preventing knee flexion	Raise height of tray
			Adjust position of footrests to allow more knee flexion
		Improper positioning in seat	Reposition pelvis (flex pelvis)
		Lap belt located too high	Lower lap belt attachment point
	Lateral tilt (weight on one buttock)	Asymmetric muscle tone	Solid base to seat
		Scoliosis with pelvic obliquity	Midline orientation by using lateral pelvic blocks
		Dislocated or subluxated hip	
		"Hammock" of wheelchair seat	Three-point pressure support of trunk and pelvis
			Contour seat to facilitate equal weight distribution
Trunk	Scoliosis	Postural	Midline pelvic orientation
		Position of pelvis not midline	Three-point support
		Hypotonia-hypertonia assymmetric muscle tone (asymmetric tonic neck reflex, asymmetric distribution of tone, hemiplegia, etc.)	Midline trunk or chest harnesses
			Recessed back or midline orientation
			Tray to help with midline orientation
			Reduce abnormal tone
			Hip angle
		Environmental or functional demands	Neck collar
			Change orientation of functional work
		Structural	Recline back to reduce effects of gravity
		Persistent asymmetric posture (fixed deformity)	
	Kyphosis	Postural	Surgery or orthotic management
		Posterior pelvic tilt	See previous solutions, pelvic tilt
		Structural	Add chest panel or bandolier harnesses
		Fixed deformity	Lumbosacral pad
			Surgery or orthotic management
Shoulder girdle	Retraction	Thoracolumbar scoliosis	Reduce extensor tone
		Extensor thrust	Roll or wedge seat
		Asymmetric tonic neck reflex	Decrease hip angle
		Instability of upper trunk	Neck collar
			Alter head position in space (gravity)
			Protract shoulders
			Tray extensions or rounded seat-back with wings
			Lower tray
			Stabilize upper trunk with straps
	Protraction	TLP	Lumbosacral pad
		Kyphosis	Raise tray height
			Chest panel
			Change attitude of body in space (gravity)
Head and neck	Hyperextension	Extensor hypertonicity	Neck collar positioned just below occipital region
		Poor flexor control	
		Headrest or neck collar positioned too low	Reduce total extensor hypertonicity at pelvis (see above)

TABLE 1 (continued)
Trouble Shooting in Postural Seating

	Problem	Possible causes	Possible solutions
		Improper neck or head support (i.e., headrest placed on occipital)	Position neckrest slightly anterior
		Thoracolumbar scoliosis	Alter position of head in space (gravity)
	Protraction	Hypotonia	Lower neckrest and align in neutral position
		Neckrest too high or too far forward	
		TLP	Raise and/or tilt tray
		Tray work too low	Low lumbosacral pad
		Kyphosis	Alter position of head in space (gravity)
	Rotation	Atonic neck reflex	Inhibit atonic neck reflex
			Midline orientation of pelvis and trunk
			Protraction of shoulders
		Sensory deficit	Thoughtful positioning for function
		Visual	Reduce general hypertonicity
		Auditory	
		Unstable spine	
		Generalized domination of primitive pathosis	
	Side flexion	Hypertonicity	Reposition of neck or headrest
		Hydrocephalus	Larger neck or headrest
		Severe retardation	More stable chest support
		Sensory deficits	Recline body in space (gravity)
Hips	Extension-adduction	Thoracolumbar scoliosis	Roll seat, with roll one finger width behind knee
		Positive supporting reaction	
	Internal rotation	Extensor thrust	Increase hip flexion by
		Dislocated hip	Higher roll
		Seat too short	Wedge
		Seat belt too long or poorly positioned	Flexing seatback anterior of vertical
			Pommel (as a last resort); keep it short enough so it is nowhere near groin area
			Platform shoes to reduce positive supporting reaction (PSR)
			Seat belt at 45° to thigh
			Alter attitude of body in space to affect tonic labyrinth supine reaction (gravity)
			Have removable footrests for initial fittings
			Caution: watch pelvis as you increase hip flexion if hamstrings are tight
	Flexion-abduction	Hypotonia	Adduction blocks with good foot position (footpads or straps)
		Adductor releases	
Knees	Flexion	Primitive patterns	Inhibit flexor tone by adjusting (roll or wedge)
		Flexion contractures	
			Position feet in neutral (if tight hamstrings, watch effect on pelvis)
			Surgery
	Extension	Extension patterns (usually dynamic response to abnormal tone)	Inhibit extensor tone with roll or wedge
			Decrease hip angle
			Neutral strapping of feet
			Shorten seat

TABLE 1 (continued)
Trouble Shooting in Postural Seating

	Problem	Possible causes	Possible solutions
Feet	Plantar flexion	Extension pattern	Check footrest height and place foot
		Positive supporting reaction	in slight dorsiflexion to inhibit PSR
		Heel cord contractures	Surgery
		Footrest too low	Inhibit tone with roll/wedge
			Platform shoes
	Inversion-eversion	Same as above	Footrest height
			Platform shoes
			Footpads or straps
			AFO[a]

[a]   AFO, ankle-foot orthosis.

Modified from Hobson, D. and Healing, A., Workshop on Seating, Memphis, November 1979.

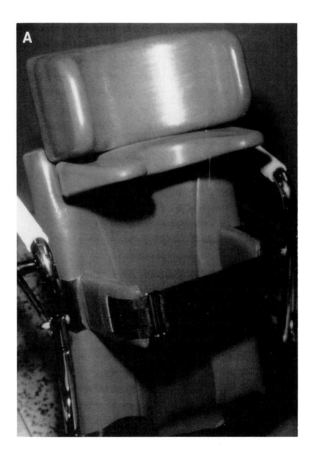

FIGURE 2.   Winnipeg head- and neckrest (A).

Tightness of the hip flexors may be counteracted to some extent by raising the front edge of the wheelchair insert 2 to 3 in. with wedges. This flexes the hips and knees more, but also prevents the child from sliding forward. In some children with spasticity resulting in hip extension contracture, proximal hamstring lengthening combined with adductor

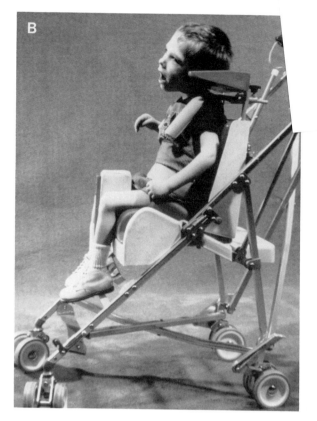

FIGURE 2 (continued).   (B) Design provides adjustable positioning
of the head.

release, and iliopsoas recession, is effective in facilitating a more normal seated position.
The presence of a spinal deformity, especially kyphosis, can sometimes be controlled effectively with an orthosis. The Soft Boston type of orthosis for this age group has been
found to be particularly effective. The seating system can then be developed around the
child with the orthosis in place.

VI. THE ASYMMETRICALLY SLOUCHED CHILD

Poor muscle tone contributes to asymmetric sitting as well as asymmetrical spasticity.
The child falls to one side because of either poor paraspinal muscle tone or spasticity that
is asymmetrical, resulting in postural scoliosis which can ultimately become fixed. For this
type of child, supportive seating with wheelchair inserts and bolsters is a necessity. This
type of posturing and deformity predisposes to hip subluxation, and the hips need to be
monitored clinically and radiographically every 6 months (Figure 11). If the adductors
become tight, tenotomy should be performed, and persistent subluxation over the age of
5 years may require varus osteotomy to avoid the disaster of a hip dislocation. Surgery for
these children at an early age should stabilize the hips, but care must be taken to avoid
excessive release, leading to abduction contractures. With present-day anesthesia and intensive care in the postoperative phase, even the most handicapped child is usually fit enough
for these procedures, and early detection of ''hip at risk'' may eliminate the need for a varus
osteotomy of the femur and avoid an impossible seating nightmare due to major fixed
deformity in adulthood.

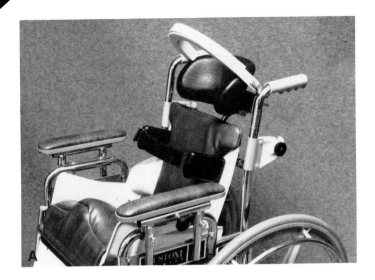

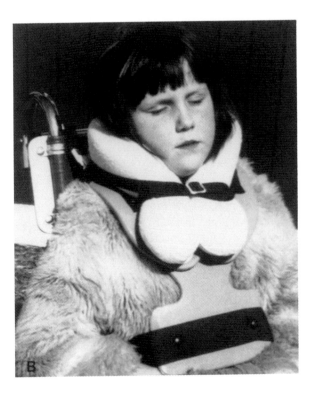

FIGURE 3.   Otto Bock head support with Winnipeg adjustable halo to keep head upright (A). (B) Hensinger head support — a foam wraparound collar designed to support the head (Danmar Products, Ann Arbor, MI).

VII. THE WINDSWEPT CHILD

Although, individually, scoliosis, pelvic obliquity, and hip contractures result in numerous seating problems, one of the most devastating is a combination of these three known as the "windswept hip syndrome". The typical deformity is a scoliosis convex away from

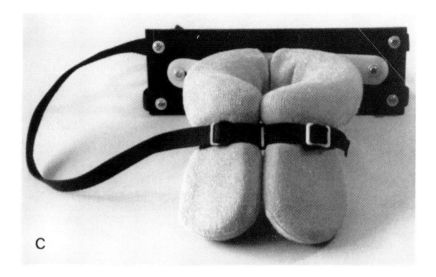

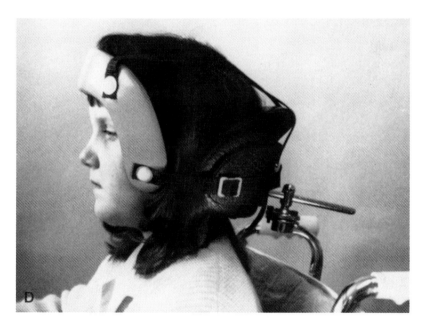

FIGURE 3 (continued). (C) Hensinger head support; (D) half-mask head support attached to the Otto Bock headrest to counteract forward thrusting of the head. Proper head positioning improves breathing and swallowing and simplifies feeding.

the side on which the hip is dislocated. The pelvis is frequently tilted upward on the side of the hip dislocation, and it becomes extremely difficult for these children to sit properly. The main thrust of the seating team should be to prevent this problem from occurring. Early surgery may minimize the development of the windswept hip syndrome by preventing dislocation of the hip, often the initiating factor in the development of the triad of pelvic obliquity, scoliosis, and hip dislocation. Needless to say, supportive seating is critical after any surgery to maintain the correction and prevent recurrence of the deformity. This difficult problem is discussed in more detail in Chapter 9.

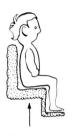
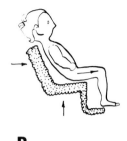
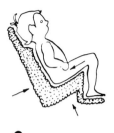
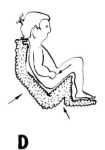

A   **B**   **C**   **D**

FIGURE 4.   Forces between the child and chair. (A) The upright seatback does not exert any force; (B) the reclined back lets some force be applied to the back, but there is a horizontal shear, so the child slips out of the chair; (C) a seat wedge and reclining back prevent forward slip, unload the spine, and permit the seatback to exert force on the child's back, but the upward gaze makes it difficult to work; (D) the angled back, proposed by Motloch, combines spinal support with forward gaze. (Reproduced with permission from Letts, M., Rang, M., and Tredwell, S., Seating the disabled, in *American Academy of Orthopaedic Surgeons: Atlas of Orthotics,* 2nd ed., C. V. Mosby, St. Louis, 1985.)

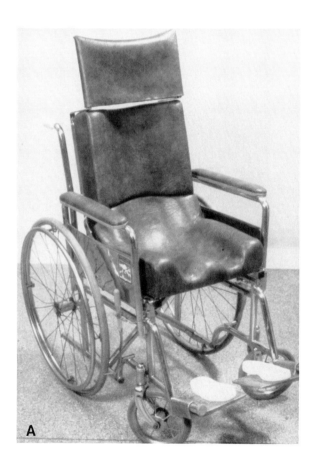

FIGURE 5.   Abduction seating built into the customized seat (A).

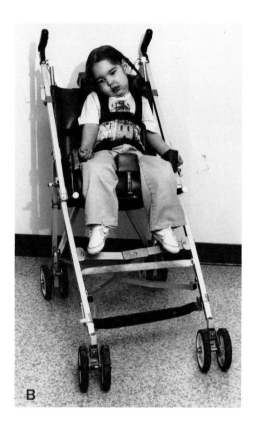

FIGURE 5 (continued). (B) Abduction seating provided by a removable pommel.

VIII. JUVENILE SEATING INSERTS

Seating inserts are frequently required in the juvenile age group for the severely handicapped individual, and such inserts, in effect, become part of the body image of the child as well as a reality of daily life for the family and caregivers. The following principles should be adhered to when choosing and designing inserts for physically disabled children:

1. The inner surface should be well padded or custom molded to the wheelchair individual.
2. The outer surface must be standardized to fit available wheelchair bases.
3. The unit needs to be adjustable for growth since the child in this age group is growing rapidly.
4. The initial fitting and subsequent adjustment should be simple and relatively easy.
5. The unit should be of single construction and relatively inexpensive.
6. The insert should be easy to use and transport by parents and staff (Figure 12).

In general, the seat surface should be a solid base rather than a hammock-type chair (Figure 13), and this is especially so for the child who tends toward an extensor reflex thrust when sitting. This type of extensor pattern can be inhibited to some extent by elevating the seat in the front to achieve hip flexion over 90°.

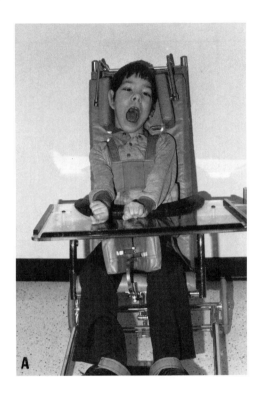

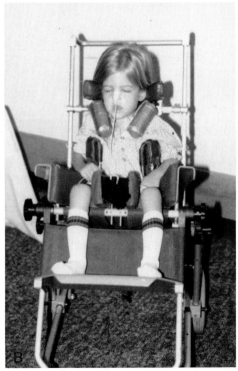

FIGURE 6. Prevention of forward slouching by (A) Otto Bock butterfly chest pad and (B) over-the-shoulder restraints in Mulholland seating system. Note abduction wings to hold legs in abduction to maintain hip stability.

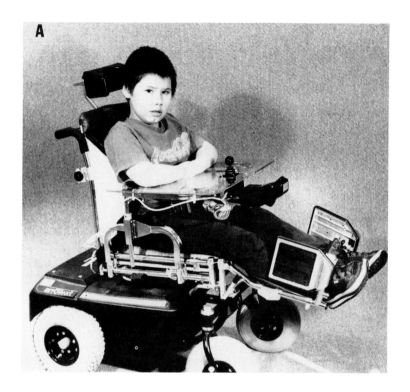

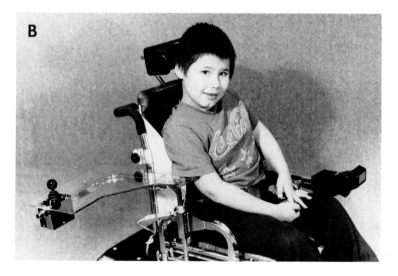

FIGURE 7. Arms supported by (A) tray with centralized joystick; (B) tray divided in middle, swings to each side to allow easy exit from chair.

Abduction seating should always be an objective, especially in those children with adductor spasticity, to maintain good hip reduction.

Pelvic instability creates major problems for the insert, and modifications may be necessary to secure pelvic fixation. The Mulholland chair illustrates some modifications needed to achieve pelvic stability (Figure 14). Three-point fixation is attained through spinal supports or bolters, with a pelvic stabilizing support being the third point. Shoulder and head restrainers are often required. For the hypotonic child who collapses into flexion, a reclining feature of the insert may be necessary up to 45°. In this instance, hip extension is desired and the

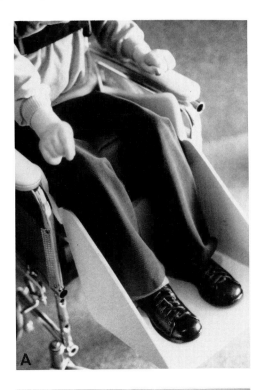

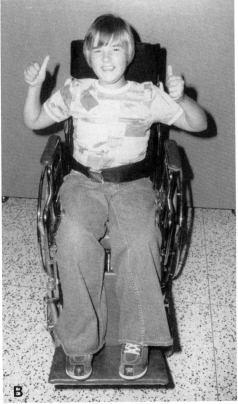

FIGURE 8.   Maintaining feet in (A) normal plantigrade position on footbox or footrests helps to ensure good sitting stability (B).

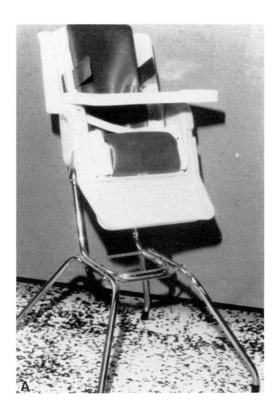

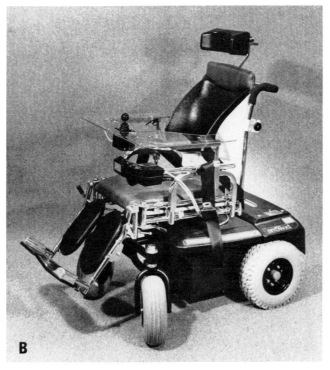

FIGURE 9. Short-term seating, as in (A) the modified highchair, is contoured with a tilt feature for ease of feeding, but has no support structure for long-term seating, as in (B) the motorized chair.

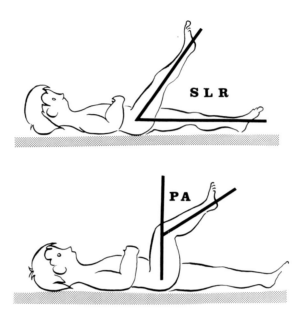

FIGURE 10. Hip extension contracture is assessed by the straight-leg raising angle and the amount of hamstring contracture by the popliteal angle of Bleck. (From Rang, M., Douglas, G., Bennet, G. C., and Koreska, J., *J. Pediatr. Orthop.*, 1, 279, 1981. With permission.)

opposite position to that of the child who goes into extensor patterning is required. Keeping the hips at about 80° of flexion often will inhibit the tendency for the child to fall into the collapsed flexed position, and sitting is facilitated with only a slight reclining of the back of the chair. Fortunately, pelvic obliquity rarely results in pressure sores in younger children, and the main objective is to stop progression of the obliquity and correct it if possible so as to avoid pressure problems when the child is older and heavier.

IX. MODULAR SEATING SYSTEMS

During rapid growth in the juvenile age group, a modular seating system may be more practical and economical. An example of this "off-the-shelf" type of seating technology is illustrated in Figure 15. Specialized components such as headrests, trays, neck supports, pommels, and chest pads can be added on as necessary. Other types of modular systems such as the Otto Bock system are available and offer considerable resiliency and economy in dealing with the changing seating requirements of size and growth.

X. SPINAL ORTHOSIS AND SEATING

During rapid growth in the juvenile age group (often associated with the juvenile growth spurt, 5 to 7 years of age), spinal curvature may develop and contribute to asymmetrical sitting. Although this can often be accommodated with bolster support, in patients with neuromuscular disease, this is often ineffectual. A spinal orthosis may provide a stable, upright spine which will facilitate good sitting posture. The Soft Boston orthosis has been found to be well tolerated in juveniles with collapsing spines secondary to spinal muscle imbalance from cerebral palsy or spinal muscular atrophy (Figure 16).

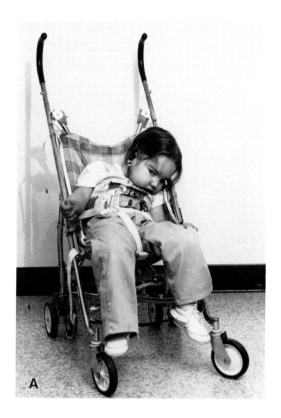

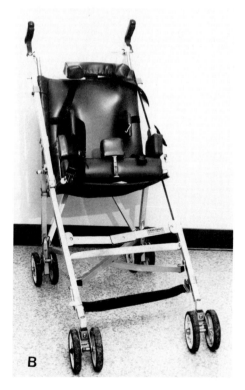

FIGURE 11.   Poor asymmetrical slouching in (A)
an unsupported stroller; (B) the Maclaren buggy with
insert and bolstering to provide stable seating.

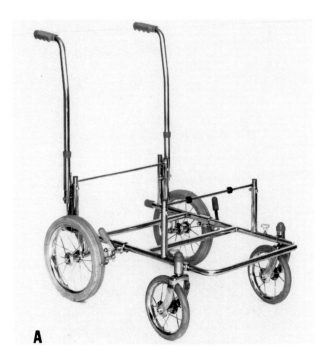

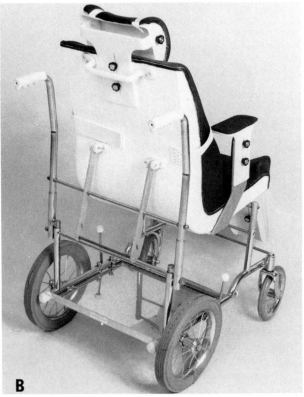

FIGURE 12.   Mooney wheelchair base (A); (B) a simple seat on the
Mooney base. Reclining the seat is easy. For travel in an automobile,
the base can be put in the trunk while the insert is used as a car seat.
(Reproduced with permission from Letts, M., Rang, M., and Tredwell,
S., Seating the disabled, in *American Academy of Orthopaedic Surgeons:
Atlas of Orthotics,* 2nd ed., C. V. Mosby, St. Louis, 1985.)

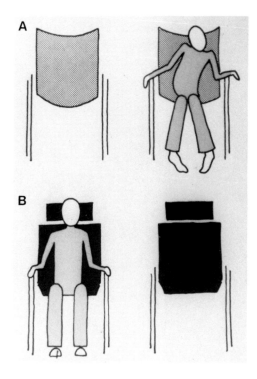

FIGURE 13. The hammock-style wheelchair seat (A) is unstable. Hands are frequently required to maintain balance. (B) A wheelchair insert provides security and stability, allowing the hands to be free for other uses. (Reproduced with permission from Letts, M., Rang, M., and Tredwell, S., Seating the disabled, in *American Academy of Orthopaedic Surgeons: Atlas of Orthotics*, 2nd ed., C. V. Mosby, St. Louis, 1985.)

XI. ALTERNATIVE SEATING DEVICES

Respite seating devices such as the pommel, corner seat, and Sleek Seat are useful additions to the seating armamentarium in the provision of good, comfortable, and stable seating for the juvenile disabled child. These devices are discussed in more detail in Chapter 19.

XII. SUMMARY

Seating the juvenile with a major disability can be a particularly rewarding experience for the seating team. The provision of a good seating system for the child will enhance the child's education, improve interrelationships with peers, and greatly enhance motor skills. The ability to sit in a comfortable position for significant portions of the day will be greatly appreciated by parents, caregivers, and teachers and will greatly enhance the ability of the child to enter adolescence and adulthood with a good sitting posture and a much more positive attitude toward a wheelchair existence. Surgery if required for increasing or recalcitrant contractures is better tolerated in this age group and should not be deferred if stable sitting is being compromised by a surgically correctable deformity.

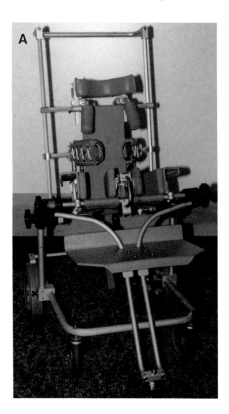 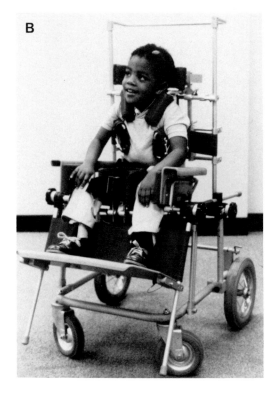

FIGURE 14.   The Mulholland seating system (A and B) provides most of the requirements for stable, comfortable seating with provision for growth and special options that can be added for head support or bolstering.

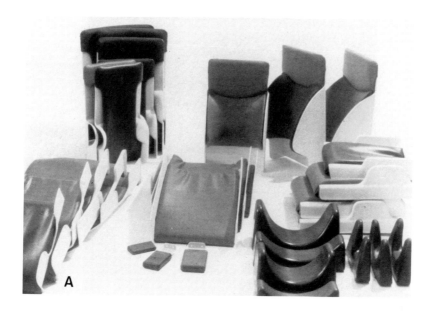

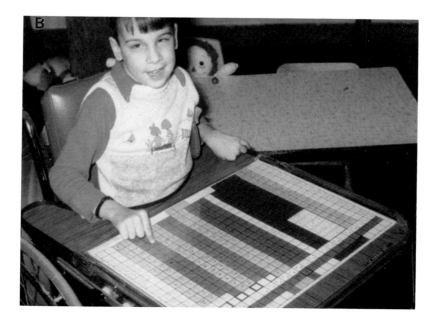

FIGURE 15. Winnipeg modular wheelchair insert system (A) illustrating the advantage of off-the-shelf fabrication of seating requirements with a change to a larger size to easily accommodate growth and special needs; (B) Bliss symbol board tray.

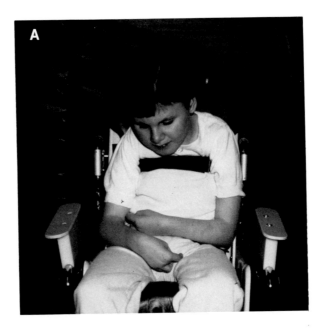

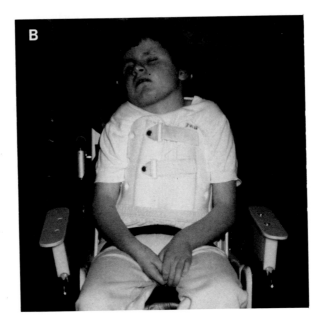

FIGURE 16.   Collapsing kypho-scoliosis (A) contributing to poor sitting in spite of a good insert; (B) sitting balance much improved with Soft Boston orthosis.

Chapter 6

ADOLESCENT SEATING

R. Mervyn Letts

TABLE OF CONTENTS

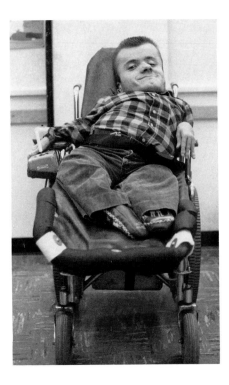

FIGURE 3. "Fixed deformities" in a teenaged osteogenesis imperfecta wheelchair user. A customized semireclining chair with powered mobility and seat control provides a functional and comfortable chair.

socialization,[6] but also to prevent the individual from becoming overweight (Figure 4). Teenagers with spina bifida and muscular dystrophy are most in danger of becoming overweight. This increased weight not only increases the pressure over bony prominences, but also makes it more difficult to maintain adequate seating support. Wheelchair inserts may have to be modified frequently, and it is advantageous to use a modular type of wheelchair system if the child is rapidly growing or changing dimensions frequently[3] (Figure 5). Several modular systems are on the market, the components of which can be interchanged, depending on the size and requirements of the child (Figure 6). Additional cushioning may be required with T-foam inserts or a ROHO® cushion to minimize the development of pressure sores. Paraplegic teenagers need a regular program of education not only about diet, but also about skin care and early signs of increasing pressure as well as hygiene and sexuality discussions. Pressure sores can usually be prevented by:

1. Even weight distribution with minimal shear
2. Regular sitting push-ups to relieve initial pressure
3. Avoidance of scars
4. Self-inspection of pressure sores with a mirror on a regular basis

IV. THE ADOLESCENT SPINE

Scoliosis is common in the seated adolescent since many of the disabilities that result in a wheelchair existence also predispose to spinal curvature. Muscle imbalance can affect not only the lower extremities, but also the paraspinal muscles, resulting in asymmetry in

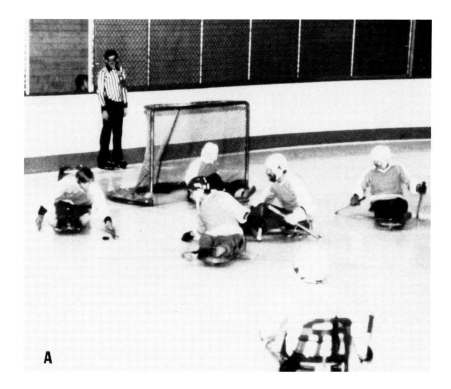

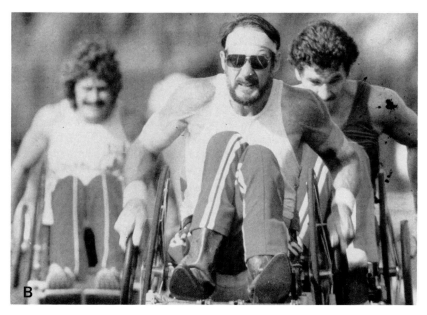

FIGURE 4.   Sports activities. (A) Sledge hockey and (B) wheelchair racing assist in keeping the wheelchair user physically fit.

strength, which, in turn, results in a spinal curvature.[9] Cerebral palsy, muscular dystrophy, quadriplegia, and myelomeningocele are a few of the many causes of both scoliosis and nonambulation in the teenager.[10] In general, it is difficult to treat spinal curvature with an orthosis in a wheelchair individual, and usually the most practical approach is to deal with

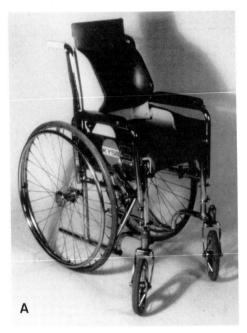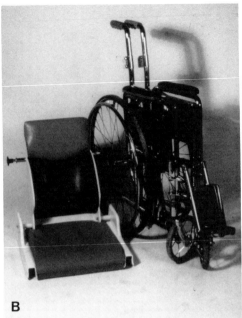

A   **B**

FIGURE 5.   Modular (A) and removable (B) wheelchair insert allowing easier transport of folding chair. Insert can be used in some instances as a supportive car seat.

the deformity surgically if the curve becomes progressive. In some seated teenagers with progressive curvatures under 45 to 50°, curve progression may be slowed with an Aliplast spinal orthosis. This so-called Soft Boston orthosis is well tolerated and improves sitting posture in those with scoliosis secondary to neuromuscular scoliosis (Figure 7). It will not, of course, correct the spinal curvature, but may buy some time until more growth occurs or the malnutrition is corrected. Most seating teams endorse the principle that a progressive curve exceeding 40° should be dealt with by surgical stabilization. The methods available are quite reliable and require little postoperative support. Sublaminar wiring with either Luque rods or segmental instrumentation have been shown to be very effective in correcting and maintaining spinal curvature in wheelchair users (Figure 8). The more recent Cotrel-Dubosset instrumentation in its initial evaluation has also been shown to be effective in maintaining curve correction.

In more severe and rigid curves, a combined anterior and posterior approach with a circumferential fusion may be required. Correcting such major curvatures not only improves sitting stability, but also extends sitting tolerance since the impingement of the rib cage on the iliac crest frequently is a source of pain and discomfort (Figure 9).

V. THE PAINFUL HIP

It is in adolescence that the dislocated or subluxated hip may become a source of pain and discomfort and limit wheelchair sitting tolerance. In some instances, this can be improved through the addition of sponge wedging or changing from a modular wheelchair insert system to a Foam-in-Place type of insert. However, in spite of this, some adolescents continue to experience considerable discomfort, primarily when the hip is subluxated rather than completely dislocated.[1] The association of spasticity seems to aggravate this problem and may result in increasing friction between the head of the femur and edge of the acetabulum in the subluxated hip. If seating adjustments do not relieve the discomfort, a muscle release consisting of adductor tenotomies and iliopsoas recessions is often effective in decreasing

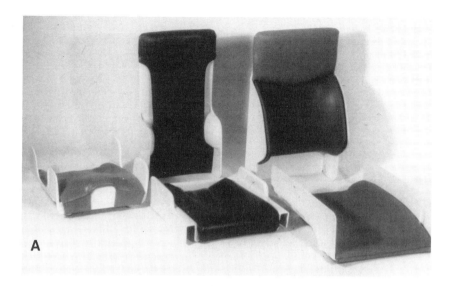

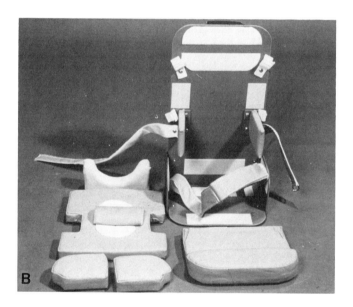

FIGURE 6. Modular seating systems. (A) Winnipeg and (B) Gillette systems allow for modifications to be made inexpensively to accommodate growth, keeping the insert functional.

the discomfort. If the acetabulum is still well developed, a varus osteotomy may provide a stable, comfortable, and permanent reduction of the hip, which, in turn, contributes to good sitting stability (Figure 10). If this is insufficient in relieving the pain, an excision of the head of the femur is carefully done so that a capsulorraphy between the remaining femur and pelvis will usually relieve the discomfort. Care must be taken in excising the head of the femur in that if too much of the femur is removed, the limb will become extremely frail and it will be difficult to seat the individual.

VI. POWERED CHAIRS

Although powered chairs are often used by younger children, it is during the teenage years that they become most functional. Powered units in school and, indeed, in the workplace

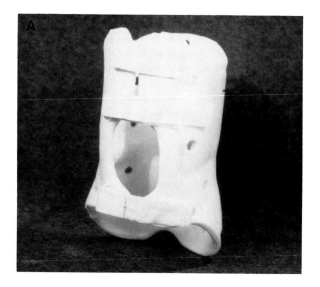

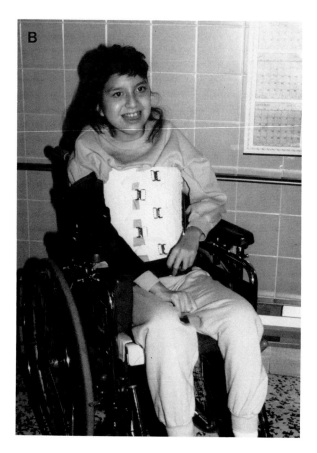

FIGURE 7. The "Soft Boston" Aliplast orthosis (A) is comfortable and effective in contributing to good sitting posture, especially for teenagers with neuromuscular scoliosis such as in the teenager with Rett's syndrome (B).

are often very practical for the teenaged wheelchair user.[2] This can be supplemented with commercially available powered scooters such as the Pony or Amigo to give the teenager more independence. Although not all wheelchair users will be capable of using powered devices, those with adequate upper extremity function should be able to use the powered chair very effectively. The power control box may have to be located in an accessible site, depending on the particular disability (Figure 11). For those with muscle weakness, a centralized control box is often preferred to allow the arms to rest on the tray and support the upper torso.

VII. SUMMARY

Seating the adolescent is a challenge that can be both frustrating and gratifying. The frustration usually centers around the rapidly changing growth that occurs at this age. The gratification comes from the knowledge that if the seating can be comfortably and functionally achieved at this age, the teenager will most likely be a good stable sitter for the rest of adult life. The combined approach of all disciplines involved in the seating team is necessary to achieve this goal, and the end result will be greatly appreciated by the wheelchair user as well as by friends and family. The spine is of major concern in this age group and the prevention of sitting imbalance because of progressive spinal curvature should be a major goal of the seating team.

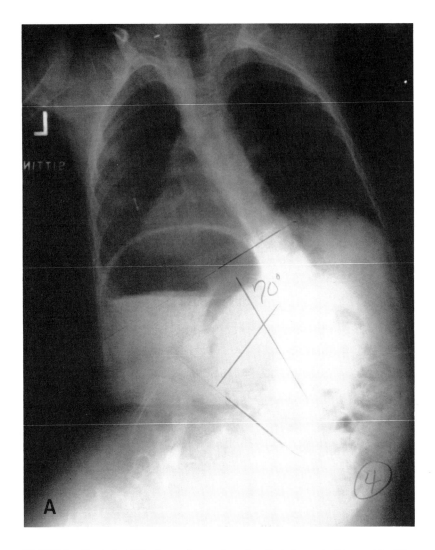

FIGURE 8.   Surgical stabilization and correction of scoliosis is required to provide sitting stability and to reduce incidence of pressure sores (A).

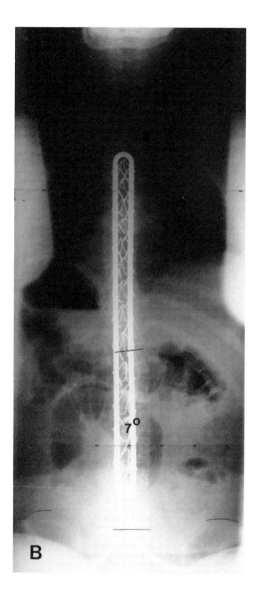
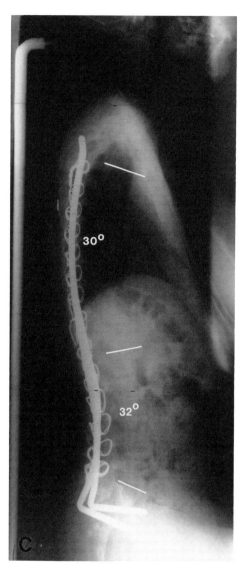

FIGURE 8 (continued).   Surgical stabilization and correction of scoliosis greatly improves and ensures good sitting posture into adulthood. (B) A Luque unit rod using the Galveston technique and segmental wiring provides an excellent correction; (C) lateral view illustrating maintenance of balanced lordosis and thoracic kyphosis by contouring the unit rod to provide excellent sitting balance. (Courtesy of Dr. Jacques D'Astous, Children's Hospital of Eastern Ontario, Ottawa.)

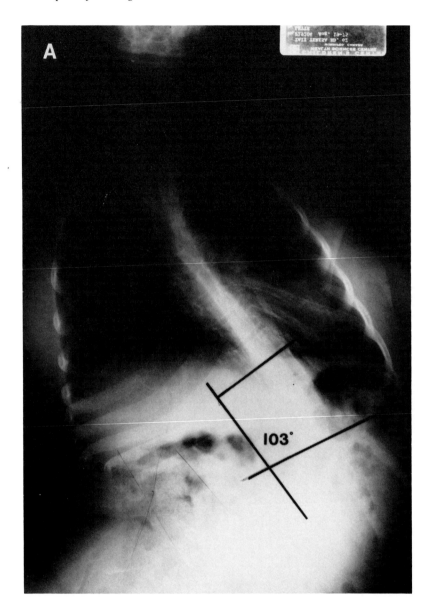

FIGURE 9. This 13-year-old girl with spinal muscular atrophy (A) was experiencing great difficulty in sitting due to pain at the site of rib cage impingement on the iliac crest.

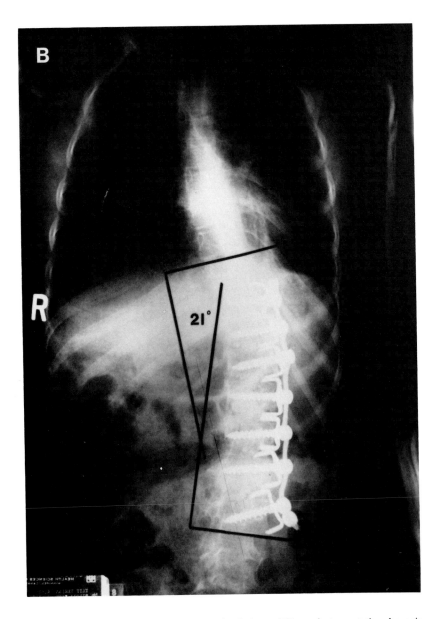

FIGURE 9 (continued). (B) Following anterior fusion and Dwyer instrumentation, her pain disappeared and sitting posture was normal.

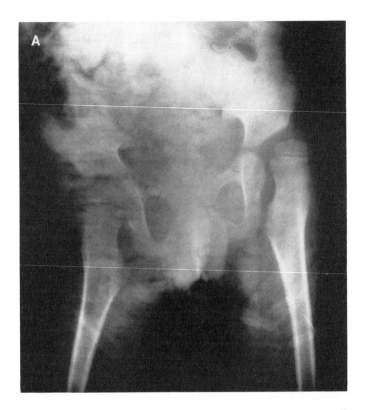

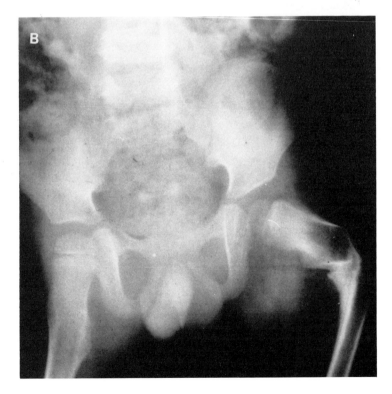

FIGURE 10. The dislocated hip (A) contributes to pelvic obliquity and sitting instability; (B) reduction contributes to a level pelvis and reduces painful sitting.

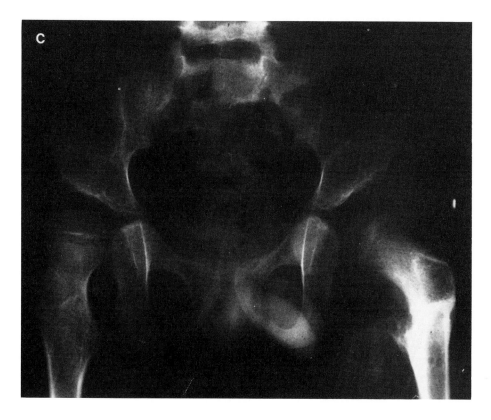

FIGURE 10 (continued).   (C) Four years following varus osteotomy, pelvis is level and hip reduction is maintained.

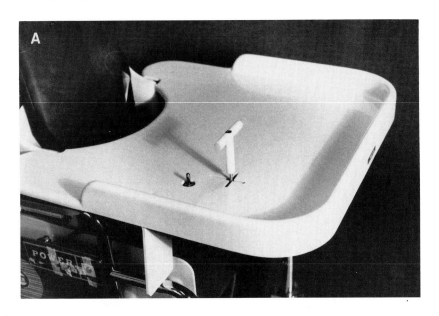

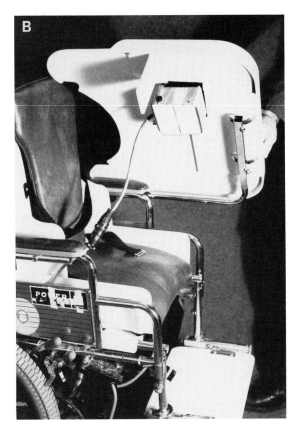

FIGURE 11. Control box mounted under the tray with joystick through the tray to allow and facilitate arm support (A and B).

REFERENCES

1. **Bodzioch, J., Roach, J. W., and Schkade, J.,** Promoting independence in adolescent paraplegics: a 2 week camping experience, *J. Pediatr. Orthop.,* 6, 198, 1986.
2. **Breed, A. L.,** The motorized wheelchair: new freedom, new responsibility and new problems, *Dev. Med. Child Neurol.,* 24, 366, 1982.
3. **Brubaker, C. E.,** Wheelchair prescription: an analysis of factors that affect mobility and performance, *J. Rehabil. Res. Dev.,* 23, 19, 1986.
4. **Coutts, K. D.,** Kinematics of sport wheelchair propulsion, *J. Rehabil. Res. Dev.,* 27, 21, 1990.
5. **DePanew, J. P.,** Sport for individuals with disabilities, *Adapted Phys. Activ. Q.,* 5, 80, 1988.
6. **Dorner, S.,** The relationship of physical handicap to stress in families with an adolescent with spina bifida, *Dev. Med. Child Neurol.,* 17, 755, 1975.
7. **Hoffer, M. M., Abraham, E., and Nickel, V. L.,** Salvage surgery at the hip to improve sitting posture of mentally retarded severely disabled children, *Dev. Med. Child Neurol.,* 14, 51, 1972.
8. **Jackson, R. and Fredrickson, A.,** Sports for the physically disabled, *Am. J. Sports Med.,* 7, 293, 1979.
9. **Robson, P.,** The prevalence of scoliosis in adolescents and young adults, *Dev. Med. Child Neurol.,* 10, 447, 1968.
10. **Silverman, M.,** Commercial options for positioning the client with muscular dystrophy, *Clin. Prosthet.-Orthot.,* 19, 159, 1986.
11. **Weiss, M. and Beck, J.,** Sport as a part of therapy and rehabilitation of paraplegics, *Paraplegia,* 11, 166, 1973.

Chapter 7

SEATING THE ELDERLY

Geoff Fernie and R. Mervyn Letts

TABLE OF CONTENTS

I. INTRODUCTION

We spend a great deal of time sitting. We may spend even more time sitting as we become older. A typical day might begin when we sit on the edge of the bed, stand up, move to the bathroom and sit on the toilet, transfer to a bath or shower seat, move to a convenient stool in the kitchen for preparing breakfast, eat breakfast from a dining room chair, take a walk and rest on a park bench, and return home to read the newspaper or watch television in a favorite reclining chair. Thus, mobility is essentially a series of movements between different chairs. The limiting factor in the mobility of many elderly is, therefore, the difficulty they may have in sitting down or rising from the chair (Figures 1 and 2).

The longevity of the population of the so-called Western world is gradually increasing due to improved disease control, nutrition, and style of living, as well as advances in the delivery of health care. Aging brings with it a number of normal physiological changes that result in a decrease in physical activity, a lessening of coordination, and increased reliance on seating devices and wheelchairs for the geriatric population group. The decreases in strength and coordination, often made more pronounced by chronic health problems, result in an ever-increasing number of the elderly population being relegated to a wheelchair existence.[7,9] The requirements for good stable sitting in this age group are often somewhat different than in the younger population, primarily since most of the elderly will not have major deformity requiring custom seating. Elderly users may be (1) ambulatory, (2) mobile nonambulatory, and (3) immobile (Table 1). Chairs need to be matched to the geriatric individual on the basis of functional mobility. A range of different seating options is required to meet the needs of the elderly on the basis of activity level. Emphasis should be placed on the ease of accessing and leaving the chair, especially in those who are partially ambulatory. For those elderly individuals who are more mobile, contoured support to accommodate poor balance and trunk strength will be required. A transfer from the chair to other surfaces and the ease of propulsion of the chair must be assured to accommodate for the weakness and functional loss that occurs with aging.

Three basic chair types — static lounge chair, reclining mobile lounge chair, and self-propelled wheelchair — will meet the needs of the types of users in the geriatric age group. In exceptional circumstances when disease or injury has resulted in severe deformity, the standard customized chairs discussed previously, such as Foam-in-Place or modular seating systems, will be required.[12]

II. STATIC LOUNGE CHAIR

This type of seating device is applicable to an elderly individual who is capable of independent ambulation with canes or crutches and can stand and sit with minimal assistance.[2] Such a person will still spend most of the time sitting, but will be capable of walking short distances. Such individuals find it extremely difficult to get up from very low, soft chairs (Figure 3). Back support is necessary and armrests are used both for support and to rise from the chair.[6] The main design criterion for such a chair is ease of access and egress from the chair (Figure 4).

III. SEAT HEIGHT, DEPTH, AND ANGLE

Getting up from low, soft seats is obviously more difficult. The seat should be high off the ground and have a shallow seat rake. The seat rake angle should be sufficient to minimize sliding forward out of the seat, but not so great that it becomes difficult to move forward in the seat for egress. The depth of the seat is important for posture and transfer. Most lounge chairs are too deep. Many lounge chairs do not provide room for users to place their

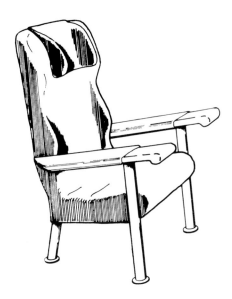

FIGURE 1. Well-designed chair. The seat is high, with modest rake and appropriate depth; the backrest provides good lateral support and emphasizes neck and head support; the armrests are broad and extended; and there is clearance for foot placement under the front of the seat. (Illustration by Stephen Reed.)

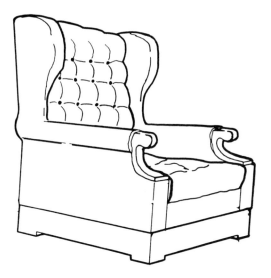

FIGURE 2. Poorly designed chair. The seat is too low, too soft, and too deep; the backrest is flat and has poor lateral support (wings are irrelevant); the armrests are too low, too short, and difficult to grasp; and there is no room for foot placement under the front of the chair. (Illustration by Stephen Reed.)

feet behind the front edge of the chair (i.e., underneath the seat). It is much more difficult to stand up if one cannot put one's heels back beneath the chair. Try it!

IV. ARMRESTS

Armrests serve two important functions during egress. The first is to help the occupant move forward to the front edge of the seat; the second is to assist the occupant in rising

TABLE 1
Types of Chairs and Users

Type of user	Type of chair	Features to be achieved
Ambulatory	Static lounge chair	Ease of ingress/egress, comfort, healthy posture
Mobile, nonambulatory	Self-propelled chair	Ease of propulsion, comfort, and safe transfer
Immobile	Mobile reclining lounge chair	Comfort and support, ease of transfer

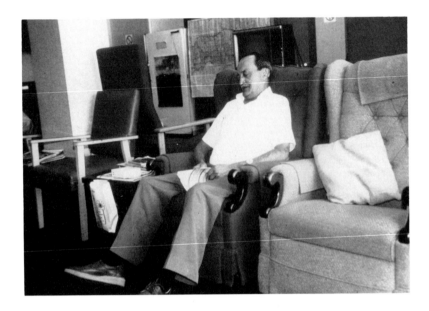

FIGURE 3.   An example of a typical geriatric lounge chair. This chair has many errors in design. One of the most significant is the inability to place the feet under the front of the chair when rising. The backrest provides no lateral support since it is flat and the wings are non-functional.

from the seat (Figure 5). Armrests that are high and come forward to the seat's front edge are therefore extremely useful. The armrest should be relatively straight and parallel to the seat surface so that it is not too high for comfortable support of the elbows when the occupant sits, but it should be as high as possible at the front edge for assistance in ingress and egress.

Armrests are frequently uncomfortable (Figure 6). People generally do not sit like the sphinx, with arms stretching forward; they sit with arms comfortably folded toward the midline. This means that the area of support on the arms is often very small, and so therapists frequently add extra padding to the armrests of chairs to increase the support area and soften it (Figure 7). Broad, lightly padded armrests are a very important additional comfort feature. The forward end of the armrest should be firm and easy to grasp (Figure 8).

V. BACKRESTS

The most important feature of backrest design for the elderly is the degree of lateral trunk support. The backrest should be curved. The classical wings often associated with geriatric chairs may be useful as limits to motion when the occupant falls asleep, but they are not adequate if they appear simply as appendages to a relatively flat seatback. In this case, the wings may only serve to isolate the occupant socially.

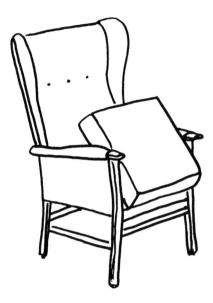

FIGURE 4.   Lifting chairs are helpful for some people. Some of these chairs are spring loaded, but the better ones are electronically operated.

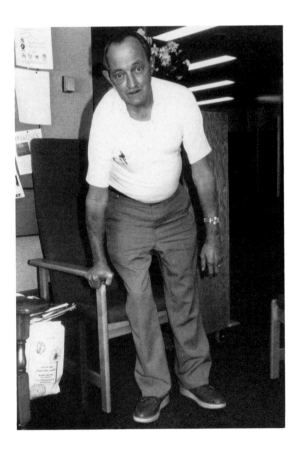

FIGURE 5.   This armrest is not high enough to assist the user to a full standing position.

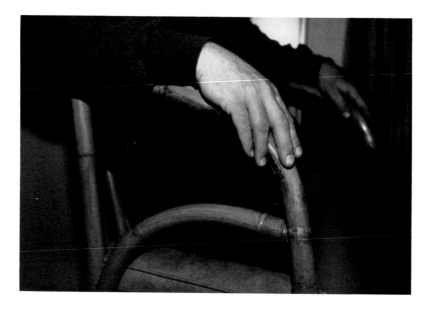

FIGURE 6.   This armrest is totally inappropriate since it is not suitably shaped to help the user move forward in the seat or to rise up from the seat.

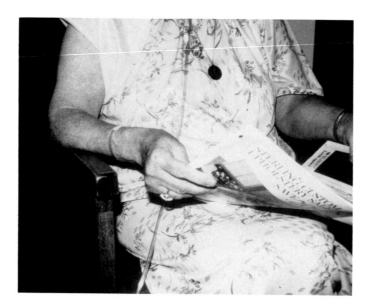

FIGURE 7.   Often, a reddened, sore patch of skin can be seen below the elbows of elderly users. Armrests should be broad and padded.

The emphasis in backrest design for younger adults is on lumbar support. In contrast, the focus of attention for the elderly must be higher in the spine. The elderly generally seem to prefer minor lumbar support, probably because of increased stiffness in extension of the spine. In fact, the elderly are often seated in a chair with too much lumbar support; as a result, they flex the pelvis on the spine and slide forward in the chair.

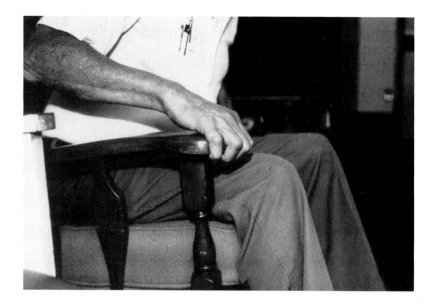

FIGURE 8.   A more appropriate armrest that provides a firm hold for pulling forward and then pushing down during egress.

VI. RECLINING LOUNGE CHAIR

This type of chair is applicable to a geriatric individual who is capable of transferring, but is not an independent walker. Physical tolerance for activity is severely compromised and more seating support is required.[20]

A method of changing the loading of various parts of the body during prolonged sitting is required, and the reclining feature accommodates this requirement. More torso support is built into this type of chair together with an adjustable headrest. A high seat will assist the occupant in transferring, but perhaps of equal importance is that it assists the caregivers and prevents back injury when assisting this type of user. Having an armrest that swings or collapses out of the way also facilitates lateral transfers. These chairs are movable on wheels, as mobility will be required. Since some of the users of this type of chair will be confused, any sharp edges need to be well padded and any removable parts of the chair need to be well fastened. Built-in holding devices for such things as urinary collection bags and blankets, and, in some instances, a tray provides more functional use for the type of individual using this form of seating device.

VII. SELF-PROPELLED CHAIR

The person who requires this type of seating device is capable of propelling the chair, but is not able to ambulate. Such an individual may have heart problems, respiratory disease, lower limb amputation, or possibly a stroke or hemiplegia.[13] Such a device is both a chair and a mobility device. Contoured seating is important to maintain a good distribution of load over the buttocks and thighs to prevent pressure sores.[23] For those where contouring is not appropriate, the provision of a gel cushion may be helpful. Ingress or egress is still important for this type of user, and it is essential that footrests be easily cleared for standing. Hydraulic devices to raise and tilt the wheelchair seat to facilitate standing and transferring have been designed[21] (Figures 9 and 10). Recent advances in wheelchair design have had particular advantages for the elderly. Conventional wheelchairs with front castors have a

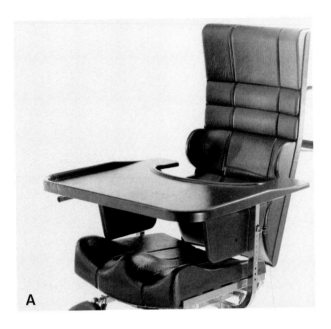

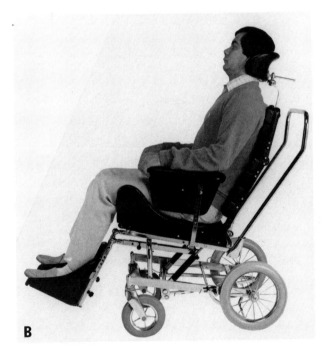

FIGURE 9. Adult seating systems. (A) Fullcare Seating System for geriatric population (Otto Bock Orthopedic Ltd., Winnipeg, Manitoba, Canada); (B) adult modular seating system which can be attached to a variety of wheel bases — tilting, standard, or power.

tendency to turn downhill when transversing a slope sideways. This increases the energy requirement by 20% for a 2° slope and tends to direct wheelchairs into the street while traversing a sloped driveway. The main cause of this problem is that the center of gravity of the system is in front of the point of contact of the large wheels of the chair.[3-5] McLaurin[19]

FULLCARE SEATING SYSTEM

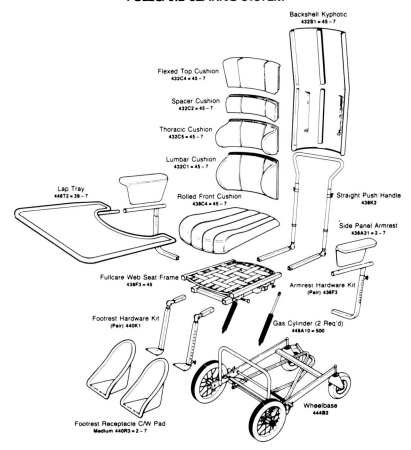

FIGURE 10. Modular geriatric seating system (Otto Bock Orthopedic Ltd., Winnipeg, Manitoba, Canada).

has designed a chair where the center of gravity is over the main wheels and castors are placed in front and behind. This design eliminates the steering problems characteristic of a standard wheelchair, which is of great advantage to a geriatric user who may be unable to exert enough strength to direct a conventional chair.

Additional features on this type of self-propelled chair include improved control of dynamic braking to control speed on a slope. Also, a device to eliminate the danger of rolling backward on an inclined plane if fatigue or motor impairment prevents adequate control is a useful safety addition.

Propulsion of chairs for the elderly is sometimes difficult. Providing a 2:1 gear ratio between the rims and the wheels results in increased efficiency at low speeds. More investigation of lever systems rather than hand rims needs to be done in the geriatric age group.[5]

VIII. POWERED CHAIRS FOR THE ELDERLY

Severe motor deficits which occur in some elderly patients may limit the variety of movements available for control of a toggle switch. Modular and programmable wheelchair control systems have been designed to accommodate individual user characteristics.[25,26] Such "smart wheelchairs" have been designed with various "intelligent" capabilities, such as ultrasonic sensor range finders to detect obstacles in the path of the chair. Newer materials are reducing the weight of these chairs and improving their portability. More work is also needed in improving standard powered chairs for the elderly population.

IX. ROBOTICS AND THE ELDERLY

The robotic work station has now been developed to the point that the robot arm is extremely versatile and flexible and can functionally operate telephones and pick up books, letters, etc. It can be programmed for tasks specific to the wheelchair through a personal computer.

X. SEATING EDUCATION FOR CAREGIVERS OF THE ELDERLY

There is probably no other group of wheelchair users who tend to be more isolated than the institutionalized elderly. Due to a combination of difficult access, inability to attend seating clinics, economic insufficiency, and a basic lack of knowledge of what is available, many elderly are denied adequate seating. As part of the seating clinic mandate, education of the caregivers for the elderly should be an ongoing responsibility. Seating clinics also should emphasize to government and insurance agencies the importance of adequate seating for this population group. There is no question that access to mobility equipment will result in a reduced cost of medical care and patient care, but this needs to be demonstrated to the agencies funding such equipment.

Equipment provided to the elderly must be cost effective and functional. Complex types of seating devices are usually not required for the geriatric population and, if provided, will often not be used properly, resulting in a failure of the program. Caregivers must be taught the importance of frequent repositioning and how good stable sitting should be ensured.[27] They need to be taught that a good sitting posture will decrease fatigue, improve respiratory and cardiac function, and assist in feeding and the overall general care of an elderly person.[10] Through proper seating, transferring to bed and toilet will be facilitated and both the caregivers and their elderly recipients will be more comfortable and happy. Medical problems such as pressure sores will be minimized through the maintenance of stable sitting postures.[23,24] Unfortunately, education in the use and availability of proper sitting devices for the elderly has not received the priority it deserves. Mobile seating clinics that can travel to geriatric institutions and deliver the care and instruction that is required on site are required since the elderly often cannot travel to seating clinics.

XI. AMPUTEE SEATING

Many of the elderly will become amputees secondary to peripheral vascular insufficiency. The loss of one or two extremities changes the center of gravity of the body, with the result that sitting stability is adversely affected. With a bilateral above-knee amputation, the center of gravity in the seated individual moves about 2.5 cm posteriorly. It is therefore prudent to have the rear wheels moved toward the rear if stability is to be ensured.[3,5] This will result in the turning radius being increased slightly; however, this can be compensated for by removing the front rigging of the wheelchair, which is usually not required unless artificial limbs are being used.

XII. THE FOOT-DRIVE CHAIR

Many elderly utilizing wheelchairs will have the use of one functional leg, such as those who have had a cerebral vascular accident and have been rendered hemiplegic. The seat for

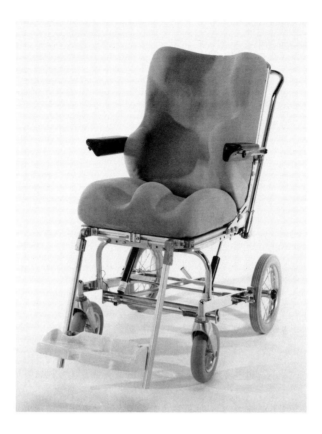

FIGURE 11. Custom seating system for severely disabled (Otto Bock Orthopedic Ltd., Winnipeg, Manitoba, Canada).

such individuals is best lowered about 2 in., with specialized front rigging to allow use of the one good leg to propel the wheelchair. This is often preferable in the elderly to allow mobility of the chair and may be preferable to the one-hand-drive chair which does require some agility and coordination to use.

XIII. MAINTENANCE OF STABLE SEATING FOR THE ELDERLY

Although many geriatric wheelchair users will be quite capable of sitting upright with minimal support, there will still be a need for some additional restraining devices for those who have a tendency to slide forward out of the chair or lose position frequently due to muscle weakness.[10] For these elderly individuals, usually with superimposed medical problems, additional measures to stabilize the pelvis to ensure stable sitting will be necessary[17] (Figure 11). Sometimes this can be ensured simply by adding a tray to the wheelchair, which provides, in its own right, a certain amount of support to the lower torso. For those with more serious postural abnormalities, more aggressive techniques may have to be utilized. However, care must be exercised to avoid increasing the agitation of confused elderly users through the application of involuntary restraining devices.

A. GEL CUSHIONS

Gel cushions provide some pelvic support and may be all that is necessary for some elderly users who have only minor postural disabilities.[22] Often, hip belts are used in conjunction with the cushions to ensure maintenance of even, balanced sitting.

B. PELVIC STRAPS

These are very commonly utilized to ensure good upright sitting and to counteract the tendency to slide forward. They need to be adjusted regularly and require application with the buttocks firmly against the seat.

C. SEAT INCLINATION

By raising the front of the wheelchair seat, the tendency to slide forward will be counteracted and stable sitting will be facilitated. In this way, gravity assists in keeping the pelvis stable (see Figure 11).

D. RIGID PELVIC RESTRAINTS

A number of more rigid pelvic restraints have been designed which may be of use where the above-mentioned methods have not been successful.[8] These include the Medical Engineering Resource Unit rigid pelvic restraint designed at the University of British Columbia by Cooper and associates.[8] This appears to be effective in holding the pelvis in a neutral position. The sub-ASIS bar developed at the University of Wisconsin by Margolis et al.[10] is another type of rigid pelvic restraint, consisting of a round, padded bar that fits below the anterior superior iliac spines. This prevents significant posterior pelvic tilt and maintains a stable sitting position. Other, more aggressive measures such as pommels and the Mulholland type of pelvic stabilizer may be effective, but for some patients are not comfortable and require removal for transferring.

XIV. CAD/CAM TECHNIQUES IN SEATING DESIGN

Computer-assisted design (CAD) and computer-assisted manufacturing (CAM) have been used for a number of years in the design and fabrication of such items as prostheses and various forms of orthosis.[11] The advantage of this type of fabrication is that it allows the design of the actual contours desired in an inexpensive manner with a short turnaround time. Seating design lends itself well to this type of automated shape assessment and if used on a large scale, has a potential to achieve low unit costs and much shorter turnaround time than can be done with manual custom fabrication (Figure 12).

A current project is assessing robot-assisted-manufacturing (RAM) in concert with CAD. Using a robot to carve out an appropriate seat mold from the CAD data has resulted in the ability to produce a complete seat and back, including a hard support surface and a molded surface for the cushion, in 40 min.

While CAD/RAM systems are still in the process of development, their postulated advantages are significant. Development of a reliable mobile simulator could lead to on-site fitting for elderly patients which would be much easier than bringing people to seating clinics and would increase caregiver and client involvement in the design.

XV. SUMMARY

The seating needs of the elderly have increased significantly over the last 2 decades and, with our aging North American population, will become much more important to seating teams. As the current disabled population ages, it will demand the same excellent service it currently receives into its later years. As the public becomes more informed regarding the availability of improved and comfortable seating devices, further demands will be made to improve the delivery of good seating care to the elderly. Education programs for caregivers to the elderly need to be developed and encouraged by seating clinic staff. This is an important and heretofore relatively neglected area that hopefully will receive the attention it deserves in the 1990s as the improved technology and resources that are being developed for the younger population are applied to the geriatric age group.

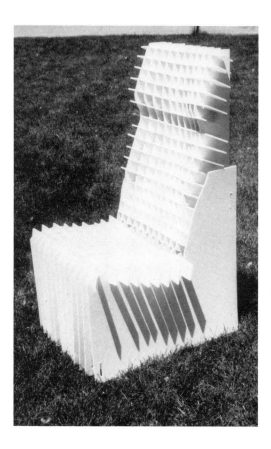

FIGURE 12. A computer-generated model of an optimal shape for a static lounge chair to fit the North American elderly population. Note the modest lumbar curvature, the more marked lateral curvature for back support, and the head and neck support.

REFERENCES

1. **Anderson, B. J. G., Ortengren, R., Nachemson, A., and Elfstrom, G.,** Lumbar disc pressure and myoelectric back muscle activity during sitting, *Scand. J. Rehabil.-Med.,* 6, 104, 1974.
2. **Atherton, J. A., Chatfield, J., Clarke, A. K., and Harrison, R. A.,** Static chairs for the arthritic, *Br. J. Occup. Ther.,* 43, 366, 1980.
3. **Brubaker, C. E.,** Wheelchair prescription: an analysis of factors that affect mobility and performance, *J. Rehabil. Res. Dev.,* 23(4), 19, 1986.
4. **Brubaker, C. E., McLaurin, C. A., and McClay, I. S.,** Effects of sideslope of wheelchair performance, in *Proc. 8th Annu. Conf. Rehabilitation Technology,* Vol. 5, Association for the Advancement of Rehabilitation Technology, Washington, D.C., 1985, 81.
5. **Brubaker, C.,** Ergonometric considerations, *J. Rehab. Res. Dev. Clin. Suppl.,* 2, 37, 1990.
6. **Brudett, R. G., Habesevich, R., Pisciotta, J., and Simmon, S. R.,** Biomechanical comparison of rising from two types of chairs, *Phys. Ther.,* 65, 1177, 1985.
7. **Cape, R. D. T.,** A concept of geriatric medicine, *Can. Med. Assoc. J.,* 115, 9, 1976.
8. **Cooper, D. G.,** Pelvic stabilization for the elderly, in Proc. Seating the Disabled, University of Tennessee, Memphis, February 1987.
9. **Cohen, J. D.,** Prospects of mental health and aging, in *Handbook of Mental Health and Aging,* Birren, J. E. and Sloane, R. B., Eds., Prentice-Hall, Englewood Cliffs, NJ, 1980.

10. **Dolan, P., Adams, M. A., and Hutton, W. C.,** Commonly adopted postures and their effect on the lumbar spine, *Spine,* 13, 197, 1988.

11. **Fernie, G., Raschke, S., Brubaker, C., and McLaurin, C.,** CADCAM: shape sensing and custom fabrication, in Proc. 6th Int. Seating Symp., Vancouver, British Columbia, February 1990.

12. **Garber, S. L.,** A classification of wheelchair seating, *Am. J. Occup. Ther.,* 39, 453, 1985.

13. **Glaser, R. M., Gruner, J. A., Feinberg, S. D., and Collins, S. R.,** Locomotion via paralyzed leg muscles: feasibility study for a leg propelled vehicle, *J. Rehabil. Res. Dev.,* 20, 87, 1983.

14. **Holden, J. M. and Fernie, G.,** Specifications for a mass producible static lounge chair for the elderly, *Appl. Ergonom.,* 20, 39, 1989.

15. **Holden, J. M., Fernie, G., and Lanau, K.,** Chairs for the elderly — design characteristics, *Appl. Ergon.,* 19, 281, 1988.

16. **Kauffman, T.,** Association between hip extension strength and stand-up ability in geriatric patients, *Phys. Occup. Ther. Geriatr.,* 1(3), 39, 1982.

17. **Kosiak, M.,** A mechanical resting surface: its effect on pressure distribution, *Arch. Phys. Med. Rehabil.,* 57, 481, 1976.

18. **Margolis, S. A., Jones, R. M., and Brown, B. E.,** The sub-ASIS bar: an effective approach to pelvic stabilization in seated positioning, in Proc. 8th Annu. Conf. Rehabilitation Engineering, June 1985, 45.

19. **McLaurin, C.,** Wheelchair development, standards, progress and issues, *J. Rehabil. Res. Dev.,* 23, 48, 1986.

20. **Munton, J. S., Chamberlain, N. A., and Wright, V.,** An investigation into the problems of easy chairs used by the arthritic and the elderly, *Rheumatol. Rehabil.,* 20, 164, 1981.

21. **Purves, W. K.,** A hydraulic seat-rise wheelchair, *J. Med. Eng. Technol.,* 7, 27, 1983.

22. **Sprigle, S., Chung, K. C., and Brubaker, C. E.,** Reduction of sitting pressures with custom contoured cushions, *J. Rehabil. Res. Dev.,* 27, 135, 1990.

23. **Taylor, V. C.,** Seating for the elderly — assessing force and contour, in Proc. 6th Int. Seating Symp., University of British Columbia, Vancouver, February 1990.

24. **Warren, C. G., Ko, M., Smith, C., and Imre, J. V.,** Reducing back displacement in the powered reclining wheelchair, *Arch. Phys. Med. Rehabil.,* 63, 447, 1982.

25. **Warren, C. G.,** Powered mobility and its implications, *J. Rehabil. Res. Dev. Suppl.,* 2, 74, 1990.

26. **Wilson, A. B. and McFarland, R.,** *Wheelchairs: A Prescription Guide,* Rehabilitation Press, Charlottesville, VA, 1986.

27. **Zacharkow, D.,** *Wheelchair Posture and Pressure Sores,* Charles C Thomas, Springfield, IL, 1984.

Chapter 8

KYPHOSIS AND LORDOSIS IN SEATING

R. Mervyn Letts

TABLE OF CONTENTS

I. KYPHOSIS AND STABLE SEATING

Children and adults with various types of cerebral palsy often have a tendency to fall forward in the wheelchair, resulting in a very nonfunctional posture and difficulty in maintaining a straight forward gaze. Butterfly chest pads have been helpful in some instances, especially in younger children, to hold them upright, together with various forms of head support (Figure 1). However, in the older child, this becomes less effective and additional measures are often necessary (Figure 2).

Tilting the wheelchair insert will be tolerated by some wheelchair users, but in others it tends to stimulate the tendency to lean forward, probably due to the righting mechanism of the inner ear that maintains upright balance (Figures 3 and 4). Use of an orthosis is sometimes effective; however, most children with this type of problem will tolerate a rigid orthosis very poorly. In this regard, the Soft Boston type of orthosis has been found to be effective in controlling this problem of forward postural kyphosis and is well tolerated by the wheelchair user (Figure 5). Augmentation with cross straps or a butterfly pad may be necessary simply for balance.

In instances where the kyphosis has become more rigid and fixed, it may be necessary to address this issue surgically. Such a decision is usually made in the teenage years to avoid a permanent kyphosis with resultant poor sitting posture. Current types of fixation such as Cotrel-Dubusset, Luque segmental instrumentation, and Drummond wiring in association with Harrington instrumentation are usually so stable that minimal orthotic management is necessary following such surgical stabilization[7,8,10] (Figure 6).

II. THE GIBBUS DEFORMITY AND SEATING

One of the most difficult problems for the seating team to deal with is the rigid, sharp kyphosis or gibbus that is frequently seen in patients with myelomeningocele. This type of deformity is very unforgiving and the skin over the gibbus is constantly in contact with the back of the chair, with the result that because of its insensate nature, it frequently breaks down from the rubbing.[11] This can be dealt with in the less severe deformities with a donut-shaped foam pad and, finally, a Foam-in-Place type of wheelchair back that is built around the entire spinal deformity (Figure 7). Adverse effects are seen in other parts of the spine, and the sitting posture is poor as a result of sacral sitting since the caudal arm of the kyphosis forces the pelvis forward and the child has to sit on the sacrum or lower part of the lumbar spine. The upper part of the spine is also affected in that there is a forward inclination and the child is constantly slouching over the wheelchair tray. This is an extremely difficult problem for the seating team to deal with and is an example of another instance where orthopedic surgical intervention can greatly facilitate the seating clinic's tasks and result in a more stable sitting posture for the patient. Stabilization of the spine and removal of the kyphosis with augmentation by segmental instrumentation is frequently helpful. A new technique developed by Dr. Joe Hyndman of Izzak Walton Killam Hospital in Halifax has provided the most effective correction of this terrible deformity to date.[6] He has perfected a technique in which the kyphosis is resected and a rod is inserted into the bodies of the caudal arm of the kyphosis and then wired segmentally to the lamina of the vertebra of the cranial arm of the kyphosis (Figure 8). This gives an excellent correction and the small step that occurs at the interface of the two spinal segments is of no consequence. This, of course, can only be done in patients who are paraplegic, but these are the individuals who frequently have the greatest problems with the fixed kyphosis deformity. Dr. Hyndman now has a 10-year experience with the procedure with little loss of correction. The spine is virtually straight and the sitting posture has been found to be excellent.

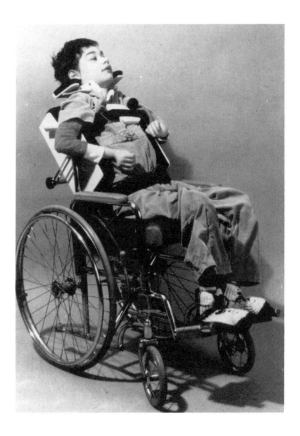

FIGURE 1.   This cerebral palsied child was constantly adopting a severe kyphotic position in the wheelchair. This was corrected by tilting the insert slightly posteriorly and using a butterfly chest strap (Otto Bock), but keeping the head positioned forward to ensure level sight using a Winnipeg modular head and neck support. (Reproduced with permission from Letts, M., Rang, M., and Tredwell, S., Seating the disabled, in *American Academy of Orthopaedic Surgeons: Atlas of Orthotics*, 2nd ed., C. V. Mosby, St. Louis, 1985.)

III. HYPERLORDOSIS

Sitting with hyperlordosis is less comfortable than with some flexion of the lumbar spine. Limited lumbar flexion reduces the compressive forces acting on the posterior annulus and apophysial joints.[1,3,5] Even the hydrostatic pressure with the disc may be higher in the lordotic, unsupported posture.[9] This is supported by Fahrni and Trueman's finding that the incidence of lumbar disc disease is very low in people who habitually sit or squat in positions that flex the lumbar spine.[4] Hyperlordosis therefore is both biomechanically and functionally a less-than-ideal position for wheelchair sitting.[12,13]

Hyperlordosis may be encountered in the sitting population secondary to neuromuscular disease — especially muscular dystrophy, spinal muscular atrophy, cerebral palsy, and, less commonly, arthrogryposis. In some spina bifida wheelchair users with lumboperitoneal shunts, the shunt itself may become a posterior tether, resulting in a progressive hyperlordosis.[12,13] This is a particularly vexing problem for the seating team and may require shunt replacement with removal of the tether if severe. In collapsing kyphoscoliosis secondary to neuromuscular disorders such as spinal muscular atrophy, lordotic support built into the wheelchair with a modular insert (Figure 9) or Foam-in-Place system (Figure 10) assists in balancing

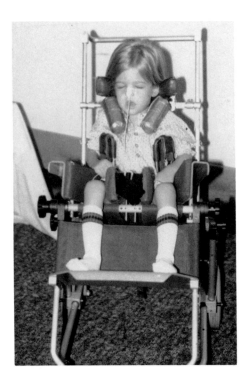

FIGURE 2.   Postural kyphosis and forward leaning may be counteracted in some children by shoulder restraints which can be added as in the Mulholland seating system.

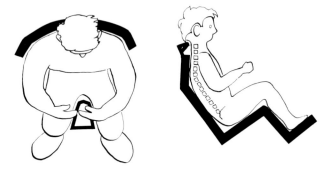

FIGURE 3.   Forward slumping with resultant kyphosis can be corrected and prevented in some children by tilting the wheelchair inserts backward slightly. (Reproduced with permission from Letts, M., Rang, M., and Tredwell, S., Seating the disabled, in *American Academy of Orthopaedic Surgeons: Atlas of Orthotics,* 2nd ed., C. V. Mosby, St. Louis, 1985.)

the spine and may allow the individual to be supported in a stable sitting position until a definitive orthosis or surgery can be instituted.

IV. HEAD SUPPORT IN THE WHEELCHAIR

Poor head control is a frequent problem that contributes to poor seating posture. The cause of chronic head flexion is frequently multifactorial and is often associated with poor

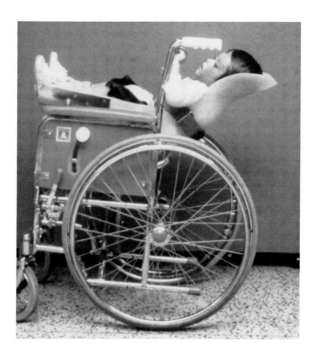

FIGURE 4. A wheelchair insert with a semireclining adjustable feature may avoid forward flopping, especially when the child is tired.

trunk stability. In certain disease entities, paracervical muscle weakness is the major contributing factor to ''chin on chest'' positions. In some wheelchair users, the head tends to follow a significant kyphosis, and the kyphosis correction may improve the head position. High spinal lesions may also create poor head control, requiring constant support. The seating team may have to come up with very innovative ways to maintain head support. A simple neck collar is often effective, but is confining and not well tolerated (Figure 11). Other methods of head support can be achieved with protective helmets (Figure 12), various bolsterings of the head (Figure 13), or forehead restrainers (Figure 14). The Winnipeg neck support is a simple and often successful method for holding the head and neck in a good position (Figure 15). Head support is an important aspect of good seating, to ensure that the seated individual can obtain maximal stimulation and information in the upright position.

V. NUTRITION, SEATING, AND SPINAL SURGERY

Many wheelchair users who have developed severe scoliosis have other major abnormalities. Many of these patients have cerebral damage and, as a result, their nutrition is very poor, resulting in poor tissue coverage of bony protuberances and a predisposition to pressure sores as well as little nutritional reserve to tolerate major spinal corrective procedures. Associated with this decreased intake is a tendency to gastroesophageal reflux, especially in patients with spasticity. We have found it very beneficial in a number of these difficult seating situations, where surgery is contemplated to improve the sitting balance through a spinal fusion, to augment the nutrition of the patients with a feeding gastrostomy and, at the same time, to perform a gastroesophageal plication to reduce or eliminate gastroesophageal reflux. This allows these children to gain weight extremely well, and as a result, they tolerate the surgery with much less morbidity. Elimination of the gastroesophageal reflux minimizes pulmonary aspiration in the postoperative period, as well as decreasing their discomfort from this annoying problem.

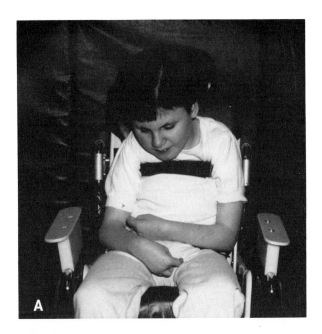

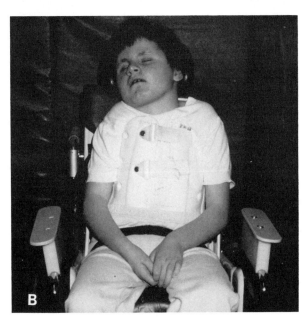

FIGURE 5. Chest pads (A) are often helpful in preventing kyphotic sitting, but in some instances more support is necessary; (B) the Soft Boston orthosis is a well-tolerated and functional orthosis for controlling postural kyphosis in handicapped sitters.

The additional subcutaneous tissue that develops is ideal for such a person, who spends a lot of time in supportive seating systems. The gastrostomy may be a bit of an annoyance if an orthosis is being used, but a talented orthotist can usually compensate for this quite satisfactorily by tailoring the spinal jacket around the gastrostomy.

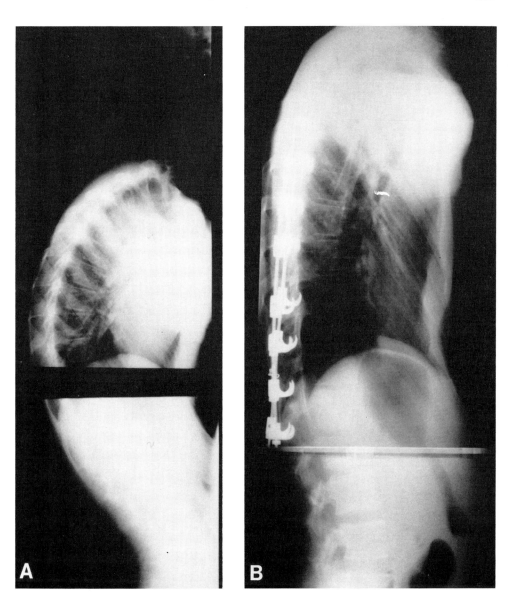

FIGURE 6. Severe kyphosis (A) which results in constant forward sitting can be corrected or improved with spinal fusion and instrumentation (B).

VI. SUMMARY

Kyphosis is a major impediment to good functional and comfortable seating. Seating innovations such as insert wedging, seat tilting, and specialized thoracic or shoulder support all have a role in preventing and correcting this postural abnormality. Where the kyphosis is rigid, progressive, or unresponsive to seating and orthotic measures, surgical correction is usually effective in solving the dilemma. Hyperlordosis is a less frequent problem to the seating team and can usually be dealt with by total contact seating such as the Foam-in-Box insert.

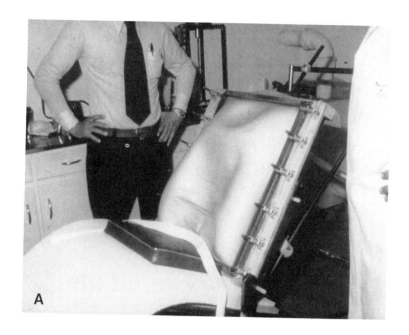

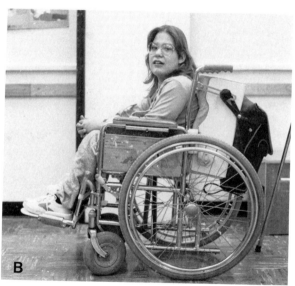

FIGURE 7. Marked kyphosis deformity of the spine can often be accommodated comfortably and excessive pressure with skin breakdown avoided by using a Foam-in-Place insert. (A) Seat being fabricated; (B) in use. (Reproduced with permission from Letts, M., Rang, M., and Tredwell, S., Seating the disabled, in *American Academy of Orthopaedic Surgeons: Atlas of Orthotics,* 2nd ed., C. V. Mosby, St. Louis, 1985.)

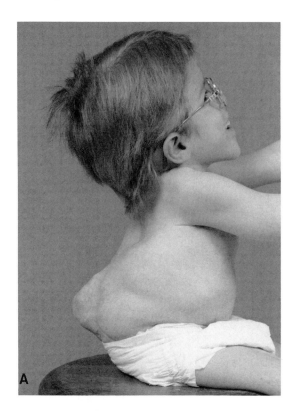

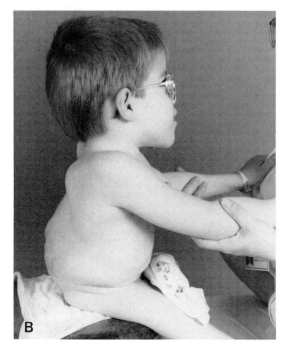

FIGURE 8.   Severe kyphosis corrected using the Hyndman technique of inserting the Luque rod into the vertebral bodies distally and wiring segmentally proximally following excision of the gibbus. (A) Preoperative and (B) postoperative patient.

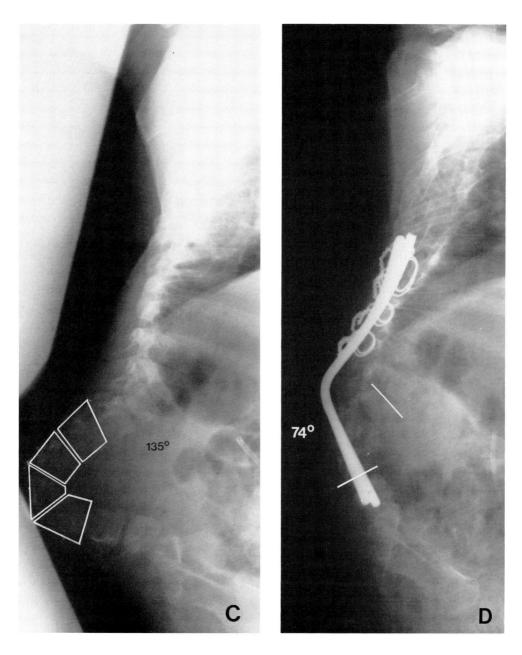

FIGURE 8 (continued).   (C) Preoperative and (D) postoperative X-rays. (Courtesy of Dr. Jacques D'Astous, Children's Hospital of Eastern Ontario, Ottawa.)

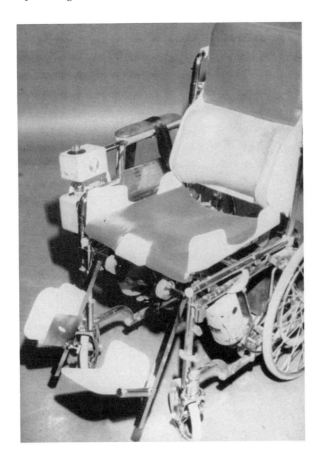

FIGURE 9. Lordosis can be supported by modular inserts, such as
the Winnipeg Modular System shown here with a lordotic bolster.

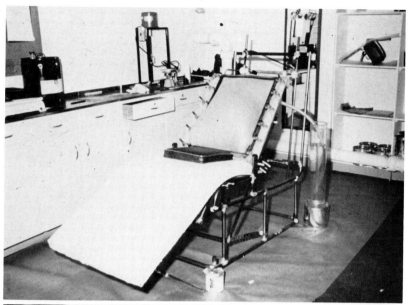

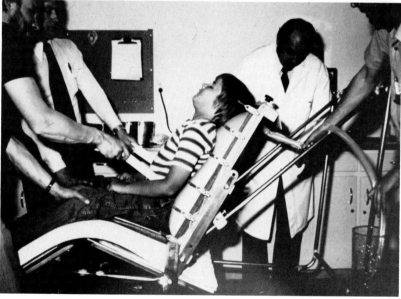

FIGURE 10. The Foam-in-Place technique is a practical and effective way to fabricate a wheelchair insert with built in lordosis. (Reproduced with permission from Letts, M., Rang, M., and Tredwell, S., Seating the disabled, in *American Academy of Orthopaedic Surgeons: Atlas of Orthotics,* 2nd ed., C. V. Mosby, St. Louis, 1985.)

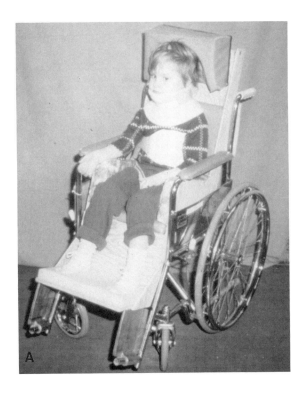

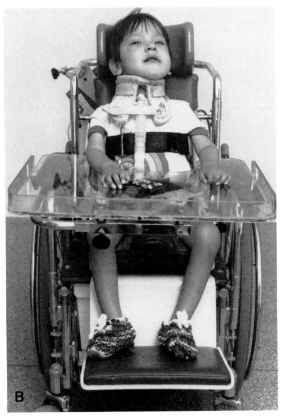

FIGURE 11.   Head supported by cervical orthosis in children with high-level quadriplegia. (A) C5 level; (B) C2 level.

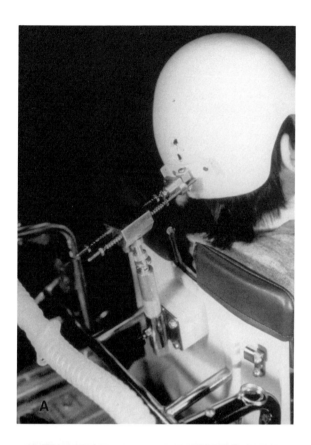

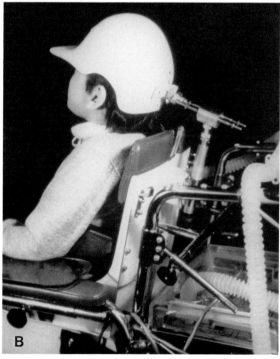

FIGURE 12.   Head supported by plastic hard hat attached to back
of wheelchair with gear system to allow rotation and adjustments
for positioning in desired amount of flexion (A and B).

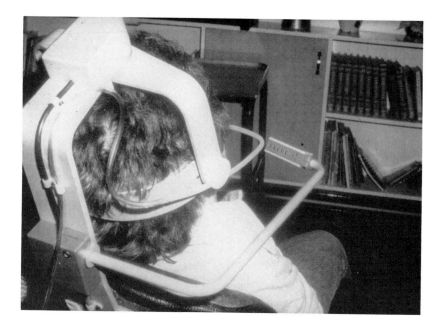

FIGURE 13. Head support with adjustable padded temporal bolsters which can be tightened to hold the head comfortably on each side.

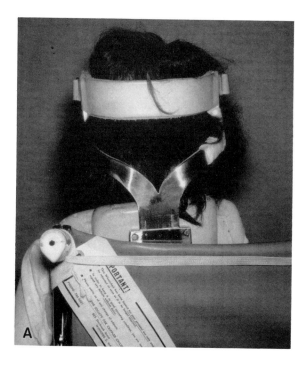

FIGURE 14. Head support attached to plastic vest (A) to prevent persistent head flexion.

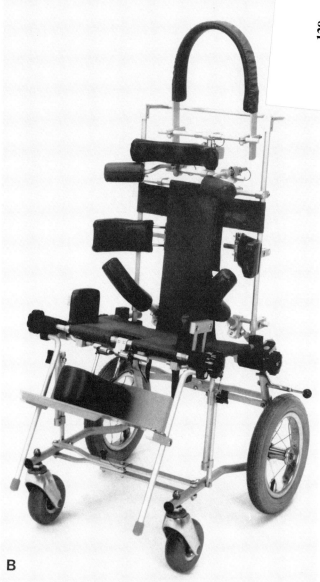

B

FIGURE 14 (continued).   (B) Adjustable forehead support on the
Mulholland Growth Guidance seating system. (Courtesy of Mulholland Positioning Systems, Inc., Santa Paula, CA.)

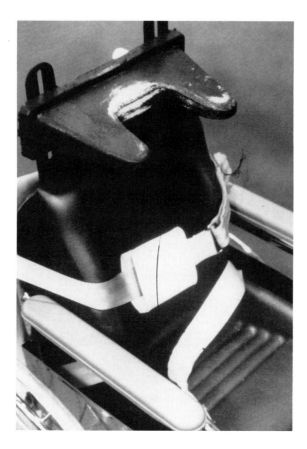

FIGURE 15.   Winnipeg neckrest which is often effective for supporting head with moderate cervical muscle weakness.

REFERENCES

1. **Adams, M. A. and Hutton, W. C.**, The effect of posture on the lumbar spine, *J. Bone Jt. Surg. Br. Vol.*, 67, 635, 1985.
2. **Caro, P. A.**, Plastic bowing of the ribs in children, *Skel. Radiol.*, 17, 255, 1988.
3. **Dolan, P.**, Commonly adopted postures and their effect on the lumbar spine, *Spine*, 13, 197, 1988.
4. **Fahrni, W. H. and Trueman, G. E.**, Comparative radiological study of the spines of a primitive population with North Americans and North Europeans, *J. Bone Jt. Surg. Br. Vol.*, 47, 552, 1965.
5. **Herring, J. A.**, Hyperlordosis, *J. Pediatr. Orthop.*, 8, 93, 1988.
6. **Hyndman, J.**, Isaac Walton Killam Children's Hospital, Halifax, Nova Scotia, Canada, personal communication.
7. **Jefferson, R. J.**, Scoliosis surgery and its effect on back shape, *J. Bone Jt. Surg. Br. Vol.*, 70, 26, 1988.
8. **Kaneda, K.**, Free vascularized fibular strut graft in the tretment of kyphosis, *Spine*, 13, 1273, 1988.
9. **Koreska, J., Robertson, D., Mills, R. H., Gibson, D. A., and Albisser, A. M.**, Biomechanics of the lumbar spine and its clinical significance, *Orthop. Clin. North Am.*, 8, 121, 1977.
10. **Kostuik, J. P.**, Combined single stage anterior and posterior osteotomy for correction of iatrogenic lumbar kyphosis, *Spine*, 13, 257, 1988.
11. **McMaster, M. J.**, The long term results of kyphectomy and spinal stabilization in children with myelomeningocele, *Spine*, 13, 417, 1988.
12. **McIvor, J.**, Complications of lumbo peritoneal shunts, *J. Pediatr. Orthop.*, 8, 687, 1988.
13. **Renshaw, T. S. and Lonstein, J.**, Neuromuscular spine deformities, *Am. Acad. Orthop. Surg. Instruct. Course Lectures*, 36, 285, 1987.

14. **Steele, H. H. and Admas, D. J.,** Hyperlordosis caused by the lumboperitoneal shunt procedure for hydrocephalus, *J. Bone Jt. Surg. Am. Vol.,* 54, 1537, 1972.
15. **Stelzer, L. and Lindseth, R. E.,** Vertebral excision for kyphosis in children with myelomeningocele, *J. Bone Jt. Surg. Am. Vol.,* 61, 699, 1979.
16. **Winter, R. B. and Carlson, J. M.,** The ''Gillette'' sitting support orthosis, *Orthot. Prosthet.,* 32, 35, 1978.
17. **Winter, R. B.,** Natural history of spinal deformity, in *Moes Textbook of Scoliosis,* W. B. Saunders, Philadelphia, 1987, 89.

Chapter 9

PELVIC OBLIQUITY AND SEATING

R. Mervyn Letts

TABLE OF CONTENTS

I. INTRODUCTION

There is probably no anatomical abnormality that makes seating more difficult than pelvic obliquity (Figure 1). It is frequently the unsolvable seating problem of most seating clinics. The oblique position of the pelvis results in marked asymmetrical sitting, with concentration of pressure over the ischium and greater trochanter of the low side of the obliquity.[8-13] This is not only extremely uncomfortable for the individual, but also predisposes to future hip dislocation, especially on the high side of the obliquity, which, in turn, causes further sitting instability. The rib cage often impinges on the high side of the oblique pelvis, predisposing to pain when sitting. Ultimately, because of the discomfort from rib impingement on the pelvis plus pressure areas over the ischium and greater trochanter, sitting becomes intolerable and a bedridden existence begins. Rigid, fixed pelvic obliquity that has been present for a long time offers an almost insurmountable seating problem for the seating clinic (Figure 2). This condition is best treated by prevention, which requires the vigilance of every member of the seating team.[14-19]

II. PELVIC OBLIQUITY DEFORMITY

The cause of pelvic obliquity may be suprapelvic, pelvic, infrapelvic, or a combination of all of these. Suprapelvic causes may result from a fixed scoliosis in which the pelvis behaves as one of the sacral vertebrae and is part of the curve itself.[28-30] This is more commonly seen in those patients with myelomeningocele, muscular dystrophy, and cerebral palsy with long C-curves which may involve the pelvis.[2-6] Pelvic causes include congenital abnormalities of the pelvis, with one hemipelvis being hypoplastic, or are secondary to partial resection for trauma. Infrapelvic causes are common in the spastic population. Iliopsoas spasticity and tightness often contribute to the genesis of pelvic obliquity and are aggravated by contracture of the adductors and hip flexors in a nonsymmetrical manner so that the pelvis becomes obliquely positioned (see Figure 2). In a study in young children of the temporal relationship between hip dislocation, pelvic obliquity, and scoliosis, it was found that frequently the hip in children with total body-involved cerebral palsy first becomes subluxed and dislocated, and this was followed by pelvic obliquity and, finally, scoliosis[19] (Figure 3). More studies of this nature are required, primarily to establish the proper methods of preventing pelvic obliquity from developing at a young age.[21] The most devastating end result of pelvic obliquity is the so-called windswept phenomenon, which is a triad of deformities consisting of fixed pelvic obliquity, scoliosis, and the so-called windswept hips in which the hip on the high side of the pelvic obliquity is usually dislocated and the leg is markedly adducted, while the opposite extremity on the low side of the obliquity is often abducted and may or may not be in joint (Figure 4). Once this syndrome has become fully established, it is a nightmare for seating teams to seat these individuals in a comfortable, functional manner without surgical correction of the major components of the deformity.[25] The emphasis must be to prevent (or minimize) the deformity from becoming fully established.

III. PELVIC OBLIQUITY AND SITTING PRESSURES

Pelvic obliquity contributes significantly to asymmetrical sitting pressures and, in the vulnerable insensate sitter, to the development of sacral and ischial pressure ulcerations.[36] It has been shown by Drummond et al. that when the posterior weight distribution becomes greater than 55% of the supported weight, the risk of skin breakdown increases significantly.[9] This may occur if the lumbar lordosis is completely eliminated by spinal fusion in which the instrumentation does not build in adequate lordosis. Weight is then transferred from the

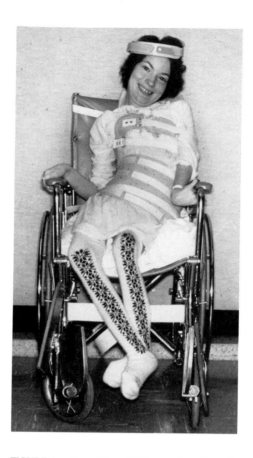

FIGURE 1.   Poor sitting stability occasioned by pelvic obliquity and the windswept hip syndrome. (From Letts, M., Shapiro, L., Mulder, K., and Klassen, O., *J. Pediatr. Orthop.*, 4, 55, 1984. With permission.)

thighs posteriorly to the ischia, resulting in a greater than 55% weight bearing over the ischia and sacral regions with subsequent pressure sore development.

Pressure measurements have shown that when the pelvic obliquity is of such a magnitude that an excess of 30% of the supported weight is borne by one ischium, the ischium becomes extremely vulnerable to skin breakdown.

In the sacral area, an increase in weight bearing over the sacrum of greater than 11% of the supported weight results in a higher incidence of skin breakdown. Abnormal pressure distribution can be avoided by correcting pelvic obliquity and ensuring that lumbar lordosis is retained during spinal fusion and instrumentation.

IV. PREVENTION OF PELVIC OBLIQUITY

The underlying principle in the prevention of pelvic obliquity is the mandatory and regular follow-up of children with spasticity from any cause, from infancy to skeletal maturity. It is only by regular follow-up and close monitoring of the hips that early subluxation secondary to tight adductors and iliopsoas, the first harbinger of pelvic obliquity, can be recognized. Early release of the adductors and iliopsoas with maintenance of abduction seating will greatly assist in minimizing and reducing the magnitude of future deformity.[23,25] The treatment algorithm seen in Figure 5 summarizes the treatment modalities that are recommended, depending upon the age of the child at the time the deformity has become

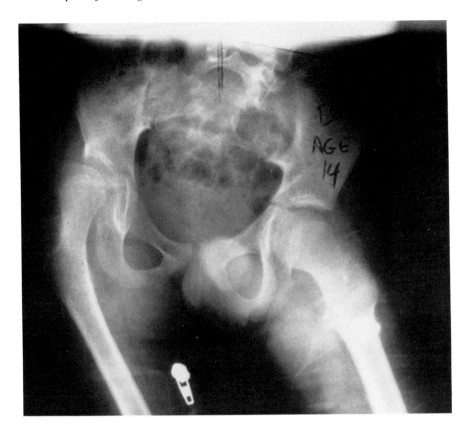

FIGURE 2.   Fixed adduction and flexion with increasing pelvic obliquity and hip dislocation.

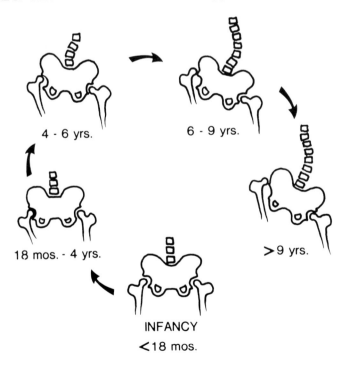

4 - 6 yrs.

6 - 9 yrs.

18 mos. - 4 yrs.

>9 yrs.

INFANCY

<18 mos.

FIGURE 3.   The genesis of the windswept hip phenomenon. (From Letts, M., Shapiro, L., Mulder, K., and Klassen, O., *J. Pediatr. Orthop.*, 4, 55, 1984. With permission.)

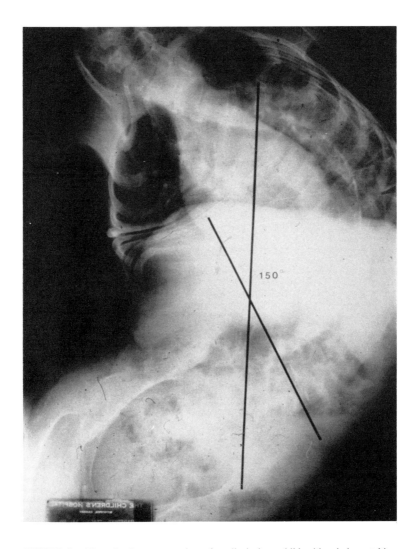

FIGURE 4. The relentless progression of scoliosis in a child with windswept hips secondary to cerebral palsy.

recognized or established. In early infancy, adductor tenotomies and iliopsoas recession may be all that is necessary, provided that this is followed up with good supportive abduction seating (see Figure 5). Indeed, children who have a tendency to develop hip contractures and pelvic obliquity should be constantly seated in abduction in all sitting devices, be it an alternative sitting device, manual wheelchair, or electric wheelchair. Abduction seating can be assisted with pommels or contoured chairs. In older children, ages 6 to 9 years, with more established pelvic obliquity and the hip having been dislocated for some time, a varus osteotomy combined with soft tissue release will be necessary in order to stabilize the pelvis (Figure 6). To facilitate wheelchair use postoperatively, the spinal hip orthosis is recommended to maintain abduction and provide spinal support (Figure 7). Stabilization of the pelvis by maintaining hip reduction frequently facilitates the management of scoliosis with an orthosis (Figure 8). Close monitoring by an orthopedic surgeon on the seating team can frequently assist in reducing the deformity to one that can be much more easily dealt with by available seating techniques.[27] Deformities that are beyond such repair will require a customized approach to seating, with the chair having to be built around the deformity. In this regard, the Foam-in-Place type of seating may provide some total contact support to

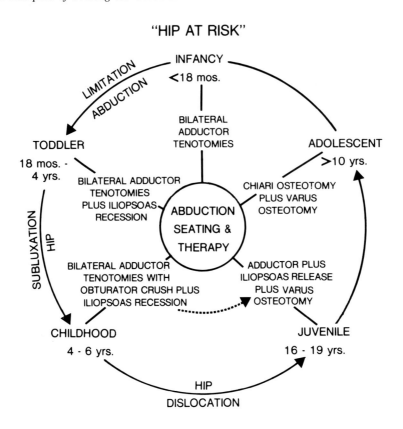

FIGURE 5.   A treatment regime for the prevention of fixed pelvic obliquity in children. (From Letts, M., Shapiro, L., Mulder, K., and Klassen, O., *J. Pediatr. Orthop., 4*, 55, 1984. With permission.)

help decrease the pressure over the low side, the obliquity, and the greater trochanter (Figure 9). A pelvic bar may be useful in those obliquities that are not completely rigid, but these may not be tolerated by the patient. The use of bolsters in an attempt to straighten the pelvis may be helpful in the mobile obliquity, but will usually be to no avail for the rigid obliquity. Unfortunately, a major rotatory component to the pelvis is frequently associated with pelvic obliquity, which compounds the seating problem (Figure 10). In some instances, the severe obliquity with the association of the windswept hip syndrome will result in the patient being completely unseatable and relegated to a mobile bean bag type of seating system.

V. SALVAGE SURGERY FOR PELVIC OBLIQUITY

In established pelvic obliquity with a painful dislocated hip, salvage resection of the proximal femur may improve sitting by eliminating a source of pain as well as a major area of pressure during sitting. Care must be taken not to simply resect the proximal femur as this will create a frail extremity which may be a problem for caregivers to manage. Resection of the proximal femur with an interposition arthroplasty is recommended. This reduces the dangers of postresection deformity and eliminates the rigid, painful bony protuberance of the dislocated hip.[24] The criteria for this procedure should be similar to those suggested by Baxter and D'Astous:[3]

1.   Severe spasticity
2.   Nonambulatory status
3.   Long-standing hip dislocation

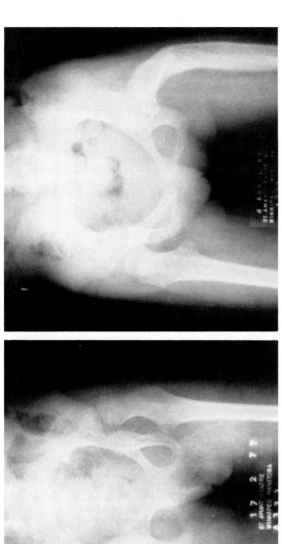

FIGURE 6. Varus osteotomy of subluxated left hip shown 8 years after the procedure with maintenance reduction and a level pelvis.

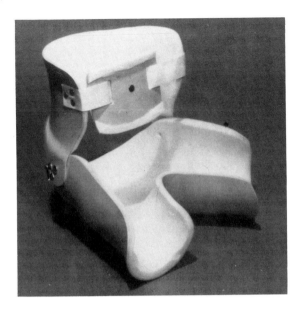

FIGURE 7. The spinal-hip orthosis is useful in the management of wheelchair users requiring a varus osteotomy. The orthosis can be worn in the wheelchair and provides spinal support as well as hip abduction. (From Letts, M., Shapiro, L., Mulder, K., and Klassen, O., *J. Pediatr. Orthop.*, 4, 55, 1984. With permission.)

4. Deterioration of sitting tolerance
5. Difficulty maintaining perineal hygiene
6. Discomfort at rest or with movement of the affected hip

Lindseth[20] designed an unique procedure to equalize the pelvis by removing a triangular segment from the low side of the pelvis and inserting it into an osteotomy on the high side of the pelvis (Figure 11).

VI. PELVIC OBLIQUITY AND SCOLIOSIS

The combination of pelvic obliquity and scoliosis may result in a devastating seating dilemma. If severe and rigid, the pain and discomfort from the rib cage impinging on the pelvis, combined with the concentration of pressure over the trochanter and buttock on the low side of the pelvis, may greatly reduce sitting tolerance. These unfortunate individuals may become bedridden, accentuating the development of pressure sores. Once the lumbar scoliosis with significant obliquity of the pelvis has developed, only surgery will offer any hope of correction and limitation of progression[22] (Figure 12). Bolstering and pelvic bars may slow the progression somewhat, but, ultimately, sitting stability can only be restored by correcting the balance between the spine and pelvis by surgical intervention.

Since the pelvis virtually becomes part of the curve, any corrective techniques must include the pelvis (Figure 13). One of the best methods with which to achieve correction and balance of both the scoliosis and pelvic obliquity is by segmental wiring using the Galveston modification of the Luque technique[1,2,28] (Figure 14). In more rigid curves, anterior correction and fusion using the Dwyer or Zielke instrumentation (Figure 15), often followed by a posterior correction and fusion, will be required. Absolute anatomical correction is not necessary to achieve considerable improvement in sitting balance and a redistribution of weight bearing over both thighs and buttocks.

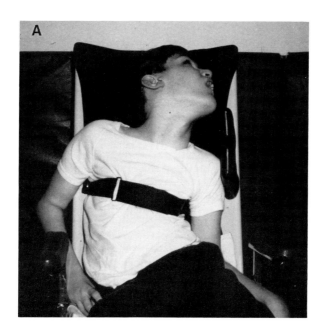

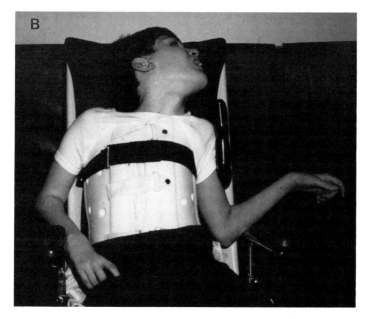

FIGURE 8. The Soft Boston orthosis is well tolerated by spastic wheelchair users (A) and is effective in facilitating sitting balance as well as curve control (B).

Children with spastic quadriplegia who are to undergo spinal correction for severe seating difficulties should be assessed preoperatively for gastroesophageal reflux and have this corrected preoperatively to reduce postoperative reflux and possible aspiration.[7,8,28]

VII. SITTING BALANCE AND POSTERIOR RHIZOTOMY

Posterior rhizotomy has been shown to be of some benefit in children with spastic diplegia to reduce spasticity.[22] The technique involves cutting the motor component of the

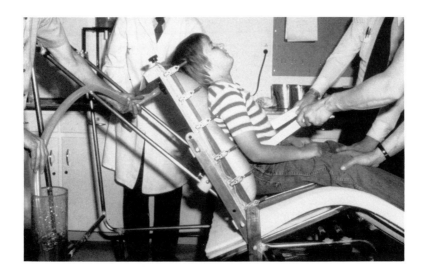

FIGURE 9.   Foam-in-Place seat being fabricated. The foam molds completely to deformity, providing soft total-contact seating support. (Reproduced with permission from Letts, M., Rang, M., and Tredwell, S., Seating the disabled, in *American Academy of Orthopaedic Surgeons: Atlas of Orthotics,* 2nd ed., C. V. Mosby, St. Louis, 1985.)

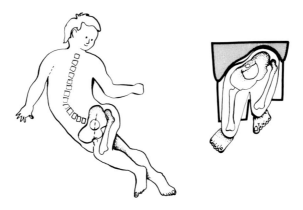

FIGURE 10.   Pelvic obliquity frequently has a rotatory component which compounds the difficulty in obtaining stable seating. (Reproduced with permission from Letts, M., Rang, M., and Tredwell, S., Seating the disabled, in *American Academy of Orthopaedic Surgeons: Atlas of Orthotics,* 2nd ed., C. V. Mosby, St. Louis, 1985.)

nerve root that has been demonstrated by nerve stimulation to contribute significantly to the spasticity of various muscle groups. This may have significant application to sitting imbalance occasioned by severe spasticity in those with spastic quadriplegia. The author's personal experience with two such children has demonstrated improved sitting stability following rhizotomy. At present, this is not an indication for rhizotomy, but the benefits to the seated population with marked spasticity and subsequent sitting imbalance needs to be assessed.

VIII. SUMMARY

Pelvic obliquity is a major disabling deformity for the wheelchair user. Wherever possible, it should be prevented with the use of judicious surgery followed up by supportive

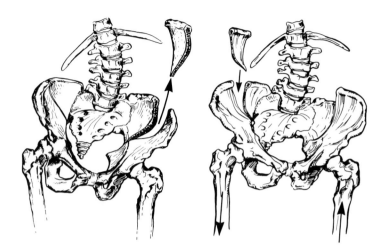

FIGURE 11. Correction of rigid pelvic obliquity by the Lindseth technique. (From Lindseth, R. E., *J. Bone Jt. Surg. Am. Vol.,* 60, 18, 1978. With permission.)

seating. The seating team must be ever vigilant for the early signs of pelvic obliquity in the seated population, and in spastic patients, the hips should be monitored closely for subluxation and dislocation and treated aggressively in younger age groups when this is identified. Prevention is the most efficient and practical way to deal with this devastating deformity.

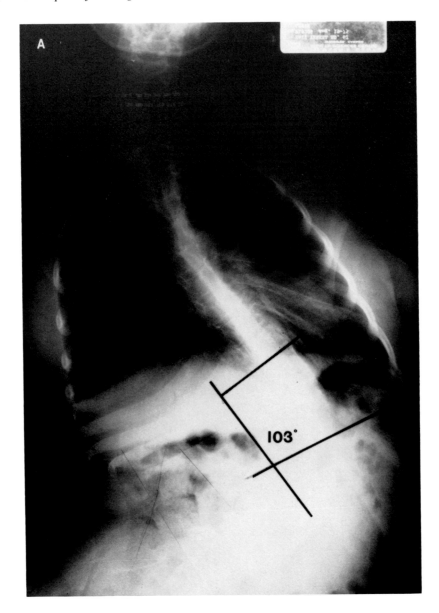

FIGURE 12.   (A) Severe scoliosis and pelvic obliquity in a 12-year-old child with spinal muscular atrophy.

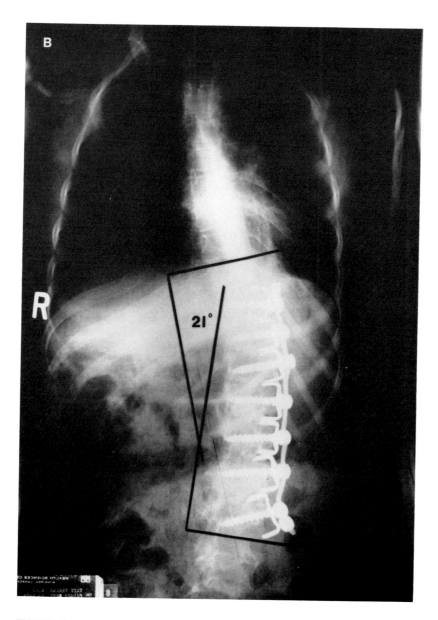

FIGURE 12 (continued). (B) Correction with soft tissue release and anterior spinal fusion.

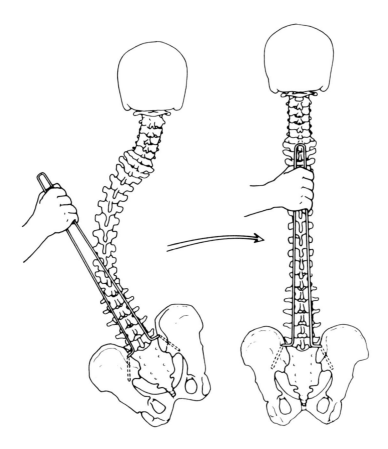

FIGURE 13. Segmental wiring with a unit rod and pelvic fixation using the rudder technique is an effective way to correct scoliosis with associated pelvic obliquity. (From Rinsky, L. A., *Clin. Orthop. Rel. Res.,* 253, 100, 1990. With permission.)

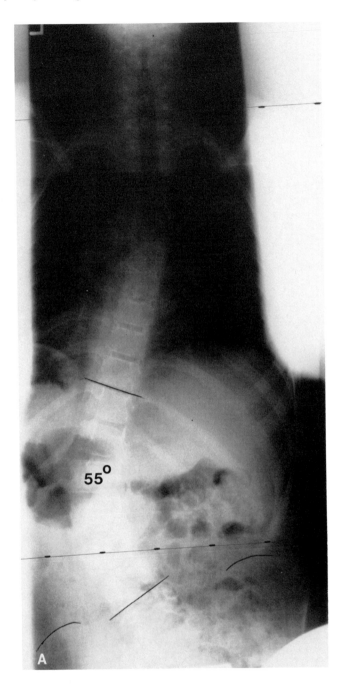

FIGURE 14.   Pelvic obliquity (A) with pelvis as part of the curve and resulting in poor sitting posture.

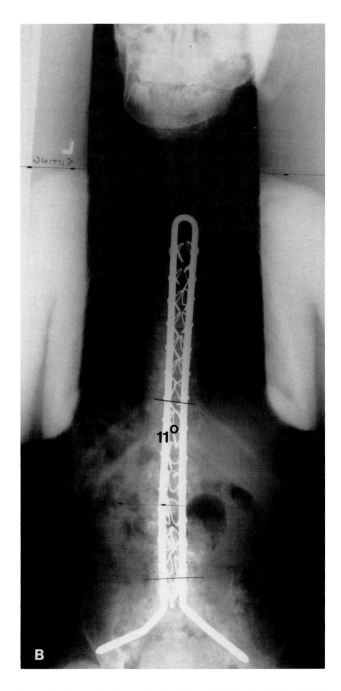

FIGURE 14 (continued). (B) Both the scoliosis and pelvic obliquity have been almost fully corrected using a unit rod and the Galveston technique with segmental wiring resulting in a stable sitting posture. (Courtesy of Dr. Jacques D'Astous, Children's Hospital of Eastern Ontario, Ottawa.)

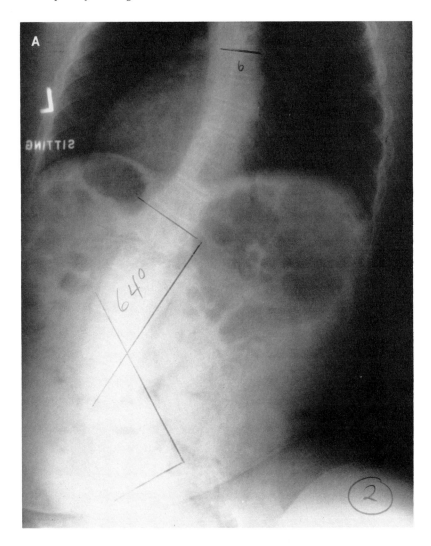

FIGURE 15. Lumbar scoliosis (A) with pelvic obliquity contributing to unbalanced sitting.

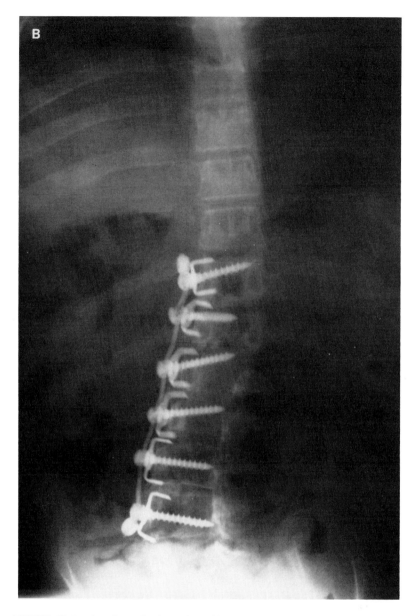

FIGURE 15 (continued).   (B) Correction with an anterior Dwyer fusion with complete correction of pelvic obliquity and provision of good sitting stability.

REFERENCES

1. **Allen, B. L. and Ferguson, R. I.,** The Galveton technique for L-rod instrumentation of the scoliotic spine, *Spine,* 7, 276, 1982.
2. **Banta, J. V., Broom, M. J. and Rensha, T. S.,** Spinal fusion augmented by Luque rod segmental instrumentation for neuromuscular scoliosis, *J. Bone Jt. Surg. Am. Vol.,* 71, 32, 1989.
3. **Baxter, M. P. and D'Astous, J. L.,** Proximal femoral resection — interposition arthroplasty, *J. Pediatr. Orthop.,* 6, 681, 1986.
4. **Beals, R. K. J.,** Developmental changes in the femur and acetabulum in spastic paraplegia and diplegia, *Dev. Med. Child Neurol.,* 11, 303, 1969.

5. **Bleck, E. E.,** Total body involvement, in *Orthopedic Management of Cerebral Palsy,* W. B. Saunders, Philadelphia, 1979, 208.

6. **Bleck, E. E.,** Where have all the cerebral palsy children gone? The needs of adults, *Dev. Med. Child Neurol.,* 26, 674, 1984.

7. **Bonnett, C., Brown, J., and Grow, T.,** Thoracolumbar scoliosis in cerebral palsy. Results of surgical treatment, *J. Bone Jt. Surg. Am. Vol.,* A58, 328, 1976.

8. **Cadman, D., Richards, J., and Feldman, W.,** Gastroesophageal reflux in severely retarded children, *Dev. Med. Child Neurol.,* 20, 95, 1978.

9. **Drummond, D., Breed, A. L., and Narechania, R.,** Relationship of spine deformity and pelvic obliquity on sitting pressure distributions and decubitus ulceration, *J. Pediatr. Orthop.,* 5, 396, 1985.

10. **Drummond, D. S., Rogala, E. J., Cruess, R., and Moreau, M.,** The paralytic hip and pelvic obliquity in cerebral palsy and myelomeningocele, in *American Academy of Orthopedic Surgeons: AAOS Instructional Course Lectures,* Vol. 28, C. V. Mosby, St. Louis, 1979, 7.

11. **Dubousset, J., Herring, J. A., and Shufflebarger, H.,** The crankshaft phenomenon, *J. Pediatr. Orthop.,* 9, 541, 1989.

12. **Ferguson-Pell, M. W.,** Seat cushion selection, *J. Rehabil. Res. Dev. Suppl.,* 2, 49, 1990.

13. **Fulford, G. E. and Brown, J. K.,** Position as a cause of deformity in children with cerebral palsy, *Dev. Med. Child Neurol.,* 305, 18, 1976.

14. **Gamble, J. G., Rinsky, L. A., and Bleck, E.,** Established hip dislocations in children with cerebral palsy, *Clin. Orthop. Rel. Res.,* 253, 90, 1990.

15. **Hobson, D. A. and Nwaobi, O. M.,** The relationship between posture and ischial pressure for the high risk population, in *Proc. 8th Annu. Conf. Rehabilitation Technology,* Vol. 5, Washington, D.C., 1985, 338.

16. **Hoffer, M. M., Abraham, E., and Nickel, V.,** Salvage surgery at the hip to improve sitting posture of mentally retarded severely disabled children with cerebral palsy, *Dev. Med. Child Neurol.,* 14, 51, 1972.

17. **Kalem, V. and Bleck, E. E.,** Prevention of spastic paralytic dislocation of the hip, *Dev. Med. Child Neurol.,* 27, 17, 1985.

18. **Lamb, D. W. and Pollack, G. A.,** Hip deformities in cerebral palsy and their treatment, *Dev. Med. Child Neurol.,* 4, 488, 1962.

19. **Letts, M., Klassen, D., Shapiro, L., and Jurenka, S.,** The windswept hip phenomenon, *J. Bone Jt. Surg. Br. Vol.,* 64, 257, 1982.

20. **Lindseth, R. E.,** Myelomeningocele, in *Lowell and Winter's Pediatric Orthopedics,* 3rd ed., Morrissy, R., Ed., Lippincott, Philadelphia, 1990, 520.

21. **Lonstein, J. E. and Beck, K.,** Hip dislocation and subluxation in cerebral palsy, *J. Pediatr. Orthop.,* 6, 521, 1986.

22. **MacEwen, G. D.,** Operative treatment of scoliosis in cerebral palsy, *Reconstr. Surg. Traumatol.,* 13, 58, 1972.

23. **Matthew, S. S., Jones, S. H., and Spirling, S. C.,** Hip derangements seen in cerebral palsy, *Am. J. Phys. Med.,* 32, 213, 1952.

24. **McCarthy, R. E., Simon, S., Douglas, B., Zawacki, R., and Reese, H.,** Proximal femoral resection to allow adults who have severe cerebral palsy to sit, *J. Bone Jt. Surg. Am. Vol.,* 70, 1011, 1988.

25. **O'Brien, J. P., Dwyer, A. P., and Hodgson, A. R.,** Paralytic pelvic obliquity. Its prognosis and management and the development of a technique for full correction of the deformity, *J. Bone Jt. Surg. Am. Vol.,* 57, 626, 1975.

26. **Oppenheim, W. M.,** Selective posterior rhizotomy for spastic cerebral palsy, *Clin. Orthop. Rel. Res.,* 253, 20, 1990.

27. **Rang, M., Douglas, G., Bennet, G. C., and Koreska, J.,** Seating for children with cerebral palsy, *J. Pediatr. Orthop.,* 1, 279, 1981.

28. **Rinsky, L. A.,** Surgery of spinal deformity in cerebral palsy, *Clin. Orthop. Rel. Res.,* 253, 100, 1990.

29. **Robson, P.,** The prevalence of scoliosis in adolescents and young adults with cerebral palsy, *Dev. Med. Child Neurol.,* 10, 447, 1968.

30. **Rosenthal, R. K., Levine, D. B., and McCarver, C. L.,** The occurrence of scoliosis in cerebral palsy, *Dev. Med. Child Neurol.,* 16, 664, 1974.

31. **Samilson, R. and Bechard, R.,** Scoliosis in cerebral palsy: incidence distribution of curve patterns, natural history and thoughts on etiology, *Curr. Pract. Orthop. Surg.,* 5, 183, 1973.

32. **Samilson, R. L., Tsou, P., Aamoth, G., and Green, W. M.,** Dislocation and subluxation of the hip in cerebral palsy pathogenesis, natural history and management, *J. Bone Jt. Surg. Am. Vol.,* 54, 863, 1972.

33. **Sarutton, D.,** The early management of hips in cerebral palsy, *Dev. Med. Child Neurol.,* 31, 108, 1989.

34. **Silver, R. L., Rang, M., Chan, J., and della Garza, J.,** Adductor release in non-ambulant children with cerebral palsy, *J. Pediatr. Orthop.,* 5, 672, 1985.

35. **Stephenson, C. T., Griffith, B., Donovan, M. M., and Franklin, T.,** The adductor transfer and illiopsoas release in the cerebral palsy hip, *Orthop. Trans.,* 6, 94, 1982.

36. **Zacharkov, D.,** *Wheelchair Posture and Pressure Sores,* Charles C Thomas, Springfield, IL, 1984.

Chapter 10

CEREBRAL PALSY SEATING

Stephen Tredwell and Lori Roxborough

TABLE OF CONTENTS

I. INTRODUCTION

The variability of expression in the cerebral palsy patient includes those with markedly exaggerated stretch reflex response (spasticity), sustained increases in muscle tone (rigidity), abnormally decreased tone (hypotonia), uncontrolled abnormal movement (athetosis), and abnormal position sense (ataxia). As combinations of the above are quite common, positioning the patient with cerebral palsy can be one of the most complex problems encountered in a seating clinic. The condition presents a group of problems that are often unique to each patient, and the array of solutions to any given problem is mind boggling. Nevertheless, there are basic principles and approaches that can assist in solving most problems.

To understand abnormal sitting well enough to offer a solution, the practitioner must first have a concept of normalcy. The act of sitting is not static. Studies carried out at Sunnyhill Hospital in Vancouver, British Columbia, during 1987 and 1988, utilizing seating surface telemetry demonstrated many unusual aspects of normal seating (Figure 1). When studied over time, normal seating was usually asymmetrical: equal upright weight bearing through both ischial tuberosities was rare (Figure 2). Most subjects tended to show a right or left dominance, although weight bearing was never exclusively unilateral. Within the right or left preference, there was a constant side-to-side oscillation of weight occurring several times a minute (Figure 3). In addition, a slower left-to-right, bi-weight shifting often occurred once or twice during a 15-min test period.

The relationship of the axis through the ischial tuberosities to the back of the chair was asymmetric, with an average slope of 0.06 (Figure 4). Increased sheer stress and weight concentration during periods of "task attentive posture" were observed, i.e., those times when the subject was concentrating on performing a specific task.

These variations help to explain the difficulties with some custom-molded solutions which do not allow movement and are therefore tolerated for only short periods. Although the variations are small, the imposition of absolute neutrality is not as comfortable for the patient as accommodating to the mild or moderate asymmetries required by a given activity. Where communication devices and other environmental controls require, the seating surface must allow the patient to shift position.

Seating for children with cerebral palsy needs to reduce secondary complications, such as muscle contracture by means of accurate placement of the child, and to minimize perceptual/cognitive deficit which may result from lack of interaction with the environment. Each seating solution should aim to maximize the child's capabilities and to provide a comfortable surface that is tolerated most of the day. Individual seating goals are established for each child based on the assessment findings and knowledge of the natural history of his/her condition. Specific goals may include:

1. Influencing muscle tone
2. Facilitating motor control by selectively controlling the degrees of freedom at various joints and progressively decreasing the degree of external support as control develops
3. Facilitating skeletal development through appropriate weight bearing and balancing of muscle forces
4. Preventing contracture through the promotion of neutral alignment and counteracting the force of gravity
5. Preventing pressure sore development by distribution of weight through support surfaces and use of materials allowing heat dissipation and moisture absorption
6. Preventing cardiorespiratory complications
7. Facilitating perceptual, cognitive, and social development through the provision of opportunities for environmental interaction

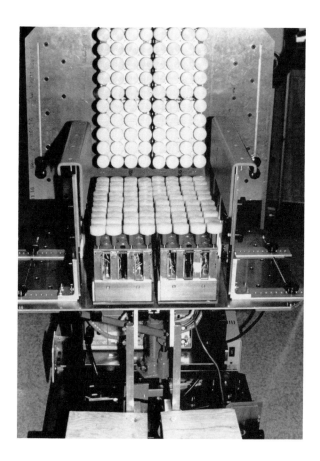

FIGURE 1.   Fully adjustable telemetrized seating surface.

The seating requirements of any child vary with age.[4] During the first year, the normal child exhibits an evolution in seating skills. From birth to around 8 weeks, there is an automatic seating response that is reflexive in nature. By 3 months of age, this is gone and the child lacks the control of trunk and hips to allow sitting. By 5 months, there is some upper trunk control along with increased control over the head and neck. By 6 months, the normal infant can be termed a "propped sitter", with extension of trunk and flexion of hips. By 7 or 8 months, most children can sit alone.

Positioning the cerebral palsy infant should concentrate on trunk support in order to stabilize the infantile kyphotic spinal alignment. Commercially available cuddle seats are usually sufficient. With the advent of increased head and neck control or head and neck tone, the more lordotic curves at the lumbar and cervical spine should be encouraged. Simple corner seats and modified highchair infant seats often suffice.

As the child matures, the seating function must adapt. A formal problem-solving approach becomes imperative for those children whose handicap dictates that the majority of their time is spent sitting. This approach must consider several factors:

1. The patient's functional ability
2. The patient's physical capability with respect to static contracture, abnormal reflexes or posturing, and predominant spastic patterns
3. The home and school environment, including the technical resources available and the experience of the people working with the child

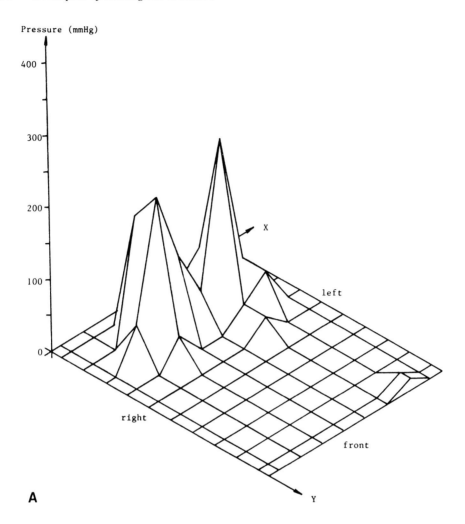

FIGURE 2.   Graphic representation of (A) ischial pressures showing left to right asymmetry.

General functional ability as modified from Hoffer's classification is useful in categorizing these children.[2]

A. THE HAND-FREE SITTER (FIGURE 5)

This patient can sit for prolonged time periods without needing the hands for support. The seat for hand-free sitters is designed primarily for mobility and to provide a stable base as well as comfort. A firm foam cushion is preferred over a commercially available hammock seat or the softer cushion which is commonly used in patients with anesthetic skin. To allow the child to perform his or her own transfers, the armrests of the chair should be removable.

B. THE HAND-DEPENDENT SITTER (FIGURE 6)

This patient needs one or both hands to maintain support while sitting. To be able to use the hands in day-to-day activities, the patient must have some form of trunk and/or pelvic support in the system. Minor modifications such as a firm contoured seat can often convert a marginally hand-dependent sitter to a hand-free state.

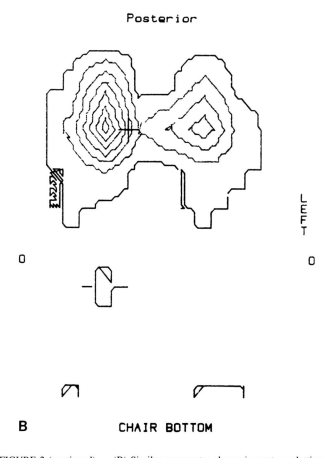

Posterior

B   CHAIR BOTTOM

FIGURE 2 (continued).   (B) Similar asymmetry shown in contour plotting.

C. THE PROPPED SITTER (FIGURE 7)

This patient, because of severe functional or structural deformity, is unable to sit without major modifications to allow for pelvic trunk and sometimes head and neck support.

II. GROUPINGS

Letts et al. have grouped the cerebral palsy patients into three major subgroups.[3] The groupings are not exact, but they can often be used as a general guide when starting to assess the patient.

A. THE SYMMETRICALLY SLOUCHED CHILD

Here, symmetrically shortened or spastic hamstrings promote posterior rotation of the pelvis, which eliminates lumbar lordosis and results in sacral sitting. When flexible, this can be managed by modification of the seating surface, but as the hamstring tightness worsens, surgery may be indicated.

B. THE ASYMMETRICALLY SLOUCHED CHILD

The individual presents with poor trunk control, asymmetric adductor tightness, and subluxation or dislocation of the hip. Although this can be accommodated early in the evolution of this deformity, careful monitoring is required to identify those children with progressive hip subluxation or dislocation.

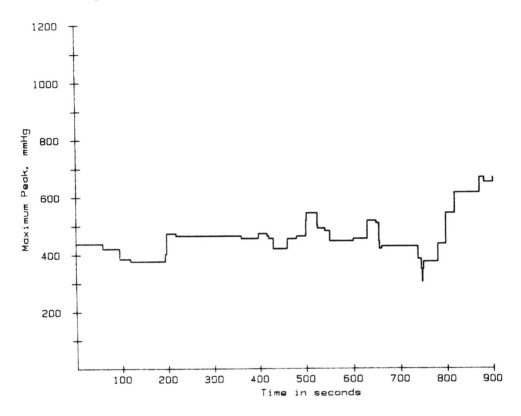

FIGURE 3.   Graphic representation of changes in seating pressure recorded over a 15-min period of relaxed sitting.

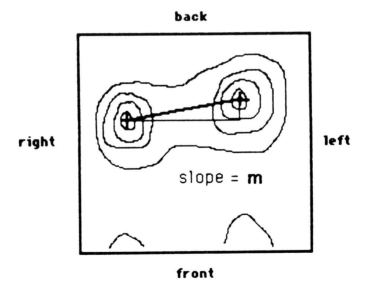

FIGURE 4.   Contour plot showing obliquity of ischial tuberosities in normal seating.

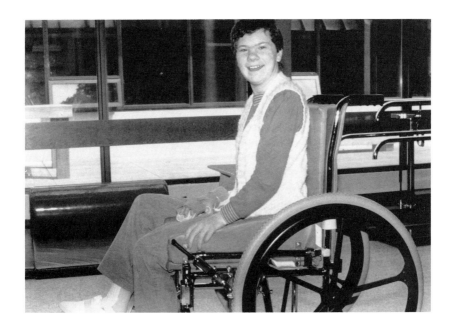

FIGURE 5. Hand-free sitter.

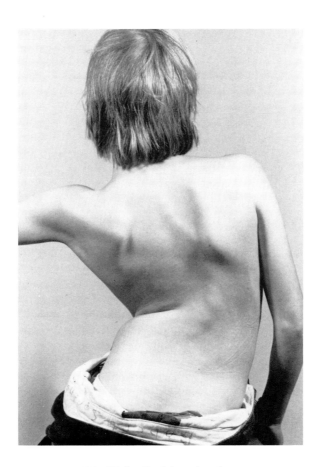

FIGURE 6. Hand-dependent sitter.

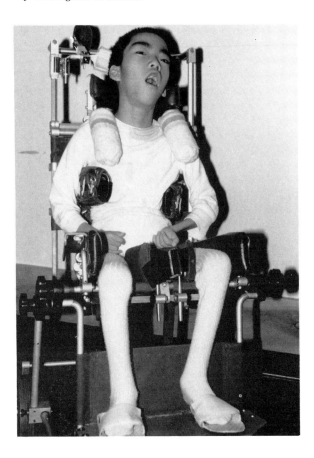

FIGURE 7.   Totally propped sitter.

C. THE WINDSWEPT CHILD

This is often the end stage of the asymmetrically slouched child. The hip is usually severely subluxed or dislocated. There is a rotatory pelvic obliquity with an apparent short thigh on the adducted side.

While the previous classification systems offer a convenient starting point when evaluating the cerebral palsy child, each case is usually unique and, in the final analysis, must be treated with an individualized solution.

III. ASSESSMENT

Participation of a multidisciplinary team in the assessment process is essential to the ultimate provision of a seating system that will fulfill the goals established for each child. Frequently, the team is comprised of community professionals working in partnership with the seating specialists in the clinic.

The seating assessment has been developed to examine the sensory, biomechanical, and neurological factors thought to be important in postural control. Important areas to consider in this assessment are discussed below.

A. SENSORY/PERCEPTUAL STATUS

Sensory organization is an important requisite for postural control in sitting. In children with cerebral palsy, faulty sensory organization may contribute to abnormal postures and difficulties in maintaining balance. Assessment of the visual, vestibular, and somatosensory systems contributes important information to the analysis of these problems and to the determination of the most appropriate seating solution. Visual perceptual miscues may lead to abnormal head alignment when the individual alters the orientation of the head in relation to the line of gravity (labyrinthine reflexes). Somatosensory difficulties may result in abnormal alignment when one segment of the body is moved in relation to another (tonic neck and lumbar reflexes) or as hypo-/hyperresponsiveness to tactile and proprioceptive stimuli. Deficits in visual, vestibular, and/or somatosensory organization may also contribute to imbalance problems, depending on the nature of the sensory system(s) affected.

Response to specific proprioceptive and tactile inputs is important in the selection of seating materials. For example, fabrication of medial thigh supports utilizing elastic materials may have the undesirable effect of stimulating stretch reflexes in the hip adductors; therefore, a nonresilient material should be selected for this application. Conversely, an elastic circumferential strap will benefit the child with truck hypotonia as it facilitates cocontraction of abdominal and spinal muscles.

B. SKELETAL DEVELOPMENT

Skeletal development frequently follows an abnormal progression in children with cerebral palsy; spastic muscles and the lack of normal weight-bearing forces influence the process of bone modeling. Common skeletal abnormalities include acetabular dysplasia, coxavalga, femoral anteversion, tibial torsion, and scoliosis. The alteration of muscle forces and provision of weight-bearing opportunities through early positioning therapy and surgical intervention may favorably influence the course of skeletal development.

Inappropriate use of seating components or failure to closely monitor seating during periods of rapid growth may increase the risk of creating iatrogenic skeletal deformities.

Assessment of this area consists of radiological and physical examinations.

C. RANGE OF MOTION

Precise assessment of joint range of motion and muscle length is required to determine the constraints on the individual and the potential degree of movement while in the sitting position. Range of motion is systematically evaluated in all joints. Diarthrodial muscle length assessments of particular interest in the seating assessment include hamstrings, tensor fascia lata, quadriceps, and gastrocnemius.

D. MUSCLE TONE

The nature, degree, and distribution of muscle tone abnormalities are noted in the assessment, with particular emphasis on the effects of position on muscle tone.

Abnormalities in muscle tone, particularly spasticity, have been thought to be a key factor in the failure of the cerebral palsy child to develop normal movement patterns. Recent advances in pharmacological and neurosurgical treatment of spasticity have offered researchers the opportunity to examine motor patterns following a dramatic reduction in muscle tone. Their findings of relatively constant synergistic patterns in both the spastic and reduced spasticity states indicate that abnormal muscle tone may not be the cause of motor control disorders in cerebral palsy, but, rather, an associated phenomenon caused by the same central lesion.

E. MOTOR DEVELOPMENT

Overall motor development is determined by the child's ability to assume, maintain, and move according to the Denver Developmental Index. The primary methods of mobility, transfer abilities, and upper limb functions are also examined during this phase of the assessment.

F. SKIN CONDITION

Examination of skin condition is undertaken to detect areas at risk from pressure sore development. Close inspection is made of weight-bearing areas (e.g., ischial tuberosities, coccyx, and sacrum), areas of bony prominence (e.g., greater trochanter and occiput), and areas where seating components may be applying pressure (e.g., trunk supports and shoulder straps). Skin is examined in terms of color, smoothness, circulation, scarring, moisture, and sensation.

G. POSTURAL CONTROL

Postural control is assessed in terms of alignment, balance, and motor control.

A segmental posture assessment is performed with the child placed in a sitting position on a firm surface. The posture of each segment is sequentially analyzed to determine whether postural abnormalities are structural or functional and whether they are primary or compensatory. Structural abnormalities need to be accommodated within the seating system, whereas functional abnormalities should be corrected by the seating system.

Many of the postural abnormalities encountered in children with cerebral palsy are compensatory. For example, a functional kyphosis may be a compensatory strategy to maintain balance and vertical head alignment in the presence of a primary posterior pelvic tilt. In this case, the seating prescription should be focused on support of the pelvis in a neutral position.

H. FUNCTIONAL ABILITIES

Assessment of functional abilities in the areas of feeding, communication, dressing, toileting, hygiene, transfers, and mobility is important in the selection of a seating system which will facilitate these daily functions.

I. ENVIRONMENTAL CONSIDERATION

Information should be gathered through interviews and site visits regarding accessibility and transportation considerations.

The specific seat prescribed will depend upon the resources available in the center and the system or systems with which the staff is most familiar. The importance of some form of simulator or trial period cannot be overemphasized.

The following sequence must be adhered to whether the seat is to be a custom design or a commercial product. The chair seat must first be fitted; then the angle between the seat and back is determined along with modifications such as medial and lateral thigh bolsters being applied to the seat as needed; and, finally, the chairback should be fixed.

1. The Chair Seat

Pelvic position is the basic foundation of any seating solution. Slight asymmetry in rotation and obliquity can be allowed, but it should be centered on the midline. Children with cerebral palsy have abnormal balance and therefore will require a firm, but not rigid surface. Soft cushions or hammock seats promote adduction of the hips and exaggerate balance problems. In addition, the proprioceptive feedback of a firm surface aids the child in maintaining an upright position. As a general rule, this seating base is slightly wedged, with the thicker part forward.

2. The Angle

Setting the angle between the seat and back may be a matter of trial and error, but generally an angle of 90° or less is preferred for those children with excessive extensor thrust or tight hamstrings. One must, however, be aware of pelvic positions with angles of less than 90° and not gain correction by inducing a lumbar kyphosis and increasing the posterior pelvic tilt. Angles of greater than 90° are useful in situations of mild hypotonia to induce a lumbar lordosis.

3. Additional Support

Medial and lateral thigh bolsters may then be considered. These should align the thigh, with the hips abducted between 20 to 30°, if possible. This will provide a stable seating base. Medial or lateral bolsters can help prevent tendencies to extremes of abduction or adduction. The medial thigh bolster can range from a simple contouring of the foam surface to the shape of the thigh to a formal pummel or anterior pelvic support.

4. Supplementary Support

Augmenting existing supports with one or more of the following can increase the patient's control of the pelvis.

The antithrust block concept was advanced by Alan Seikman at Stanford University in 1978.[7] This seat cushion was designed to help control the pelvic position and depends on layers of foam of varying density, which allows the ischia to sink down in the posterior part of the cushion, but meet the resistance of the increasing stiffness of the foam as the ischia move forward with attempts at posterior pelvic rotation.[1]

Supports can also be placed under the anterior superior iliac spine. The commercially available pelvic hooks can provide some stability. The sub-ASIS bar design by David Cooper at the University of British Columbia is useful in patients with an excessive tendency to posterior pelvic rotation.

In patients with flexibility, a posterior sacral bolster (not lumbar) may also decrease posterior tilt. This support was designed by the Chailey Heritage Hospital and Craft School in East Sussex and has been used by the rehabilitation engineering program at the University of Tennessee. This posterior bolster comes no higher than the L4 or L5 level. In flexible patients, it is used in association with a 45° lapbelt; in more rigid patients, it is used with an anterior knee block and belt.

5. The Chair Back

Given adequate pelvic position by whatever means, the trunk must be addressed next. In the totally involved cerebral palsy patient, some trunk support will be necessary. With any degree of asymmetry, a scoliosis will tend to develop; therefore, asymmetrically spinal support pads should be used, with the pad on the concave side of the curve being placed as high as the patient will tolerate it. The support pads allow a three-point system to work against the curve, the third point being the pelvic fixation. Although these pads will help center the patient, they probably do not prevent an increase of curvature.

Totally molded back surfaces can be of some help in the severe scoliotic curve, but will usually require that the seating surface be rotated in space to slightly recline the patient and ''load'' the molded surface. This is even more important in the symmetrically slouched, kyphotic patient.

In patients with truncal hypotonia, we have found that a lightweight, flexible polypropylene underarm brace (thoracolumbar sacral orthosis, TLSO) molded to induce a lumbar lordosis is often an appropriate solution. This brace allows a more standard back component to be used in the chair, usually along with some form of belt system.

This concept has been reviewed more formally by Yamashita and Letts,[8] using a TLSO of Aliplast termed a Soft Boston orthosis.

6. Lower Extremity Position

With the pelvis well centered and the spine stable, the lower extremities need to be addressed. The feet should always be supported. In those patients with excessive valgus and external tibial torsion, where the externally rotated foot becomes the hazard, a well-molded ankle-foot orthosis (AFO) that fits within the shoe often makes positioning easier. The knee should be flexed to 90°. Patients with excessive hamstring tightness may have the seat pad beveled back slightly to allow more knee flexion; however, in this type of patient, surgical lengthening of the hamstrings is often preferable.

J. ROLE OF SURGERY

While the chair remains the primary treatment mode for cerebral palsy patients, surgery can be a powerful adjunct in the management of seating problems. In cerebral palsy, surgery should be viewed as an aid to maximizing potential, avoiding impending disaster, and in selected cases, to salvaging an end-stage situation.

The decision to operate cannot be made in isolation. Knowledge of the patient's current functional ability, including his/her sitting tolerances and communication skills, as well as other environmental control needs, a survey of the patient's change in function over the past several years, and attendants' reports are essential parts of an appropriate evaluation. Pain is often difficult to document in this group, but it is often a common accompaniment of dislocation of the hip. Even harder to document is the difficulty in maintaining an adequate body weight in those children who have severe feeding problems because of trunk distortion.

As a general guideline, increasing needs for straps and/or add-on supports to the chair should stimulate a review *vis à vis* surgical intervention. For example, the patient who reports a need for increased straps to prevent posterior pelvic rotation and a constant sliding out from underneath these restraints in the chair coupled with hamstring tightness greater than 90° may be more simply helped with a limited hamstring lengthening than with the additional straps and/or knee blocks that add to the complexity of the care and, in the end, may only add a temporary respite from the problem (Figure 8).

Surgery is neither indicated nor uniformly successful in all cases of hamstring tightness, scoliosis, or pelvic obliquity. Equal to preoperative evaluation in importance is choice of surgical procedure.

As stressed earlier, a stable pelvis is the first requirement for a stable seating function. Increased adduction contracture narrows the seating base and, in a patient with already compromised control of his/her equilibrium seating balance, can be even more compromised. When adduction contracture is asymmetrical, a pelvic rotation is usually observed clinically as asymmetry of thigh length (apparent shortening on the adducted side) (Figure 9). This so-called windswept position can have several etiologies: the asymmetrical adduction contracture mentioned previously, an asymmetrical abduction contracture described by Sussman, hip dislocation, and/or scoliosis. Determining which came first often proves to be a difficult task.

Increasing adduction contracture can lead to progressive subluxation and eventual dislocation of the hip on the adducted side. Samilson reported that the average age of hip dislocation in the severely involved spastic quadriplegic is 7 years.[6] Hip dislocation then becomes a secondary event and, although part of the natural history of the untreated cerebral palsy patient, should be modifiable by therapy. Reimers has shown that subluxation up to 40% can be controlled by adductor myotomy.[5] Rang suggests that subluxation of up to 50% may be amenable to soft tissue surgery. Provided an adequate seating program is in place, subluxation that progresses to between 40 and 50% is a candidate for bilateral adductor release. In the absence of a good seating program, the child should be seated first and then observed to follow his/her progress. Soft tissue surgical intervention should take place in patients with subluxations of less than 50%. In a child with greater than 50% subluxation, a primary intertrochanteric femoral derotation osteotomy coupled with open reduction of the hip is indicated. This is followed by revision of the seating orthosis.

Hamstring tightness can also produce pelvic rotation, but in the transverse plane. This posterior pelvic tilt causes sacral sitting loss of the lumbar lordosis and difficulty in knee positioning. When the deformity is early and flexible, a seating orthosis may control the

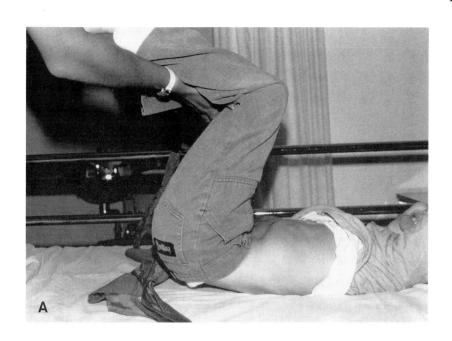

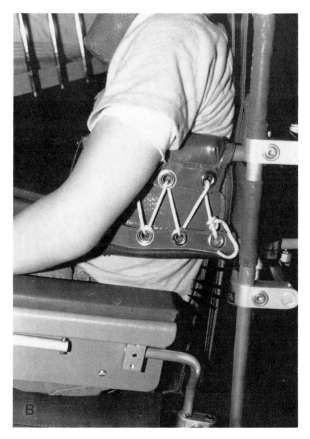

FIGURE 8.   Clinical demonstration of hamstring tightness (A); (B) same patient in totally supported seating orthosis showing early sacral sitting.

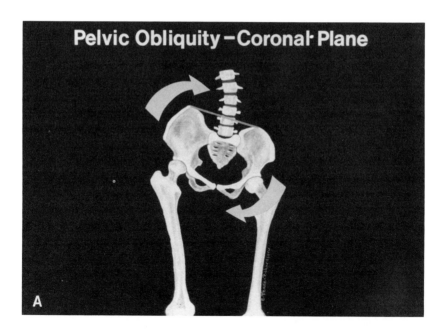

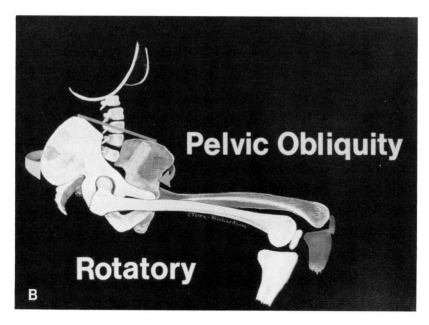

FIGURE 9. Classical pelvic obliquity (A) viewed in the coronal plane can be caused by pathology above the pelvis such as scoliosis or asymmetric abdominal wall spasticity, by abnormal forces crossing the pelvis such as iliopsoas spasticity, or from forces below the pelvic brim, such as adduction contracture, abduction contracture, or dislocation of the hip; (B) in the seated position, infrapelvic causes of obliquity in the upright position produce a rotatory obliquity and apparent asymmetry of thigh length.

problem. When it is progressive and nonresponsive to moderate seating changes, or when it becomes rigid, hamstring lengthening is preferred.

Collapsing spine deformity can also compromise the patient's ability to sit (Figure 10). In addition, severe distortion of the trunk may result in difficulties in feeding, resulting in aspiration as well as exaggerating the esophageal reflux which is common in this group.

Solutions to the problem of scoliosis may involve modification of the support pads and a flexible TLSO. Often overlooked and of help to some patients is a simple feeding gastrostomy. This is especially useful in the patient who is difficult to feed, whose weight is poor, and where aspiration and reflux are a problem.

If, however, more moderate solutions fail to halt the deterioration of seating function, i.e., increasing time required by the caregiver, decreasing chair time, increasing bed time, or decrease in communication skills, then spinal instrumentation should be considered. It should be noted that a 16-year-old patient with a 75° spinal curve controlled with a TLSO who experiences no decrease in function is not a candidate for surgical intervention. The patient's functional ability must be the indicator for surgery, not the parameters of his/her handicap.

Extremity surgery can also benefit the seated patient. To improve the patient's upper body function, flexor-carpi ulnaris transfer increases control over the power chair and facilitates the use of communication devices. In more severe cases, wrist fusion may also benefit the patient. In the lower extremities, failure of an AFO to control foot and leg alignment can place a child at risk by catching the externally rotated foot on the bed or doorway or, in the more severe case, by causing pressure areas over the apex of a severely deformed cavovarus foot. A triple arthrodesis often solves these problems as well as making shoe or slipper wear and chair positioning easier. A simple procedure such as tendoachilles lengthening or tibialis posterior tenotomy plus AFO may also suffice.

With the advent of the selective posterior dorsal rhizotomy, some totally involved patients have been helped, with a general decrease in muscle tone making more standard seating options viable. This is an area of surgery that is in its infancy and patients for this must be carefully selected.

ACKNOWLEDGMENT

The authors gratefully acknowledge the editorial assistance provided by Lawrence A. Davis, M.A.

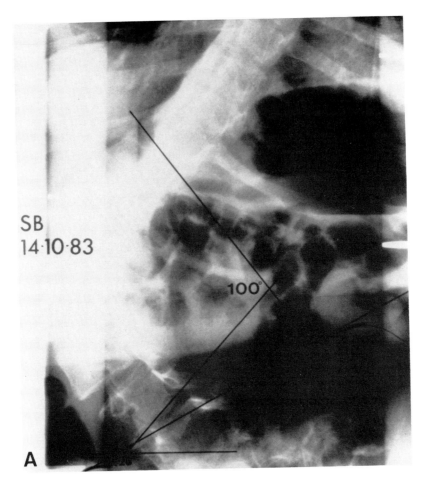

FIGURE 10.   Scoliosis in pelvic obliquity (A) associated with decline in seating function and the ability to use communicating equipment. (From Tredwell, S. J., *Spine State Art Rev.*, 1(2), 252, 1987. With permission.)

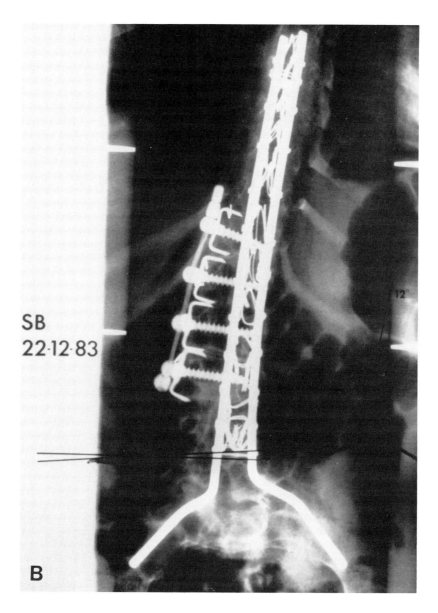

FIGURE 10 (continued).   (B) Following surgical correction. (From Tredwell, S. J., *Spine State Art Rev.*, 1(2), 252, 1987. With permission.)

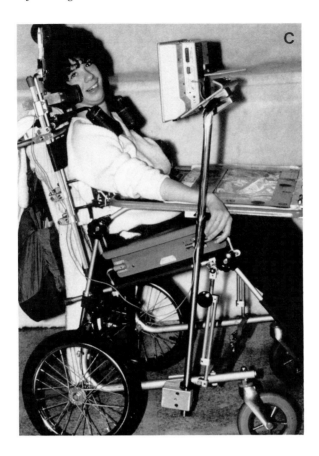

FIGURE 10 (continued).   (C) The patient following surgery in seating orthosis with communication aids.

REFERENCES

1. **Cooper, D.,** Biomechanics in postural control, in 6th Int. Seating Symp., University of British Columbia, Vancouver, February 1990.
2. **Hoffer, M. M.,** Basic considerations and classifications of cerebral palsy, in *American Academy of Orthopedic Surgeons: Instructional Course Lectures,* Vol. 25, C. V. Mosby, St. Louis, 1976.
3. **Letts, M., Rang, M., and Tredwell, S. J.,** Seating the disabled, in *American Academy of Orthopaedic Surgeons: Atlas of Orthotics,* 2nd ed., C. V. Mosby, St. Louis, 1985.
4. **Martin, M.,** The first year of life in 4th Int. Seating Symp., University of British Columbia, February 1988.
5. **Reimers, J.,** The stability of the hip in children, *Acta Orthop. Scand.,* Suppl. 184, 49, 1980.
6. **Samilson, R. L., Tsou, P., Aamoth, G., and Green, W. T.,** Dislocation and subluxation of the hip in cerebral palsy, *J. Bone Jt. Surg. Am. Vol.,* 54, 863, 1972.
7. **Seikman, A.,** The antithrust cushion — a twelve year retrospective review, in 6th Int. Seating Symp., University of British Columbia, February 1990.
8. **Yamashita, T. and Letts, M.,** Use of the Soft Boston orthosis in seating, in 6th Int. Seating Symp., University of British Columbia, February 1990.

Chapter 11

SEATING IN MUSCULAR DYSTROPHY

Richard D. Beauchamp, William G. Mackenzie, and Alison Kelly Stewart

TABLE OF CONTENTS

I. INTRODUCTION

The muscular dystrophies are categorized into various types based on their clinical progression, distribution of weakness, and patterns of inheritance. Duchenne's muscular dystrophy (DMD) is one of the categories of muscular dystrophy that is genetically determined, sex-linked recessive, in which the muscle deterioration proceeds relentlessly throughout the boys' lives.[15] Duchenne first described the invariable progression and fatality of the disease in his articles in the 1800s. To these children, their families, peers, and members of the clinical management team, the progression of the disease is manifested in a series of crises that usually occur in a predictable, stepwise fashion.[2]

The first crisis occurs at about the age of 3 years when the diagnosis is initially made; the second is at about the age of 10 years, when the boy is no longer able to continue walking. The third crisis occurs in the late teenage years when spinal deformity and respiratory compromise may cause the child to become bedridden, and, finally, death occurs in the 20s.

Unfortunately, DMD is one of the most common and most severe types of dystrophies. The disease can not only result in severe physical deformity, but also in profound psychological distress to the child and family, further complicating the management process. Positive management of DMD requires a great deal of empathy, patience, and support by members of the clinical team.[12]

II. HISTORICAL BACKGROUND

One of the most severe consequences resulting from the progressive muscle weakness in DMD is the development of spinal deformity. Prior to 1975, the standard method for mobility was the manually propelled wheelchair with a sling seat and back. Most nonambulatory children (approximately 90%) with DMD will develop severe deformities of the spine in a relatively short period of time. The onset of the deformity usually occurs between the ages of 10 to 12 years, with rapid progression taking place between 12 to 14 years of age.[3,7] Without intervention, spinal curvature will progress relentlessly toward a severe structural deformity with inherent problems of reduced cardiopulmonary function, pelvic obliquity, difficulty with seating, pressure sores, and subsequent reduced mobility and independence. Conventional orthotic devices, including thoracic suspension jackets and simple corsets, have proven ineffective in controlling the progression of the deformity as well as unacceptable to most of the DMD patients due to discomfort. The orthotic approach has been successful in arresting other types of spinal deformity due to the "active" nature of the application, i.e., the user "actively" moves away from the areas of discomfort and therefore generates intrinsic corrective forces. Due the paralytic nature of DMD, this "active intrinsic" principle does not apply. Also, the discomfort from external forces necessary to generate effective spinal support without the intrinsic contribution from active muscles is above the acceptable tolerance level for most individuals and rejection is therefore inevitable.[19]

Surgery to correct and prevent progression of scoliosis was advanced significantly with the introduction of the rigid internal fixation by Harrington.[9] Prior techniques of *in situ* fusions achieved little correction and were followed by long immobilization — leading to devastating results for the DMD patients. The newer techniques using Luque and Cotrel-Dubousset instrumentation are stronger, more effective, and do not require postoperative immobilization.[22,23]

However, this was not the case in 1975, at which time the majority of patients were not benefiting from surgical intervention or appropriate seating and mobility devices. The clinical atmosphere was one of teenage boys presenting with relentlessly collapsing spines,

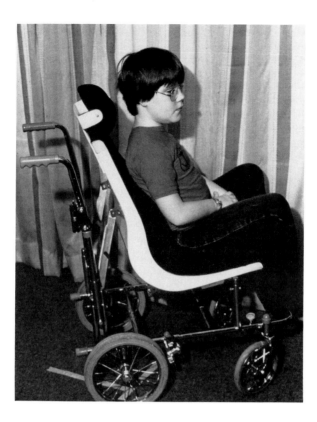

FIGURE 1. Spinal support system.

manifesting extreme physical discomfort combined with overpowering psychological implications, with limited means of providing adequate home and community support in terms of appropriate seating and mobility and devices for activities of daily living. It is important to realize that it is within this milieu that the concept of a spinal support system (SSS) was conceived and clinically applied. The SSS was initially developed at the Hospital for Sick Children in Toronto by Dr. Donald A. Gibson, orthopedic surgeon, and Mr. Jan Koreska, a biomedical engineer, in 1975.[7,24] The SSS was originally designed to prevent progressive deformity in a flexible and unstable spine (Figure 1). It was observed that a small percentage of children diagnosed as having DMD appeared to spontaneously acquire a lordotic posture of the lumbar and thoracic spines without any significant subsequent lateral or rotational deformities.[20] This observation suggested that lumbar lordotic posturing may prevent the onset of lateral deformity for all seated children with DMD. Furthermore, it set the stage for theoretical development of a seating system that would:

1. Arrest the progression of scoliotic deformity by extending the spine through use of custom-contoured seat components
2. Facilitate midline positioning and support of the body segments, as required, through the use of appropriate head, arm, and foot supports
3. Provide a seating and mobility system that is comfortable, functional, reproducible, affordable, and esthetically acceptable through use of available materials, components, and fabrication techniques

This has all led to the development of numerous seating devices initially spurred on by the spinal support system in 1975 in Toronto. Most of these systems include the incorporation of a lumbar lordotic pad to maintain lumbar and thoracic extension, the concept being that if the spine is going to become fused, or rigid spontaneously, it will adopt a stiff extended alignment rather than a flexed kyphotic attitude which may promote the development of scoliosis. Some researchers have disagreed with this concept of the lumbar pad.[26] There is no orthotic or seating system in use today that will prevent the majority of these children from developing a scoliosis. Even in the few cases in which the result is a stiff extended spine, the contribution of the seating system toward that outcome is probably only minimal.

Spinal surgery is a tremendous undertaking and must be offered to the patient and parents with full knowledge of the potential complications. The patient's pulmonary reserve must be sufficient to withstand the surgery and, hence, the surgery should be done early on in the nonambulatory phase of the disease.[1] The rationale for surgical intervention may be difficult to accept by the parents when the scoliosis is not severe. Posterior spinal fusion and instrumentation will stabilize the spine, making the seating problems easier for the management team. However, even when surgical stabilization is undertaken, usually at curves greater than 30°, appropriate seating systems are still required as the patient still requires pelvic support, appropriate upper and lower limb alignment, head support, and mobility.[8]

III. SPECIAL SEATING GOALS IN DUCHENNE'S MUSCULAR DYSTROPHY

1. Provide support and comfort as muscular weakness increases
2. Prevent pressure sores
3. Prevent or retard development of contractures (scoliosis probably excluded)
4. Provide for upright position as long as possible to delay respiratory problems, to assist functional abilities and maintain quality of life
5. Aid independent mobility in standard or power wheelchairs
6. Provide proximal stability to increase distal mobility and function
7. Facilitate ease of management and transport

IV. ASSESSMENT

Participation of the multidisciplinary team in the assessment process is essential to the ultimate provision of a seating system which will fulfill the goals established for each child. Frequently, the team is comprised of community professionals working in partnership with the seating specialists in the clinic.

The seating assessment has been developed to examine the biomechanical, neuromuscular, and sensory factors thought to be important in postural control. Important areas to consider in this assessment include:

1. Cardiac and pulmonary function — Postural compression can compromise vital capacity. Assessment of this area consists of physical examination and review of pulmonary function studies.[18]
2. Skeletal development — As the trunk muscles weaken, trunk and pelvic instability increase, with scoliosis and spinal collapse. Significant scoliosis correlates with deterioration of pulmonary and cardiac function. Assessment of this area consists of a review of radiological findings and a physical examination.[4,13] Inappropriate use of seating components or failure to closely monitor fit during periods of rapid change may contribute to iatrogenic skeletal deformities.
3. Range of motion — Contractures and deformities may compound the effect of muscle weakness and limit functional activities. Precise assessment of joint range of motion

and muscle length is required to determine the possible constraints on positioning the individual in sitting and the range of motion available for movement within the sitting position. Typical contractures found in the DMD children include hip and knee flexion, hip abduction, equinovarus foot deformities, shoulder internal rotation, elbow flexion, and forearm pronation.

4. Muscle tone and strength — The nature, degree, and distribution of muscle tone, strength, and weakness are noted in the assessment, with particular emphasis on the proximal vs. distal muscle strength and the effect of gravity in movement of the upper and lower extremities. The muscle weakness is usually symmetrical.[4]

5. Motor development — Overall gross and fine motor development is determined by the child's ability to assume, maintain, and move within developmental positions, as well as position tolerance. The primary method of mobility, endurance, transfer abilities, and compensatory strategies as well as upper limb dominance and patterns of movement are also examined.

6. Skin condition/sensation — Sensation is usually intact, but due to muscle wasting, there is a significant risk for pressure problems over bony prominences. The ischial tuberosities may be at the greatest risk. Many other areas may also be at risk such as the greater trochanters, spinous processes, and areas where seating components may be applying pressure such as the armrests and trunk supports. Examination of skin condition is undertaken to detect areas at risk for pressure sore development. Close inspection is made of weight-bearing areas. Skin is examined in terms of color, smoothness, circulation, scarring, moisture, and sensation. Pressure transducers may also be used bilaterally and simultaneously for specific pressure readings in areas of greatest concern.

7. Postural control — Postural control is assessed for alignment, balance, and motor control. A segmental posture assessment is performed with the child placed sitting on a firm surface. The posture of each segment is sequentially analyzed to determine whether postural abnormalities are structural or functional and whether they are primary or compensatory. Structural abnormalities should be accommodated within a seating system, whereas functional abnormalities should be corrected by the seating system.

8. Perceptual/cognitive status — This area is an important consideration when addressing safety while considering prescription of a power or manual wheelchair. The literature suggests that approximately one third of all Duchenne boys have less than average IQ.[17]

9. Psychosocial status — The preservation of mobility and function, either with a manual or power wheelchair and aids, can help prevent social isolation and increase independence, which is especially important during adolescence.

10. Functional abilities — Again, endurance and ability are assessed during functional activities such as toileting, dressing, hygiene, feeding, and communication. Methods of interacting with the environment, such as the ability to control light switches, the computer, and the telephone, are also important considerations in the selection of a seating system which will facilitate these daily functions.[21]

11. Environmental considerations — Information is collated through reports by team members, interviews, and site visits regarding accessibility and transportation considerations. Independent living is often a common goal which requires close contact for frequent reassessment of ability and equipment servicing. This may help to identify when changes are needed to ensure safety.

Although each child with DMD will have the same goals whether or not there has been spinal instrumentation, the seating prescription will vary, depending on the stage of the disease and specific problems a child is experiencing. The following are points to consider when matching a child's postural problems with appropriate seating solutions.

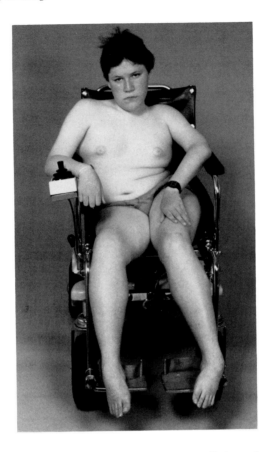

FIGURE 2.   Marked pelvic obliquity, scoliosis, and equinovarus foot deformities. Note the inadequate sling seat and back support.

V. SEATING SOLUTIONS FOR POSTURAL DEFORMITIES

Pelvis — Pelvic instability with obliquity and posterior pelvic tilt are common problems, often also seen with pelvic rotation (Figure 2). Lateral pelvic supports, firm back and firm seat positioned at 90°, and hip belt over anterior superior iliac spines to prevent anterior movement of the upper pelvis, or set at 45° to help prevent lower pelvis shifting forward, are provided. In fixed deformities, accommodation can be achieved through custom contouring the seat surface with pressure relief foam such as Sunmate. In these cases, the benefits of contouring are compromised when a material is placed over the cushion that does not stretch to meet the specific shape, such as a sheepskin.

Pressure — Pressure is an ongoing problem due to the lack of weight-shift abilities, with the most common occurrence being redness over the ischial tuberosities. Shear stress also occurs from drifting over the seat surface.[26] Relief can be obtained with the use of a firm seat, a contoured cushion, or one designed for its pressure relief qualities, such as the Jay® gel cushion. The use of a tilt-in-space option to approximately 40° can shift weight to relieve pressure.[14]

Trunk — Scoliosis and trunk rotation are the spinal deformities frequently seen in the DMD patient. Depending on the severity, some correction, maintenance, or accommodation can be achieved with the use of asymmetrical lateral trunk supports for a lateral spinal curve and curved lateral trunk supports for rotation. In theory, a lumbar pad may improve spinal alignment (and pelvic stability). The use of a tilt-in-space position, while maintaining seat-to-back angle, may relieve gravity's influence on the kyphosis (Figure 3). The recline position may also be used to unload the spine, but shearing forces preclude the use of a contoured back and lateral trunk supports in most positions.[16] A custom-contoured back support can accommodate severe, fixed deformities (Figure 4).

Hip/knee — Hip abduction and hip and knee flexion contractures as well as knee-ankle-foot orthoses (KAFOs) pose positional problems. Hip abduction can be well controlled with long lateral pelvic supports. KAFOs can be locked at the knee and used with elevated leg rests to avoid flexion contractures at the knee in the transition between the ambulatory and nonambulatory stage[10] (Figure 5). It is important to allow room in the seating system for KAFOs and to carefully review the seating when KAFOs are no longer used. If fixed hip and/or knee flexion contractures are present, accommodation of range can be achieved with additional wedging, ensuring that footrests can be fitted high enough. Elevating legrests are contraindicated when positioned beyond muscle length as the pelvis will shift.

Ankle/foot — Equinovarus is the most common foot deformity. Use of ankle-foot orthoses (AFOs) and pressure on the footrest in plantigrade are effective for those developing the equinovarus position, but surgery is also frequently needed.

Upper extremities — Shoulder internal rotation, elbow flexion, and forearm pronation is often a posture Duchenne patients assume. The scapulae should be well supported to allow maximum function. Also, the weight of the arms (and trunk), especially during activity, may pull the trunk forward and laterally such as when maneuvering a joystick on a power chair. Full-length, padded armrests of correct height and width from the patient can help support the trunk, while improved postural control can free the upper extremities.[25] A mobile arm support may be a useful aid for increased independent function. A central joystick may also be useful in centering the trunk.

Head/neck — The neck usually loses mobility and strength over time as well; therefore, it is important to provide support in as upright a position as possible to facilitate the use of vision. The provision of a sturdy neckrest or headrest can provide support during travel, especially if the child travels in a front-facing position. The use of a tilt-in-space or reclining wheelchair can also support the head and neck by eliminating the influence of gravity.

VI. SEATING SYSTEM SELECTION

Selecting the appropriate seating system for each child is a process of matching needs with available technology. For the child with mild seating problems, modular seating systems consisting of standard components are often selected. Multiadjustable seating systems are generally prescribed for individuals with moderate to severe motor disorders in the absence of severe deformities. Custom-contoured systems are used for individuals with severe structural deformities. A number of commercial manufacturers produce seating systems within each of the aforementioned categories.[11] The ever-changing range of components available precludes an exhaustive list in a text of this nature.[6]

Those concerned with the patient should contribute to the objectives and specifications of the seating system and wheelchair. This would include parents, orthopedic surgeon, pediatrician, occupational therapist, physiotherapist, rehabilitation engineer, and school teacher. Patients themselves provide much valuable feedback on the seating system and wheelchair to be prescribed.

VII. SOME SEATING SYSTEMS AVAILABLE FOR DUCHENNE'S MUSCULAR DYSTROPHY PATIENTS

A. SPINAL SUPPORT SYSTEM

The spinal support system has indicated the limitations of any type of external support system, clarifying the role of early surgical intervention. It has emphasized the importance

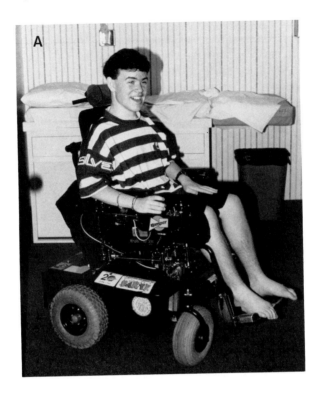

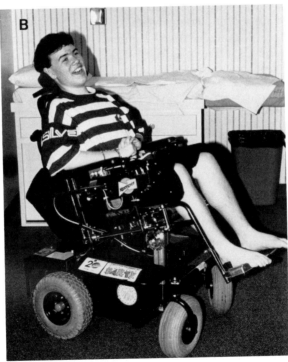

FIGURE 3.   Typical power chair with tilt-in-space capabilities (A).
Note extended lateral leg supports to control excessive hip abduction;
(B) with wheelchair tilted.

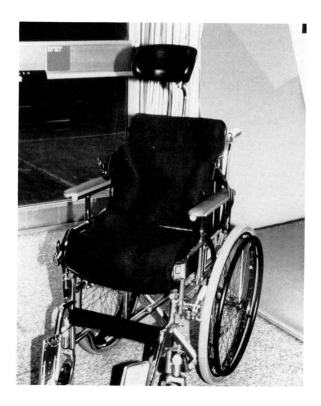

FIGURE 4. Custom seating system fabricated for an 18-year-old boy with severe scoliosis and pelvic obliquity. Spinal surgery was refused.

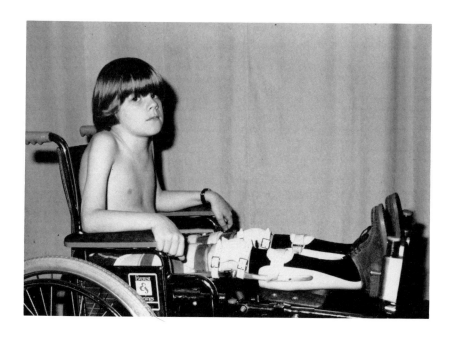

FIGURE 5. Elevated legrests are important to accommodate for KAFOs.

of powered mobility for these individuals and popularized the concept of providing both manual and powered mobility options. Although rarely used in clinical situations for DMD, the spinal support system has proven to be a very important background in the formation of other seating systems. Unique adaptations of the spinal support system are being seen in all other aspects of specialized seating.

B. SHAPEABLE MATRIX SEATING SYSTEM

The shapeable matrix seating system was developed at the Medical Engineering Resource Unit at the University of British Columbia. This device is now being clinically applied and used in European and North American countries. The shapeable matrix system consists of a two-dimensional matrix of plastic modules strung on a stainless steel wire cable. The potential advantages include the ease of adjustability to accommodate growth and realignment. Unfortunately, it is difficult to make adjustments and it is not possible to be intimately contoured when small-radius curvatures are necessary.

C. FOAM-IN-PLACE AND FOAM-IN-BOX SYSTEMS

The Foam-in-Place system was conceived at the Rehabilitation Centre for Children in Winnipeg and has undergone further development at the University of Tennessee in Memphis. It is a system based on the polymerization reaction of two-component flexible polyurethane foams. The materials are mixed and injected into a vacuum-formed plastic tray. The system is readily interchangeable between most standard manual and powered bases. Its advantage lies in the rapid fabrication of the intimately fitting components and accommodation for bony prominences. However, the limitations involve modifications, sometimes requiring replacement of the supporting module itself.

D. VACUUM CONSOLIDATION SYSTEMS

These systems are based on the vacuum consolidation principle popularized in Europe in the 1960s. The principle involves the evacuation of a flexible container filled with small, low-density particles.

Bead-seat system — The bead-seat system is a more recent development, again from the University of Tennessee, Memphis. The bead-seat shell is reusable, easy to upholster, and reinforced and includes mounting hardware for interface systems.

DESMO system — The DESMO system uses a large weather balloon as the flexible container and is now being produced and marketed in the U.S. It can provide a firm, custom-contoured support surface in 4 to 8 h. The final product is relatively lightweight. There is some concern about its durability and excessively firm surface. Shape alterations usually necessitate refabrication of the seat or back module.

E. STANDARD FOAM MODULAR SYSTEM

Prefabricated flexible foamback modules and seat systems are currently being designed and produced by a variety of manufacturers. Otto Bock Industries in Winnipeg produces preshaped modules compatible with the various sizes of standard wheelchair. It is a quick and inexpensive method for providing spinal support early in the nonambulatory phase. Multiple sizes, headrests, and lateral trunk supports make this a flexible, easily modified system.

F. FOAM AND PLYWOOD SYSTEM

Perhaps the earliest modular system involved plywood bases with foam and fabric or synthetic coverings. It is still useful in some early stages of DMD, but requires technical expertise to produce and has limited adaptability. However, these systems are relatively inexpensive and the materials may be more readily available when other products are not.

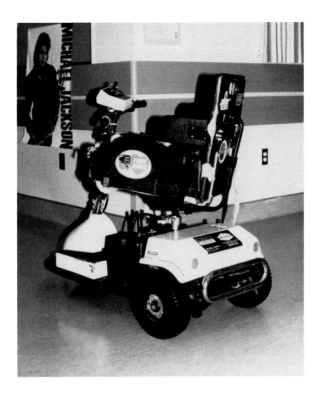

FIGURE 6. Typical three-wheeled scooter which has limited in-
dications in children with Duchenne's muscular dystrophy.

VIII. WHEELCHAIR SELECTION

Often, a manual and power wheelchair base are required. To prevent interruption of a child's active life, a power chair is usually introduced when ambulation ceases. This may mean that a manual and power chair are prescribed at the same time.

A manual chair is an important back-up system in the event the power chair is unexpectedly malfunctioning, which is a frequent occurrence. Environment is a critical factor when considering wheelchair selection. A power base with wide front and rear wheels may be a necessity when living in rugged terrain, whereas a standard power wheelchair would be adequate for roads, level ground, and indoors.

The three-wheeled scooter is probably inappropriate for some children due to the lack of seating options, spatial orientation, microcomputer control, and instability during transport. It may be useful in limited situations in the late ambulatory stage (Figure 6).

To ensure that a durable and appropriate wheelchair is selected, the following points should be considered when selecting a manual or power wheelchair:

1. Meets performance standards (no current Canadian standards)
2. Cost-effective maintenance and repair
3. Cost-effective "growability"
4. Multiadjustable axle plate to increase a fixed tilt-in-space
5. Narrower width to allow correct upper extremity position on armrests, for neutral alignment of trunk
6. Center-mounted joystick to encourage centering of trunk
7. Caregivers demonstrate understanding of daily use and maintenance
8. Caregivers able to transfer child

9. If needed, ventilator, batteries, oxygen, and suction machine can be mounted under frame without compromising stability, safety, or turning radius
10. User demonstrates ongoing, complete understanding of safety and use of device in all environments
11. Adequate durable tray on flat work surface available to interface with wheelchair to support computer or other technical aids or wheelchair can be positioned under table or desk at correct height
12. Specific prescribed technical aids or assistive devices such as a mobile arm support can be mounted on a frame or tray (Attention should be drawn to those technical aids the user may need in the future.)
13. Any technical aids needed to interface electronically with driving controls are possible
14. Transfer board or lift can be easily used with seating system and wheelchair
15. Future changes are possible for determining function: (1) in position of frame, i.e., tilt and recline, and (2) alternate access, i.e., head and tongue controls
16. Restraint system and separate tie downs, approved by Canadian Department of Transport, are used in all methods of transport, i.e., family van and taxi[5]
17. Durable for recreation as desired, such as ''motor soccer''
18. Pressure relief cushion can be used in both chairs

There are now a multitude of seating devices on the commercial market. Many have esthetic appeal, but lack scientific research in their design and marketing. We recommend the use of a system that is versatile, practical, and economical. One must be familiar with the device, including its options, match to the client, ease of use, and maintenance. There is probably no single recommended seating system designed for all DMD patients. It is our role as members of the seating clinic team to review the patient's needs and the resources available and to blend them together in providing the most appropriate seating device at that point in the patient's disease and not to be afraid to change if the product is not suitable to those needs.

Frequent reassessment and modifications are required for the seating system, including pressure relief and the manual and power mobility systems due to skeletal and size changes and progressive deterioration of development (Figure 7).

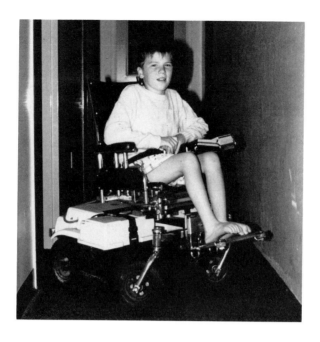

FIGURE 7.   Frequent reassessment is important. This child needs adjustment for growth as well as a more appropriate seating insert.

REFERENCES

1. **Begin, R., Bureat, M. R., Luprin, L., and Lemiene, B.,** Control of breathing in Duchenne muscular dystrophy, *Am. J. Med.,* 64, 221, 1980.
2. **Brooke, M.,** *A Clinician's View of Neuromuscular Diseases,* 2nd ed., Williams & Wilkins, Baltimore, 1986.
3. **Cambridge, W. and Drennan, J.,** Scoliosis associated with Duchenne muscular dystrophy, *J. Pediatr. Orthop.,* 7, 436, 1987.
4. **Case-Smith, J., Fisher, A., and Bauer, D.,** An analysis of the relationship between proximal and distal motor control, *Am. J. Occup. Ther.,* 43(10), 657, 1989.
5. Department of Transport, Motor Vehicle Safety Act, Motor Vehicle Safety Regulations — Amendment (Schedule 1141), *The Canada Gazette, Part 1,* 3401-14, August 20, 1988.
6. **Enders, A. and Hall, M.,** *Assistive Technology Sourcebook,* RESNA Press, Washington, D.C., 1990.
7. **Gibson, D. A., Koreska, J., Robertson, D., Kahn, A., and Albisser, A.,** The management of spinal deformity in Duchenne's muscular dystrophy, *Orthop. Clin. North Am.,* 9(2), 437, 1978.
8. **Gilsdorf, P., Patterson, R., Fisher, S., and Appel, N.,** Seating forces and wheelchair mechanics, *J. Rehabil. Res.,* 27(3), 239, 1990.
9. **Harrington, P. R. and Dickson, J. H.,** An 11-year clinical investigation of Harrington instrumentation: a preliminary report on 518 cases, *Clin. Orthop.,* 93, 133, 1973.
10. **Heckmott, J. Z.,** Prolongation of walking in Duchenne muscular dystrophy with lightweight orthoses: review of 57 cases, *Dev. Med. Child Neurol.,* 27, 149, 1985.
11. **Henderson, B.,** *Seating in Review: Current Trends for the Disabled,* Otto Bock Orthopaedic Industry of Canada Ltd., Winnipeg, Manitoba, 1989.
12. **Hobson, D., Desrosier, F., Beauchamp, R., and Martel, G.,** *The SSS and Other Approaches to Specialized Seating for Duchenne Muscular Dystrophy Patients: A Review Report,* sponsored by the Muscular Dystrophy Association of Canada, 1983.
13. **Hoppenfeld, S.,** *Physical Examination of the Spine and Extremities,* Appleton-Century-Crofts, New York, 1976.
14. **Hulme, J. B., Gallacher, K., Walsh, J., et al.,** Behavioral and postural changes observed with use of adaptive seating by clients with multiple handicaps, *Phys. Ther.,* 67(7), 1060, 1987.

15. **Ketenjian, A. Y.,** Muscular dystrophy, diagnosis and treatment, *Orthop. Clin. North Am.,* 9, 25, 1978.
16. **Lee, W. A.,** A control system framework for understanding normal and abnormal posture, *Am. J. Occup. Ther.,* 43(5), 291, 1989.
17. **Marsh, G. G. and Munsat, T. L.,** Evidence for early impairment of verbal intelligence in Duchenne muscular dystrophy, *Arch. Dis. Child,* 49, 118, 1974.
18. **Miller, F., Moseley, C. F., Koreska, J., and Levison, H.,** Pulmonary function and scoliosis in Duchenne muscular dystrophy, *J. Pediatr. Orthop.,* 8, 133, 1988.
19. **Seeger, B. R.,** Orthotic management of scoliosis in Duchenne muscular dystrophy, *Arch. Phys. Med. Rehabil.,* 65, 83, 1984.
20. **Seeger, B. R. and Sutherland, A. D.,** Lumbar extension in Duchenne muscular dystrophy: effect on lateral curvature, *Arch. Phys. Med. Rehabil.,* 66(4), 236, 1985.
21. **Staller, J.,** *Philosophy of Adaptive Seating,* PPD Approved Programs for Persons with Disabilities, New York.
22. **Sussman, M. D.,** Advantage of early spinal stabilization and fusion in patients with Duchenne muscular dystrophy, *J. Pediatr. Orthop.,* 4, 532, 1984.
23. **Sussman, M.,** Role of surgery in the treatment of children with developmental disabilities, Partners in Progress: Seating the Disabled (Syllabus), in 6th Int. Seating Symp., Vancouver, February 15 to 17, 1990, 3.
24. **Wilkins, K. E. and Gibson, D. A.,** Patterns of spinal deformity in Duchenne muscular dystrophy, *J. Bone Jt. Surg. Am. Vol.,* 58, 24, 1976.
25. **Yasuda, Y., Bowman, K., and Hsu, J. D.,** Mobile arm supports: criteria for successful use in muscle disease patients, *Arch. Phys. Med. Rehabil.,* 67(4), 253, 1986.
26. **Zacharkow, D.,** *Wheelchair Posture and Pressure Sores,* Charles C Thomas, Springfield, IL, 1984.

Chapter 12

SEATING IN MYELOMENINGOCELE

Jacques L. D'Astous, Linda Kealey, and Barry Mason

TABLE OF CONTENTS

I. INTRODUCTION

The principal goal of seating in spina bifida is to achieve a stable, "hands-free" sitting posture in order to allow optimum upper extremity function. This stable, "hands-free" sitting posture is essential even in the very young to facilitate play activities and manipulation of objects necessary for normal childhood development. It also is important to provide mobility and promote independence for these young children in order that they may explore their environment and socialize with their peers.

The actual design of the seat and mobility aid will of necessity be quite different for a preschool child than for an adolescent or an adult, but the basic requirements are identical. These requirements are as follows:

- Stable, "hands-free" sitting posture
- Patient comfort
- Ease of transfer
- Avoidance of pressure sores
- Esthetic acceptability

II. SPECIAL CONSIDERATIONS

A. LEVEL OF PARALYSIS

As a general rule, it may be said that the higher the level of paralysis, the lesser the trunk control and, the consequently, the more support required. Also, children with high thoracic level spina bifida, hydrocephalus, and delayed development may require a special head support as well as extensive trunk support.

B. INSENSITIVE SKIN

Patients with spina bifida are at a very high risk of developing decubitus ulcers as a consequence of the absent sensation in the skin overlying the buttocks and the lower extremities. This is especially true if spinal and lower limb deformities are present. The seating insert can help by providing even weight distribution with minimal shear forces, but no matter how sophisticated and well designed the seating insert, this alone is not enough to prevent the occurrence of decubitus ulcers. The child and his/her family should be educated about skin care and taught to identify and avoid pressure areas over the sacrum, greater trochanter, ischia, and the apex of the kyphos. In addition, the child should be taught to do regular sitting push-ups, relieving the weight from the ischium and sacrum for 15 sec every 30 min in order to allow adequate blood circulation. Also, getting out of the chair for 15 to 30 min at midday, again to relieve the pressure from the buttock area as well as self-inspection with a mirror, should be strongly encouraged.[9]

C. URINARY AND FECAL INCONTINENCE

Although urinary and fecal incontinence are almost always present, with a good intermittent catheterization program and a good bowel protocol, the patients can be kept dry. If incontinence is not well controlled, the moist environment and chemical irritation leads to skin maceration and a much higher incidence of skin breakdown.

D. FIXED DEFORMITIES

Spinal deformities such as scoliosis, kyphosis, or lordosis, combined with pelvic obliquity, may result in an uneven pressure distribution and localized areas of increased pressure over the ischial tuberosities, greater trochanter, or coccyx, which, in turn, may lead to decubitus ulcers. Patients with a severe kyphosis are prone to skin breakdown over the apex

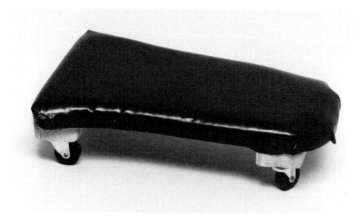

FIGURE 1. "Skate board".

of the kyphos. It also must be remembered that the lower limbs are insensitive and that excessive pressure on the outer border of a rigid equinovarus foot or pressure on the lateral calf from the post supporting the footrests may lead to serious pressure sores. The role of the orthopedic surgeon therefore is to prevent or correct deformities of the spine, hip, and feet in order to facilitate sitting and thereby make the patient as functional as possible.

III. CHANGING SEATING REQUIREMENTS AT DIFFERENT AGES

In the infant and young child, sitting, balance, and function are compromised when the level of the lesion is high lumbar or thoracic. Without functional hip extensors, and weak trunk muscles, there is no pelvic or trunk stability. For these children, the use of a "floor sitting support" or corner seat is indicated. Supported sitting is also frequently required for use in strollers, highchairs, and car seats. Accommodation for poor head and trunk control is achieved with customized seats and special headrests, lateral supports with chest straps, and cushions. Care must be taken to ensure that the head and neck support does not impinge on the ventricular peritoneal shunt. Occasionally, some of the very severely involved children may require a tracheostomy and ventilatory support, necessitating the use of a highly customized seating insert and mobility base. When a respirator is required, the wheelchair or stroller base must be of a sturdy construction and have enough space for a pan to safely support the respirator with its batteries.

As the infant becomes developmentally ready to crawl, the use of a low platform on wheels can be used to allow the child to "crawl" by pulling with the upper extremities and preventing abrasions of the knees and feet (Figure 1). Between the ages of 9 months and 2 years, the caster cart permits the child to be mobile and explore his or her environment and promotes the development of the muscles of the upper extremities as well as a sense of spacial awareness (Figure 2). It also prevents the children from scooting around on their bottoms, which may lead to skin breakdown over the coccyx. The caster cart can be supplemented with a postural seating device for those children who lack trunk and head control or have severe spinal deformities such as a kyphosis.

Other devices have also been used to provide mobility, and these include hand-propelled tricycles (Tara Cycle) and wheelchair bicycles (Figure 3). These are important for the children's self-esteem and independence as they permit them to have a tricycle like other able-bodied children of their age.

By the age of 3 or 4 years, the child is ready to start school and wheelchair skills for community mobility become essential. The child is assessed with respect to his/her seating

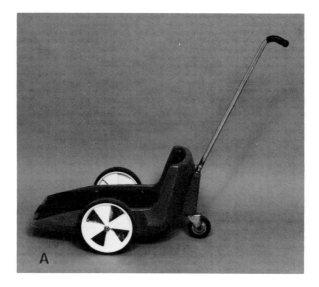

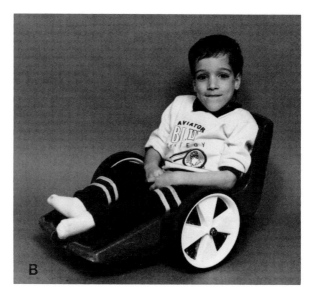

FIGURE 2.   Caster carts (A and B).

needs by a team consisting of an orthopedic surgeon, occupational therapist, physiotherapist, and seating technician. Depending on the needs, the final product may be as simple as a lightweight wheelchair with base cushion or as complex as a motorized wheelchair with an elaborate seat, back, lateral support, headrest, and sometimes even a respirator. As these children approach adolescence, they spend more and more time in the wheelchair, their body weight increases, scoliosis and pelvic obliquity may progress, and they may ignore their sitting push-ups, all of which may increase the frequency of pressure sores. In the adolescent, seat design must accommodate for deformities in the spine, hips, and legs, prevent tissue trauma, allow easy transfers, and, finally, be esthetically pleasing.

IV. BIOLOGY AND BIOMECHANICS

It is known that pressure sores develop in areas which are subjected to high tissue pressures and shear. The role of the seat cushion therefore is to decrease or equalize pressures

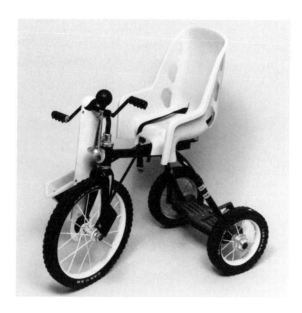

FIGURE 3.   Hand-propelled tricycle (Tara Cycle).

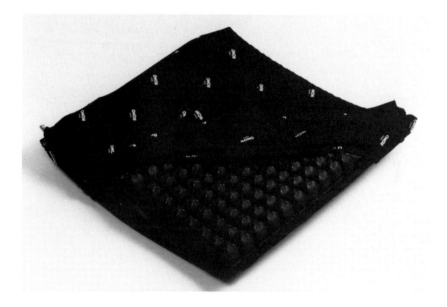

FIGURE 4.   ROHO® cushion inflated with air.

over bony protuberances and to decrease shear. In general, seating cushions can be subdivided into three types:

1. Those that equalize support pressures with fluid-based designs (air, fluid, and gel), i.e., ROHO® cushion (Figure 4)
2. Those that redistribute the pressures, i.e., Temperafoam and cutout foam cushions (Figure 5)
3. Those that combine equalization and redistribution of pressures such as custom-contoured cushions, i.e., Jay® cushion, Foam-in-Place (Figure 6)

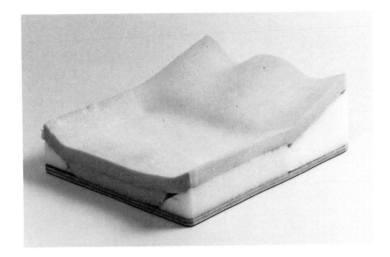

FIGURE 5.   Temperafoam cushion.

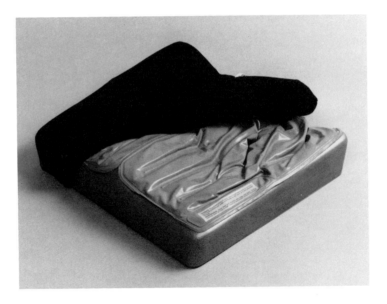

FIGURE 6.   Jay® cushion with individual gel packs.

Irrespective of the cushion used, it is important to put this cushion on a solid base to prevent the hammock effect which leads to uneven pressure distribution and pelvic obliquity (Figure 7).

Normally, in the absence of fixed pelvic obliquity, the pressure is usually evenly distributed over both ischia and posterior thighs (Figure 8). With severe pelvic obliquity, two-point sitting may be converted to a one-point sitting centered over the greater trochanter. With moderate pelvic obliquity, two-point sitting may be restored, with the pressure divided between the ischium and the greater trochanter on the same side (Figure 9). If the pelvic obliquity is incompletely corrected, this may result again in a one-point sitting, in which almost the entire weight is borne through one ischium (Figure 10).

Similarly, loss of normal lumbar lordosis will result in a straight lumbar spine with a vertical sacrum, causing increased pressure at the tip of the sacrum and more pressure posteriorly over the ischia, with less pressure being borne through the thighs (Figure 11).[5,12]

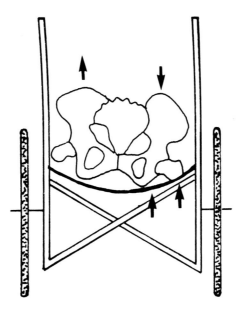

FIGURE 7.   Hammock effect of wheelchair sling seat. Note uneven pressure distribution.

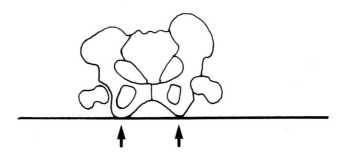

FIGURE 8.   Solid seat base. Note even pressure distribution on both ischia.

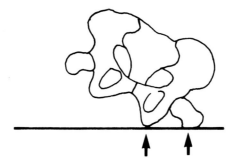

FIGURE 9.   Moderate pelvic obliquity. Note pressure divided between ischium and greater trochanter.

In this instance, one can try using an ischial bar (Figure 12) fabricated with a denser foam in order to transfer some of the weight to the thighs and, by leaving the footrest a bit longer, using the weight of the legs to exert a lever effect to decrease the pressure on the ischial tuberosities.

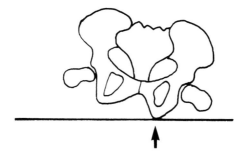

FIGURE 10.   Incompletely corrected pelvic obliquity. Note increased pressure over ischium on the low side.

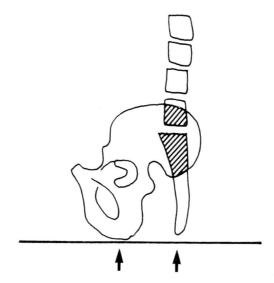

FIGURE 11.   Loss of lumbar lordosis. Note increased pressure posteriorly over ischia and coccyx.

In the presence of a kyphosis, the weight is usually borne over the sacrum and thighs, resulting in a fairly broad surface area for weight bearing. There is, however, a posterior force at the apex of the kyphos which increases the pressure and, combined with shear forces at this level, may lead to skin breakdown (Figure 13).

A. PRESSURE MEASUREMENTS

Various techniques of measuring pressures in seating devices have been used, and these are useful as an adjunct to measure pressures and identify sites at risk of developing pressure sores. The following methods have been used to measure pressure:

1.   Visual (With a patient sitting on a glass table and using an inclined mirror, one can see the areas of high pressure which correspond to the areas of blanching. Using edge lighting techniques, areas of higher pressure can be identified as brightly illuminated zones.)
2.   Dynamic pneumatic systems (air cell transducers), i.e., Oxford pressure monitor
3.   Miniature electronic transducer, i.e., pressure scanner[5]
4.   Infrared (IR) color thermography (This method can identify sites that are at risk of breaking down.)

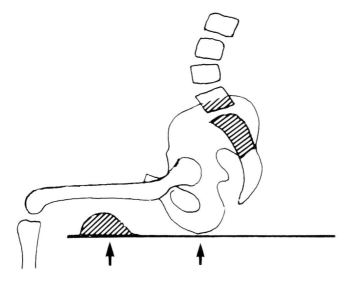

FIGURE 12.   Effect of ischial bar. Weight of legs counterbalances and decreases the weight borne on the ischia.

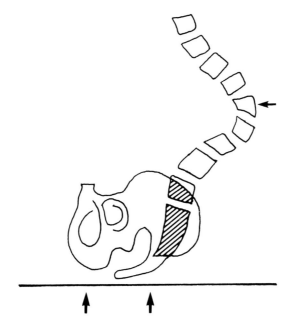

FIGURE 13.   Effect of kyphosis. Weight borne over sacrum, posterior thighs, and apex of kyphos.

5.   Pressure-sensitive paper
6.   ''Hands on'' or, more appropriately, ''hands under the buttocks'' technique

In our experience, the first five methods of measuring pressure are useful for quantitating the degrees of pressure in various areas, but in practice, putting a hand under the buttocks of the seated patient enables areas of high pressure to be easily identified by both the surgeon and the seating technician. This simple technique provides very helpful information that can be incorporated into the seat design.

V. CUSTOM SEAT DESIGN

The basic design of the seating system for spina bifida patients begins with the goal of placing a level pelvis on a stable base and then working distally down the legs and proximally up the trunk. The seat is built on a rigid base to decrease the hammock effect. By selectively using viscoelastic foams under the ischial tuberosities and coccyx and firmer foams distally under the thighs, it is possible to distribute the pressure more evenly between the thighs and the ischial tuberosities (see Figure 12). It is imperative, however, that the footrests be barely supporting the feet in a neutral position. If the footrests are too high, the thighs will be unweighed and the pressure will be transferred more posteriorly over the ischial tuberosities and the coccyx. The patients must also be warned not to cross their legs as they can significantly alter the pressure distribution, which may lead to the development of pressure sores.

With respect to the back of the insert, frequently the sling back on the wheelchair will be sufficient. If the patient has a bony prominence in the back, a firm back with a soft foam cushion can be used. For the patient with a rigid kyphosis, it may be necessary to cut out a large "keyhole" to allow the foam cushion to bulge out and take on the shape of the kyphos in order to evenly distribute the pressure. It is unwise to completely remove the foam or lining from the "keyhole" as this might produce areas of high pressure at the edges which may lead to skin breakdown (Figure 13).

In patients with a lack of truncal stability, lateral thoracic supports and a chest strap may be added to the back of the seating insert or to the wheelchair. Custom-molded spinal orthoses and thoracic suspension orthoses may also be used to improve the truncal stability.[4] Unfortunately, any attempt at increasing truncal stability by orthotic means decreases the ability for independent transfers. For patients with poor head control, a prefabricated or custom-made headrest may be added to the rigid back of the seating insert.

Ideally, the seating insert should have a seatback angle of 90° and the entire insert should be on a slight recline in the wheelchair (approximately 10°). Reclining the seating insert on the wheelchair may also help decrease the pressure on the ischial tuberosities; for every degree of recline, up to 45°, there is a weight transfer of 1.1% of the body weight from the buttocks to the back.

A. COVERING MATERIALS

Most custom-made seating systems are constructed with an open-cell foam. These foams are sensitive to ultraviolet (UV) light and moisture and will degrade very rapidly when exposed. It is necessary to ensure that moisture, in the form of perspiration or urine, does not penetrate into these foams. The use of a latex barrier (Dental Dam) or silicone-based paint will keep the foams dry, as will the use of a vinyl- or rubber-impregnated nylon. Removable, washable terry cloth covers can be used to decrease the build-up of humidity and keep the skin cooler and drier in warm weather. The use of three-way stretch fabrics has also been advocated for use as a cushion cover in order to decrease the shear at the skin/seat interface. As a final point, the patients should be warned against putting objects such as combs and coins in their back pockets and they should make sure that their clothes don't bunch up under their buttocks, in order to decrease the possibility of developing pressure sores.

VI. ROLE OF ORTHOPEDIC SURGERY IN SEATING FOR SPINA BIFIDA

The goal of the orthopedic surgeon is to maintain or restore "hands-free" sitting balance by centering the head and trunk over the pelvis. In doing so, one can hope to maximize upper extremity function, decrease the incidence of decubitus ulcers, improve self-image, and perhaps exert potential beneficial effects on respiratory, gastrointestinal (GI), and genitourinary functions.

A. SCOLIOSIS AND PELVIC OBLIQUITY

It is generally agreed that scoliosis in the myelomeningocele patient combined with pelvic obliquity should be treated by an anterior and posterior spinal fusion because of the poor bone stock posteriorly.[11,15,16] Dwyer and Zielke instrumentation may be useful in older adolescents (>12 years old) with severe fixed pelvic obliquity, providing that the vertebral bodies are large enough and that the bone is not too osteoporotic (Figure 14). Recent developments in posterior spinal instrumentation, such as segmental fixation with sublaminar wires, Drummond buttons, and pedicle screws, have decreased the need for postoperative immobilization and anterior spinal instrumentation (Figure 15).[1,3,6,11,13,15-17] In correcting spinal deformities, it is important to try to correct the pelvic obliquity as completely as possible and to maintain lumbar lordosis.

Incomplete correction of pelvic obliquity may result in changing someone who was two-point weight bearing on the ischium and greater trochanter to someone who now bears weight only on one ischium. Ideally, complete correction of the pelvic obliquity would lead to even weight distribution over both ischia. Similarly, maintenance of lumbar lordosis is important so that the weight can be taken on the back of the thighs and not on the tip of the coccyx or ischial tuberosities, as one sees with loss of lumbar lordosis when the pelvis is retroverted and the sacrum becomes vertical. Drummond et al. have implicated the use of anterior Dwyer instrumentation as one of the causes of loss of physiologic lordosis, leading to development of decubitus ulcers.[5] Osebold et al. report a surprising lack of correlation between pelvic obliquity, sitting balance, and pressure sores.[15] Gillespie and Wedge report failure of the surgery to improve sitting posture, pressure sores, and appliance fit even when good correction and solid fusion were achieved.[7] Letts reports that "caution must be exercised in fusing the spine down to the sacrum lest pelvic obliquity and loss of lumbar lordosis transform a patient who before fusion was ulcer free into one who after fusion becomes prone to development of pressure sores."[10] It is generally felt, however, that surgery does improve sitting balance, restores trunk height, and increases the volume of the abdominal cavity, with potential beneficial effects on respiratory, GI, and genitourinary functions.[2,12]

For the child with residual pelvic obliquity causing pressure sores after spinal surgery, Lindseth has described a technique of double pelvic osteotomy in order to correct the pelvic obliquity.[11] Some pressure sores will also respond quite well to subtotal ischiectomy and primary excision of the ulcer. Similarly, pressure sores at the tip of the coccyx, secondary to loss of lumbar lordosis and a vertical sacrum, can be eliminated by excision of the coccyx and the distal sacrum.

B. KYPHOSIS

The treatment of kyphosis remains more controversial. Historically, kyphectomy has been associated with a very high complication rate, including pseudoarthrosis, recurrence of deformity, and even death. With the advent of improved spinal instrumentation, such as segmental fixation with wires and pedicle screws, it has become technically possible to stabilize the spine after a kyphectomy without the need for prolonged plaster immobilization and bed rest (Figure 16).[8,14] The benefits of kyphectomy include correction of deformity, decreased incidence of pressure sores at the apex of the kyphos, restoration of trunk height, and increased volume of the abdominal cavity.

Patients with severe kyphosis are prone to ulceration at the apex of the kyphos. However, Drummond has shown in his series that none of the four patients with thoracic-level paralysis and thoracolumbar kyphosis had an excessive pressure distribution posteriorly over the ischia

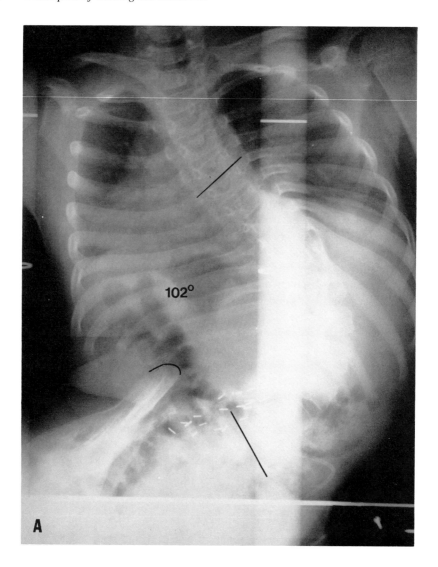

FIGURE 14.   A 9 + 5 girl with thoracic level spina bifida. (A) Preoperative; note severe
pelvic obliquity.

and coccyx and that all were ulcer free. It is possible that after correcting the kyphosis,
more pressure may be distributed posteriorly, with the appearance of skin breakdown at the
tip of the coccyx and over the ischium.[5]

For the patient with a flexible kyphos, anterior strut grafting and fusion may be all that
is required to correct and stabilize the spine.[16] In the young child, however, despite a solid
fusion, the fused segment can bend, leading to a progressive recurrence of the kyphosis.

In patients with a very rigid kyphosis, excision of the kyphos starting just distal to the
apex of the kyphos and extending proximally into the lordotic thoracic spine is advocated.[8,14,16] This is combined with excision of the spinal cord, localized anterior and posterior
spinal fusion, and rigid internal fixation.

VII. SUMMARY

Seating a child with a fixed pelvic obliquity or rigid kyphosis can challenge the skills
and imagination of the best seating clinic team, despite the fact that the requirements for

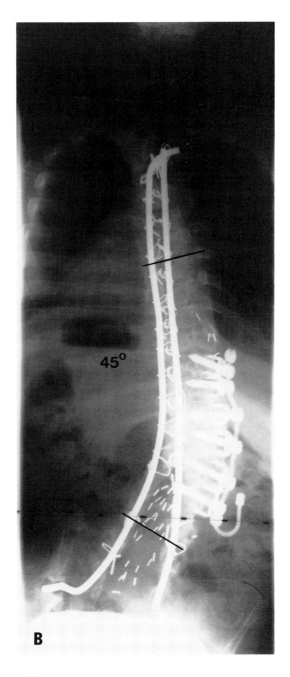

FIGURE 14 (continued).   (B) Postoperative; note residual
pelvic obliquity.

the seating inserts are quite straightforward. A better understanding of seating biomechanics
and the pathophysiology of pressure ulceration, combined with the advent of new materials
and technology, has facilitated this sometimes difficult task. Nevertheless, the orthopedic
surgeon continues to play a very active and important role in the treatment of severe, fixed
spinal and pelvic deformities. Perhaps a more aggressive surgical approach prior to the
adolescent growth spurt will make it possible to more completely correct the rigid kyphosis
or pelvic obliquity and therefore optimize the pressure distribution, leading to greatly improved sitting stability and a decreased incidence of pressure ulcerations.

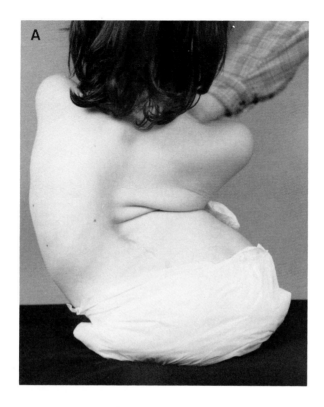

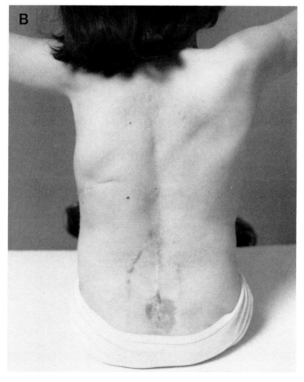

FIGURE 15. A 8 + 9 girl with L2 level spina bifida. (A) Preoperative
photograph; (B) postoperative photograph. Note improvement in truncal
balance and pelvic obliquity.

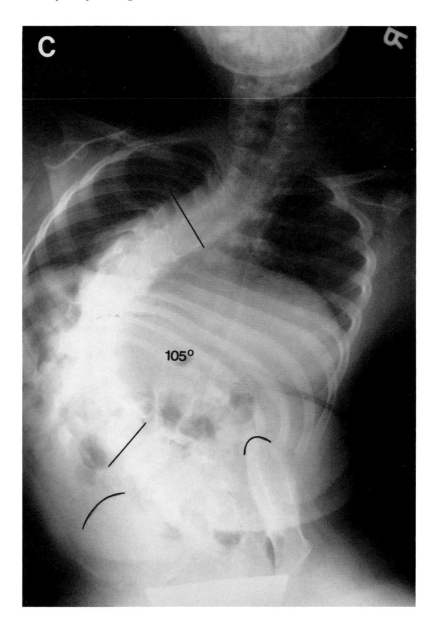

FIGURE 15 (continued).   (C) Preoperative X-ray.

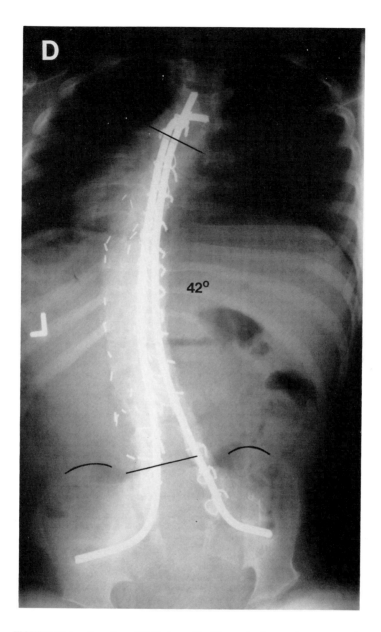

FIGURE 15 (continued). (D) Postoperative X-ray. Again note improvement in pelvic obliquity and sitting stability.

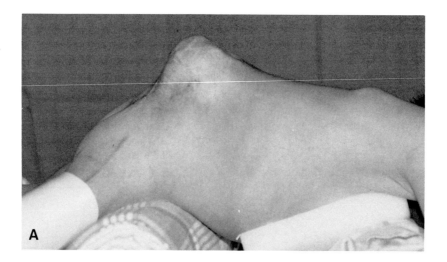

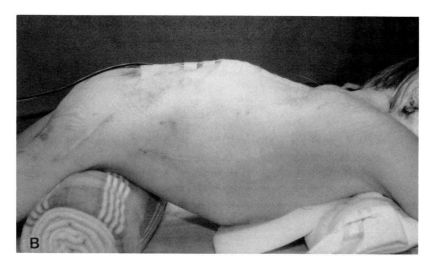

FIGURE 16.   A 4 + 6 boy with spina bifida and severe thoracolumbar kyphosis. (A) Preoperative photograph; (B) postoperative photograph.

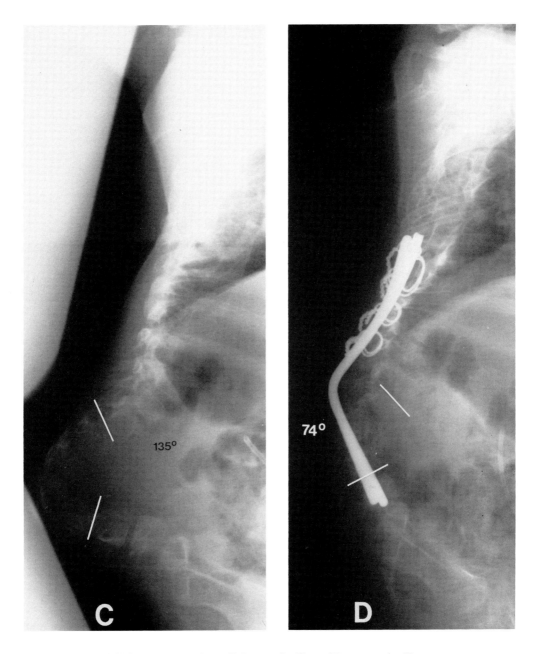

FIGURE 16 (continued).   (C) Preoperative X-ray; (D) postoperative X-ray.

REFERENCES

1. **Allen, B. L., Jr. and Ferguson, R. L.**, The operative treatment of myelomeningocoele spinal deformity — 1979, *Orthop. Clin. North Am.*, 10, 845, 1979.
2. **Banta, J. V. and Park, S. M.**, Improvement in pulmonary function in patients having combined anterior and posterior spine fusion for myelomeningocoele scoliosis, *Spine*, 8, 765, 1983.
3. **Broom, M. J., Banta, J. V., and Renshaw, T. S.**, Spinal fusion augmented by Luque-rod segmental instrumentation for neuromuscular scoliosis, *J. Bone Jt. Surg. Am. Vol.*, 71, 32, 1989.
4. **Drennan, J. C.**, Myelomeningocele, in *Orthopaedic Management of Neuromuscular Disorders*, 3rd ed., Lippincott, Philadelphia, 1983, chap. 9.
5. **Drummond, D., Breed, D., and Narechania, R.**, Relationship of spine deformity and pelvic obliquity on sitting pressure distributions and decubitus ulceration, *J. Pediatr. Orthop.*, 5, 396, 1985.
6. **Ferguson, R. L. and Allen, B. L., Jr.**, Staged correction of neuromuscular scoliosis, *J. Pediatr. Orthop.*, 3, 555, 1983.
7. **Gillespie, R. and Wedge, J. H.**, The problems of scoliosis in paraplegic children, *J. Bone Jt. Surg. Am. Vol.*, 56, 1767, 1974.
8. **Heydemann, J.-S. and Gillespie, M. B.**, Management of myelomeningocele kyphosis in the older child by kyphectomy and segmental spinal instrumentation, *Spine*, 12, 37, 1987.
9. **Kosiak, M.**, Etiology and pathology of ischemic ulcers, *Arch. Phys. Med. Rehabil.*, 40, 62, 1959.
10. **Letts, M., Rang, M., and Tredwell, S.**, Seating the disabled, in *American Academy of Orthopaedic Surgeons: Atlas of Orthotics*, 2nd ed., C. V. Mosby, St. Louis, 1985, chap. 24.
11. **Lindseth, R. E.**, Myelomeningocoele, in *Lovell and Winter's Pediatric Orthopaedics*, 3rd ed., Morrissy, R. T., Ed., Lippincott, Philadelphia, 1990, chap. 14.
12. **Mazur, J., Menelaus, M. B., Dickens, D. R. V., and Doig, W. G.**, Efficacy of surgical management for scoliosis in myelomeningocoele: correction of deformity and alteration of functional status, *J. Pediatr. Orthop.*, 6, 568, 1986.
13. **McMaster, M. J.**, Anterior and posterior instrumentation and fusion of thoracolumbar scoliosis due to myelomeningocoele, *J. Bone Jt. Surg. Br. Vol.*, 69, 20, 1987.
14. **McMaster, M. J.**, The long-term results of kyphectomy and spinal stabilization in children with myelomeningocoele, *Spine*, 13, 417, 1988.
15. **Osebold, W. R., Mayfield, J. K., Winter, R. B., and Moe, J. H.**, Surgical treatment of paralytic scoliosis associated with myelomeningocoele, *J. Bone Jt. Surg. Am. Vol.*, 64, 841, 1982.
16. **Winter, R. B.**, Myelomeningocoele, in *Moe's Textbook of Scoliosis and Other Spinal Deformities*, 2nd ed., Bradford, D. S., Lonstein, J. E., Moe, J. H., Ogilvie, J. W., and Winter, R. B., Eds., W. B. Saunders, Philadelphia, 1987, chap. 14.
17. **Ward, W. T., Wenger, D. R., and Roach, J. W.**, Surgical correction of myelomeningocele scoliosis: a critical appraisal of various spinal instrumentation systems, *J. Pediatr. Orthop.*, 9, 262, 1989.

Chapter 13

SEATING IN OSTEOGENESIS IMPERFECTA

R. Mervyn Letts

TABLE OF CONTENTS

I. SEATING FOR OSTEOGENESIS IMPERFECTA

Osteogenesis imperfecta (OI) is an heritable disorder of connective tissue with a very high mutation rate. Individuals with this disorder present many additional problems to the seating team due to the extreme fragility of the bones. In the more severe cases of OI, handling and transfers as well as stable seating can be very difficult.[12,16]

It is the more severe type of OI that results in frequent fracturing secondary to severe osteoporosis and results in extreme apprehension, not only for the patients suffering from the disorder, but for all of the caregivers.[15] The Silence classification of OI (Table 1) has categorized several pedigrees with consistent clinical features.[13] In the more severe forms of OI, fracturing occurs much more frequently at a very young age. The major goals in seating management include prevention of such fractures and the maintenance of the extremities in an anatomical, functional position. This facilitates rehabilitation, especially in the teenage years when the fracturing becomes less frequent and both sitting stability and ease of transferring improves.

II. SEATING THE INFANT WITH OSTEOGENESIS IMPERFECTA

In the more severe forms of OI, sometimes termed "osteogenesis imperfecta congenita", fractures may occur *in utero* or shortly after birth. The bones are so fragile that even rolling over or changing diapers may result in a fracture of a major long bone. In early infancy, the main seating requirements are (1) well-padded infant seats, (2) transferring devices to minimize handling, and (3) avoidance of external pressure or sudden motion. This can usually be accomplished with foam inserts and padded infant carriers. Because children with OI often have very hypotonic ligaments and muscles, since all connective tissue is basically involved in the abnormality, the normal motor milestones of development are often delayed. Thus, the child usually does not sit at 5 to 6 months of age and will require supportive seating for a much longer period of time than normal infants (Figure 1).

The Cozy Seat has been found to be a particularly adaptable type of seating device for OI children since it can be reclined and padded and the addition of a head support and bolsters provides additional support for the infant with brittle bones (Figure 2). Parents soon learn to handle the infant utilizing this type of seating device, and the infant gains confidence and a sense of protection. Feeding is facilitated with the Cozy Seat and is much safer for the OI infant (Figure 3). Head support for these children is particularly important due to the fact that (1) the head, relative to body size, is quite large in children with OI and (2) the cervical musculature is hypotonic and often cannot support the head for long periods of time, requiring assistive head support in sitting. Bathing the OI infant and child can be a harrowing experience for parents and caregivers. The portable bath seat (Figure 4) allows safe and easy transport and bathing of a child prone to fracturing. Toileting these children can also be very challenging. Good support to allay anxiety is essential (Figure 5), and during childhood, supportive attachments to the toilet are helpful (Figure 6).

Children with severe OI often grow at a very slow rate, and most will be quite small in stature compared to their peer groups. The Cozy Seat or some of the commercial infant seats can thus be used until even 3 to 4 years of age.

III. SEATING THE OLDER CHILD WITH OSTEOGENESIS IMPERFECTA

As the child with OI matures in age, the need to interact with their environment and participate in schooling increases. In the very severe OI patient, powered chairs with hydraulic modifications to the seat to facilitate change of position with minimal outside intervention

TABLE 1
Osteogenesis Imperfecta Classification

Type	Inheritance	Clinical features
I	Autosomal dominant	Bone fragility, blue sclerae, onset of fractures after birth (most preschool age); type A, without dentinogenesis imperfecta; type B, with dentinogenesis imperfecta
II	Autosomal recessive	Lethal in perinatal period, dark blue sclerae, concertina femurs, beaded ribs
III	Autosomal recessive	Fractures at birth, progressive deformity, normal sclerae and hearing
IV	Autosomal dominant	Bone fragility, normal sclerae, normal hearing; type A, without dentinogenesis imperfecta; type B, with dentinogenesis imperfecta

After Silence, D., *J. Bone Jt. Surg. Am. Vol.,* 41, 137, 1959.

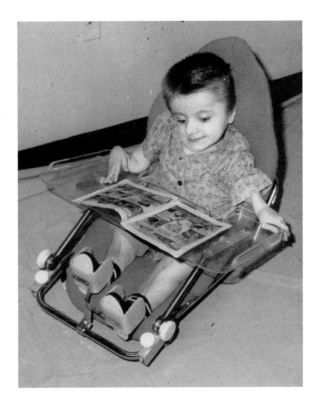

FIGURE 1.   Well-padded supportive seating to allow easy transfer from one place to another facilitates care in OI.

may be required (Figure 7). Care must be taken to avoid constant pressure from bolsters, which can actually deform rib cages.[4] Spinal curvature that may occur in older children with OI is extremely difficult to treat by orthotic means or by any form of wheelchair bolstering. In most instances, it is best managed by fusion *in situ* of the spine, and this will facilitate future stable and upright sitting as well as prevent further progression of the scoliosis.[2,7]

In attempts to improve the ossification of the lower extremities to facilitate future weight bearing, the stand-up wheelchair (Figure 8) and the vacuum pant orthosis (Figure 9) may allow Wolf's law to be harnessed to improve bone mass, i.e., bone is deposited in areas of

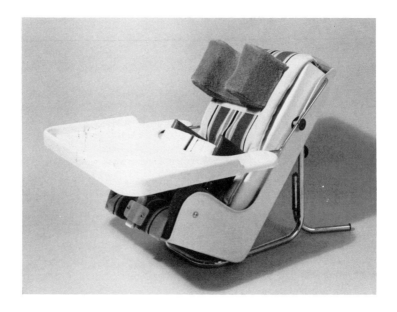

FIGURE 2.   Well padded Cozy Seat with head support for OI infant.

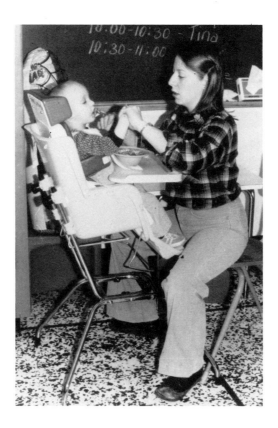

FIGURE 3.   The OI infant is easily moved from one location to another in the Cozy Seat or removable wheelchair
insert, facilitating feeding. (Reproduced with permission
from Letts, M., Rang, M., and Tredwell, S., Seating the
disabled, in *American Academy of Orthopaedic Surgeons:
Atlas of Orthotics,* 2nd ed., C. V. Mosby, St. Louis, 1985.)

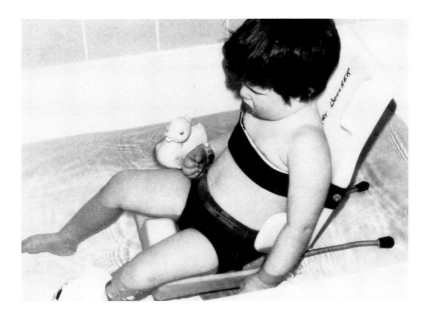

FIGURE 4. The portable bath seat facilitates bathing for the OI infant. (Reproduced with permission from Letts, M., Rang, M., and Tredwell, S., Seating the disabled, in *American Academy of Orthopadedic Surgeons: Atlas of Orthotics,* 2nd ed., C. V. Mosby, St. Louis, 1985.)

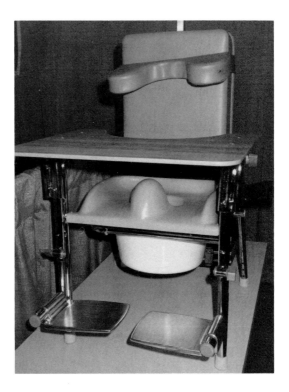

FIGURE 5. Infant toileting device with head support and tray to facilitate trunk support for the OI child.

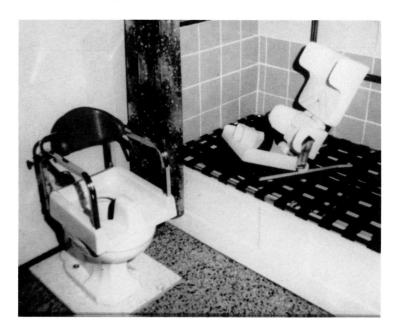

FIGURE 6.   Child toileting attachment which provides good support for the older OI child. Note the bath frame to facilitate shower bathing and the portable bath seat for the smaller OI child.

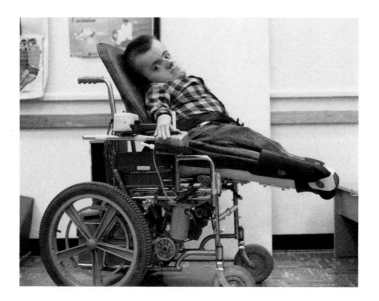

FIGURE 7.   An OI child extremely prone to fracturing using a specially designed electric wheelchair with a custom hydraulic, well-padded polypropylene seat. (Reproduced with permission from Letts, M., Rang, M., and Tredwell, S., Seating the disabled, in *American Academy of Orthopaedic Surgeons: Atlas of Orthotics,* 2nd ed., C. V. Mosby, St. Louis, 1985.)

stress and removed in areas of reduced stress.[5] This has been shown to be possible using the vacuum pant splint which also provides a sense of security for children with severe OI and facilitates standing (Figure 10).[8,9] Modular seating systems which allow the wheelchair insert to be easily transferred with the patient are an advantage for patients with OI. In some instances, specially designed, molded transfer seating devices may be of benefit to reduce

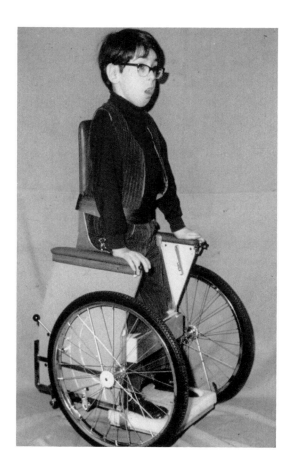

FIGURE 8. The stand-up wheelchair allows controlled weight bearing which stimulates ossification for the OI child. (Reproduced with permission from Letts, M., Rang, M., and Tredwell, S., Seating the disabled, in *American Academy of Orthopaedic Surgeons: Atlas of Orthotics,* 2nd ed., C. V. Mosby, St. Louis, 1985.)

fracturing and allay anxiety (Figure 11A and B). The correction of bowing in the extremity long bones by the Sofield technique using intramedullary rods will greatly facilitate seating (Figure 11C and D) in these fragile children.[14] The rodding not only maintains extremity length, but will also protect against further fractures.[11] The child will sit in a more functional position and transfers will be safer and easier.

Because the OI child is somewhat disproportionate in trunk height and extremity length, special modification of the insert may be necessary to accommodate the short size. Care must also be taken to protect the child in the chair from any external trauma that might be encountered if the chair bumps a wall or doorway. Lightweight pediatric chairs are particularly useful for the OI group, even in the teens and adult years.

IV. WHEELCHAIR MOBILITY IN OSTEOGENESIS IMPERFECTA

Most children with OI will not be able to manually wheel a chair for long periods of time. The danger of upper extremity fractures sustained in trying to maneuver the chair is often not worth the risk. The strength of the upper extremities in such children is just not

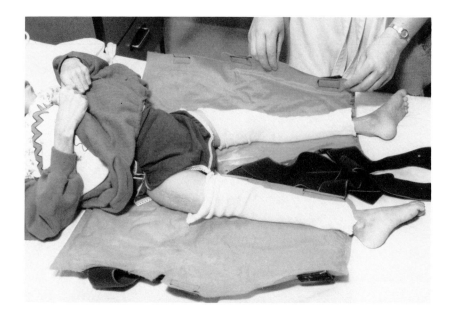

FIGURE 9.   Vacuum pants filled with styrofoam beads are easily applied to the OI child. When the air is evacuated, the beads coalesce to form a rigid splint. (From Letts, M., Monson, R., and Weber, K., *J. Pediatr. Orthop.*, 8, 454, 1988. With permission.)

sufficient to properly use a hand-driven chair. A powered wheelchair is really the most practical and functional type of mobility for the OI child[1] (Figures 12 and 13). Some of the milder cases of OI who are nonambulatory will be able to use a manual chair in the older age group, but even in those individuals, it is probably best to have both a powered device and a manual chair with an interchangeable wheelchair insert system. Depending on the size and strength of the individual with OI, positioning of the joystick may be better in a centralized position, similar to muscular dystrophy seating (see Figure 13). This allows the sitter to lean forward on the joystick support system and provides a more practical and efficient method of using the steering control system with either hand. To minimize pelvic and spinal compression fractures, a well-padded foam seat to minimize shocks and bumps should be used for seating in OI.[10]

As patients with OI reach their mid-teens, the number and severity of fractures decreases. This allows much greater freedom of motion and an increased confidence. Some OI patients will actually become ambulatory during this stage, provided care has been taken to keep their lower extremities and joints functional so that weight bearing is possible with lightweight orthosis.[3,6]

V. SEATING THE ADULT WITH OSTEOGENESIS IMPERFECTA

The seating requirements of the adult with OI decrease with skeletal maturity. The lightweight sports wheelchair with a short back is often ideal for the small-statured OI sitter (Figure 14). Powered chairs with alternate powered mobility devices, such as the Pony™ or Amigo™ (Figure 15), will often allow the OI person to pursue further education and training as well as function more efficiently in the work place.

In adult OI, much more interest in transferring to cars, vans, and the workplace environment is possible because of the decreased chances of injury. In this instance, the wheelchair must be lightweight and easily transportable and one from which transfers can be made with ease. Electric wheelchairs often are still the most practical and blend well with the use

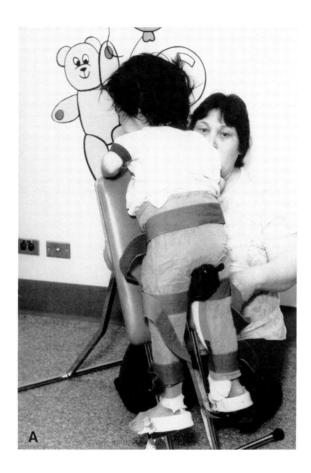

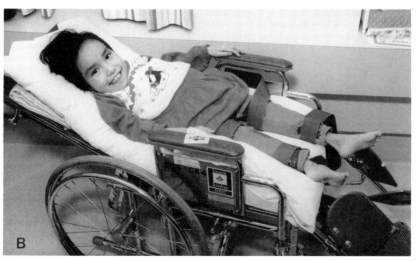

FIGURE 10. Vacuum splint (A) allows the OI child to stand, here facilitated by a prone board. (Reproduced with permission from Letts, M., Rang, M., and Tredwell, S., Seating the disabled, in *American Academy of Orthopaedic Surgeons: Atlas of Orthotics,* 2nd ed., C. V. Mosby, St. Louis, 1985.) (B) Use of the splint in the wheelchair facilitates handling. (From Letts, M., Monson, R., and Weber, K., *J. Pediatr. Orthop.,* 8, 454, 1988. With permission.)

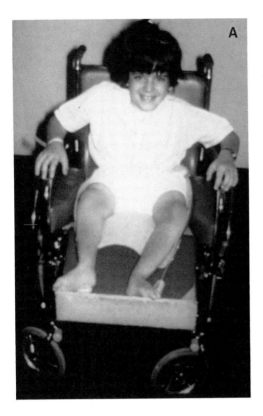
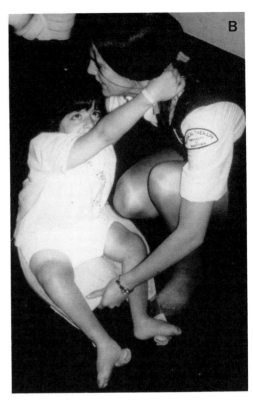

FIGURE 11. This child was sustaining numerous extremity fractures during transfers (A). A molded transfer seat was fabricated in which the child could sit in the wheelchair; (B) transfers into and out of the wheelchair with the transfer seat greatly decreased the fracturing.

of modified vans. In this way, these individuals can become gainfully employed in spite of their disability.

VI. SUMMARY

Adequate seating for the OI clientele can greatly alleviate much suffering and assist in rehabilitation as well as prevention of injury and deformity. These special modifications of the chair, as previously discussed, will provide caregivers with a much easier method of caring for these patients, and the OI children especially will gain confidence and security with such seating and be able to devote more time and effort to participating in peer group activities as well as school activities.

C

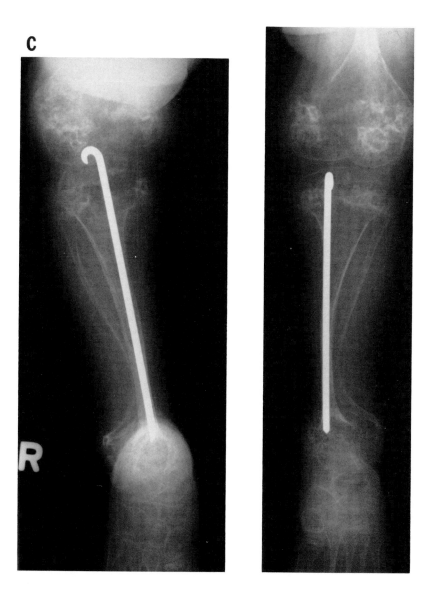

FIGURE 11 (continued).   (C) Intramedullary rodding of the long bones (tibia) in OI patients maintains alignment and facilitates stable sitting.

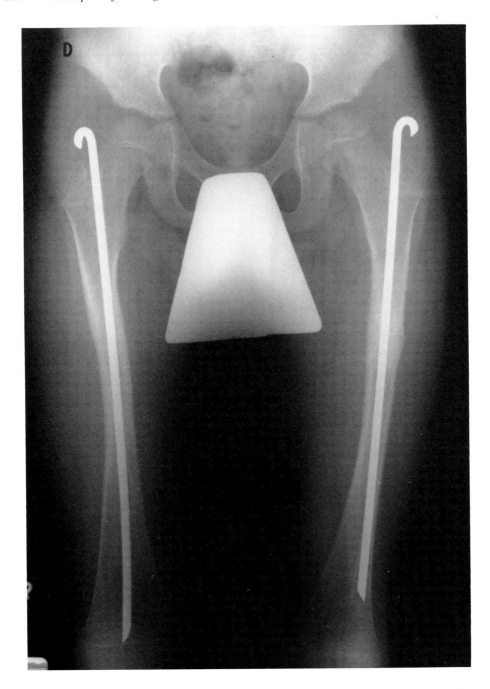

FIGURE 11 (continued).   (D) Intramedullary rodding of the long bones (femur) in OI patients maintains alignment and facilitates stable sitting.

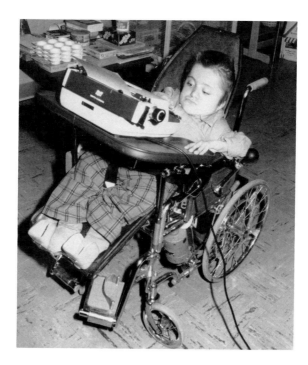

FIGURE 12. The powered wheelchair is most practical in the school environment, allowing more independence and participation.

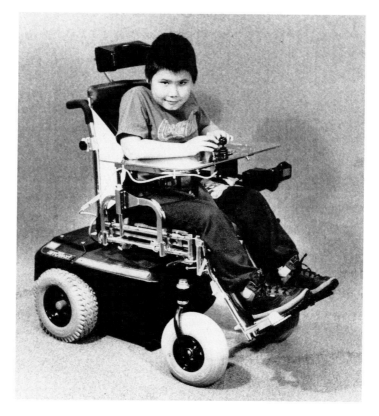

FIGURE 13. Electric wheelchair with centralized joystick and tray. Heavy-duty construction with balloon tires was designed for a northern environment with few sidewalks.

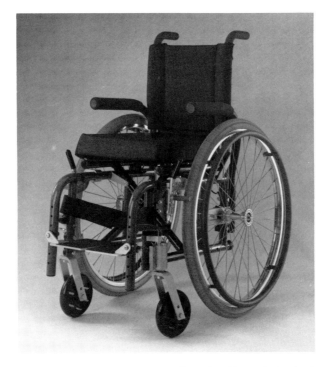

FIGURE 14.   A light-weight, adjustable, well-padded pediatric wheel-chair (Quicki Designs, Inc.), ideal for small OI users.

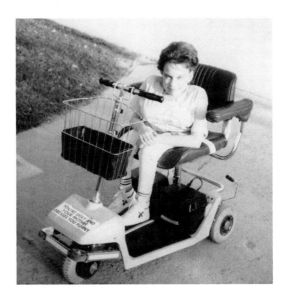

FIGURE 15.   The Pony™ powered mobility device provides excellent transport for the older OI person.

REFERENCES

1. **Breed, A. I.,** The motorized wheelchair, new freedom, new responsibility and new problems, *Dev. Med. Child Neurol.,* 24, 366, 1982.
2. **Cristofaro, R. L., Hock, K. J., Bonnett, C. A., and Brown, J. C.,** Operative treatment of spine deformity in osteogenesis imperfecta, *Clin. Orthop. Rel. Res.,* 139, 40, 1979.
3. **Cole, W. G.,** The orthopedic and medical treatment of osteogenesis imperfecta, *Ann. N.Y. Acad. Sci.,* 543, 157, 1988.
4. **Caro, P. A.,** Plastic bowing of the ribs in children, *Skel. Radiol.,* 17, 255, 1988.
5. **Frasca, P. and Alman, B.,** Fracture failure mechanisms in patients with osteogenesis imperfecta, *J. Orthop. Res.,* 5, 139, 1987.
6. **Gertner, J. M. and Root, L.,** Osteogenesis imperfecta, *Orthop. Clin. North Am.,* 21, 151, 1990.
7. **Hanscom, D. A.,** The spine in osteogenesis imperfecta, *Orthop. Clin. North Am.,* 19, 449, 1988.
8. **Letts, M., Monson, R., and Weber, K.,** The prevention of recurrent fractures of the lower extremities in severe osteogenesis imperfecta using vacuum pants, *J. Pediatr. Orthop.,* 8, 605, 1988.
9. **Morel, G. and Houghton, G. R.,** Pneumatic trouser splints in the treatment of severe osteogenesis imperfecta, *Acta Orthop. Scand.,* 53, 547, 1982.
10. **Moore, S., Bergman, J. S., and Edwards, G.,** Custom molded seating for the severely disabled persons, *Phys. Ther.,* 62, 460, 1982.
11. **Ryoppy, A., Alberty, A., and Kaitla, I. E.,** Semiclosed intramedullary stabilization in osteogenesis imperfecta, *J. Pediatr. Orthop.,* 7, 139, 1987.
12. **Sharpiro, F.,** Consequences of an osteogenesis imperfecta diagnosis for survival and ambulation, *J. Pediatr. Orthop.,* 5, 456, 1985.
13. **Silence, D.,** Osteogenesis imperfecta: an expanding panorama of variants, *Clin. Orthop.,* 159, 11, 1981.
14. **Sofield, H. A. and Miller, E. A.,** Fragmentation, realignment and intramedullary rod fixation of deformities of long bones in children, *J. Bone Jt. Surg. Am. Vol.,* 41, 137, 1959.
15. **Shea-Landry, G. L. and Cole, D. E.,** Psychosocial aspects of osteogenesis imperfecta, *Can. Med. Assoc. J.,* 133, 977, 1986.
16. **Stoltz, M. R., Dietrich, S. L., and Marshal, G. J.,** Osteogenesis imperfecta: perspectives, *Clin. Orthop.,* 242, 1120, 1989.

Chapter 14

SEATING OF THE ARTHROGRYPOSIS MULTIPLEX CONGENITA GROUP

R. Mervyn Letts

TABLE OF CONTENTS

I. SEATING CHALLENGES IN ARTHROGRYPOSIS

Arthrogrypotic individuals often have many fixed contractures of joints, presenting specific problems to the seating team.[1,5,7] Not only do they present contractures and deformities of the hip and lower extremities, but the upper extremities are frequently involved as well, resulting in difficulty in accomplishing the activities of daily living in the wheelchair that are usually taken for granted in most seating situations.[2,13] There is a wide variety of severity in these disorders, which include numerous syndromes whose main features are associated with congenital contractures secondary to muscle fibrosis. Spinal curvature may add to the seating difficulties and occurs in about one third of patients.[6,9] Frequently, the curves are not severe, but when progression occurs beyond 40°, surgical stabilization of the spine is preferable to maintain good sitting stability.[10]

The more severe forms of arthrogryposis will necessitate a wheelchair existence since ambulation is often severely compromised (Figure 1). In some instances, joint contracture release at the knees to facilitate seating and at the hips to correct extension contractures may be required to improve sitting stability.[11,12] In older children, osteotomies of the humerus, to facilitate a hand-to-mouth function, or of the tibia, to permit shoe wear in fixed equinus, may also be indicated.

II. FOOT SUPPORT IN ARTHROGRYPOSIS

Although the child with arthrogryposis may be a permanent wheelchair user, it is important not to neglect severe foot deformities. Although these types of foot deformities are often severe, many will respond to club-foot release and/or talectomy to allow a more plantigrade foot, which will facilitate shoe fitting.[4,13] This also makes it easier for persons with this affliction to keep the feet secure on the wheelchair foot supports and contributes to more efficient and stable sitting. This should be accomplished in early childhood, and the benefits will be reaped into adulthood.

III. UPPER EXTREMITY FUNCTION IN THE WHEELCHAIR

Unfortunately, many persons with arthrogryposis have fixed elbow extension, which necessitates orthopedic and orthotic intervention to improve wheelchair utilization. In some instances, the elbow may respond to a triceps transfer to the radius or biceps tendon to provide some flexion when the elbow joint is mobile. This will facilitate use of an electric wheelchair and allow improved feeding. Since many of these individuals will not have good muscle function, assistive devices may be necessary for play communication and activities of daily living. The placing of the control box for electric wheelchairs will depend on the deformities that exist in the upper extremity. In some instances, a centralized box will be found to be the most appropriate if elbow flexion is present, but in fixed extension contractures of the elbow, a lowered side control stick is more functional (Figure 2). In other instances, the seating team will be called upon for unique solutions (Figure 3).

IV. HYPERLORDOSIS

Patients with severe arthrogryposis may have a fixed hyperlordosis of their lumbar spine, necessitating a lumbar insert to provide comfort and support for prolonged sitting (Figure 4). A Foam-in-Place type of seating for the severely deformed may be more appropriate and provide a total contact support for the back (Figure 5). For severe deformity, including scoliosis, it is recommended that consideration be given to correcting the deformities surgically to facilitate seating, since seating around the deformity will be a lifelong difficulty.[8]

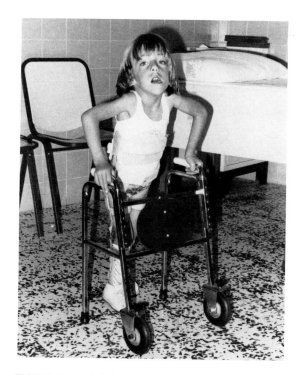

FIGURE 1. Ambulation in a child with severe lower extremity arthrogryposis using a reciprocating orthosis. A wheelchair was required 90% of the time.

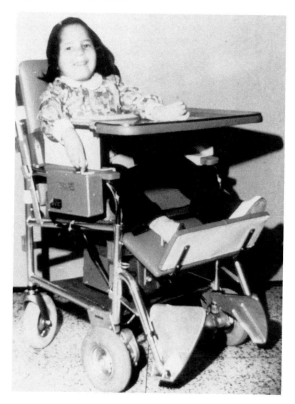

FIGURE 2. Control box lower than seating height to facilitate use by an arthrogrypotic girl with fixed elbow extension, but excellent hand function.

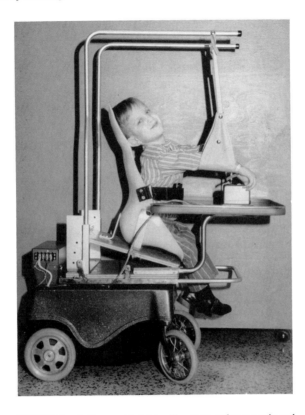

FIGURE 3.   A 5-year-old child with severe arthrogryposis and fixed elbow extension contractures. With the assistance of the shoulder girdle, muscles in the hands could be positioned over the centralized control box with the aid of arm slings.

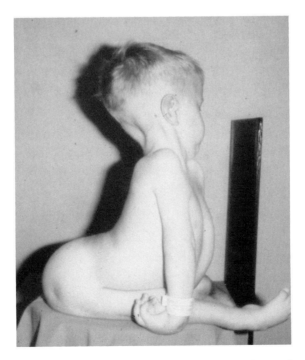

FIGURE 4.   Fixed lordosis in child with arthrogryposis as well as wrist flexion contractures and elbow extension contractures.

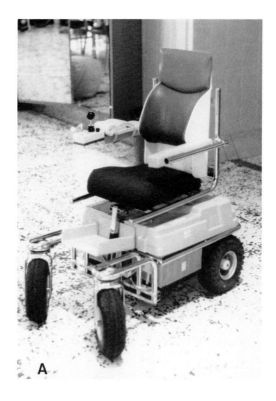

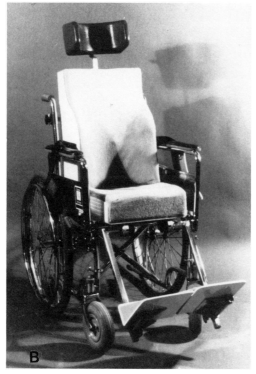

FIGURE 5. Examples of lordotic support built into the wheelchair to accommodate for hyperlordosis. (A) Modular insert; (B) Foam-in-Place wheelchair insert.

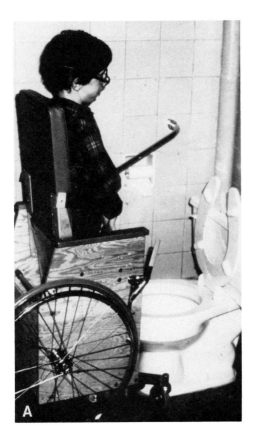
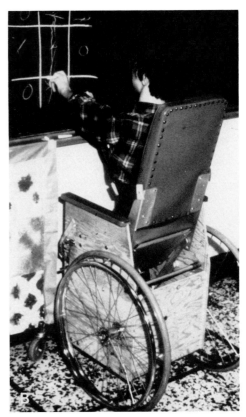

FIGURE 6. (A and B) The stand-up wheelchair may facilitate some functions as in this 11-year-old boy with arthrogryposis affecting primarily his lower extremities. (Reproduced with permission from Letts, M., Rang, M., and Tredwell, S., The orthotics of myelomeningocele, in *American Academy of Orthopaedic Surgeons: Atlas of Orthotics,* 2nd ed., C. V. Mosby, St. Louis, 1985.)

V. PHYSIOTHERAPY IN ARTHROGRYPOTIC SEATING

The arthrogrypotic patient may have severe contractures, but maintenance of the range of motion that remains is important. These wheelchair users should receive regular physiotherapy directed at improving and maintaining their sitting stability by ensuring adequate flexion of ankles, knees, and hips to allow good seating. This should, of course, also always follow any surgical procedure in the seated arthrogrypotic patient. Occasionally, it may be appropriate to use a stand-up wheelchair to allow the arthrogrypotic patient to exercise the lower extremities as well as to participate in a number of standing activities (Figure 6).

VI. SUMMARY

Arthrogryposis will pose unique and difficult problems for the seating team and may require some ingenuity to improve the function of the seated individual with permanent contractures. However, judicious use of orthopedic surgery combined with wheelchair innovations and an interested occupational therapist can make most of these wheelchair users useful members of society, quite capable of attending school and, ultimately, being gainfully employed in the work force.

REFERENCES

1. **Brown, L. M., Robson, M. J., and Sharrard, W. J.,** The pathophysiology of arthrogryposis multiplex congenital neurologica, *J. Bone Jt. Surg. Br. Vol.,* 62, 291, 1980.
2. **Carroll, R. E. and Hill, N. A.,** Triceps transfer to restore elbow flexion, *J. Bone Jt. Surg. Am. Vol.,* 52, 239, 1970.
3. **Dias, L. S. and Stern, L. S.,** Talectomy in the treatment of resistant talipes equinovarus deformity in myelomeningocele and arthrogryposis, *J. Pediatr. Orthop.,* 7, 39, 1987.
4. **Doyle, J. R., James, P. M., Larsen, L. J., and Ashley, R. K.,** Restoration of elbow flexion in arthrogryposis multiplex congenita, *J. Hand Surg.,* 5A, 149, 1980.
5. **Drennan, J. C.,** Neuromuscular disorders, in *Lovell and Winters Pediatric Orthopedics,* 3rd ed., Morrissy, R. T., Ed., Lippincott, Philadelphia, 1990, 451.
6. **Drummond, D. S. and Mackenzie, D. A.,** Scoliosis in arthrogryposis multiplex congenita, *Spine,* 3(2), 146, 1978.
7. **Gibson, D. A. and Urs, L. D.,** Arthrogryposis multiplex congenita, *J. Bone Jt. Surg. Br. Vol.,* 52, 483, 1970.
8. **Herring, J. A. and Banta, J. V.,** Arthrogryposis, *J. Pediatr. Orthop.,* 8, 353, 1988.
9. **Herron, L. D., Westlin, G. W., and Dawson, E. G.,** Scoliosis in arthrogryposis multiplex congenita, *J. Bone Jt. Surg. Am. Vol.,* 60, 293, 1978.
10. **Shapiro, F. and Bresnan, J.,** Orthopedic management of childhood neuromuscular diseases, *J. Bone Jt. Surg. Am. Vol.,* 64, 949, 1982.
11. **Staheli, L. T., Chew, D. E., Elliot, J. S., and Mosca, V. S.,** Management of hip dislocations in children with arthrogryposis, *J. Pediatr. Orthop.,* 7, 681, 1987.
12. **Thomas, B., Schopler, S., Wood, W., and Oppenheim, W. L.,** The knee in arthrogryposis, *Clin. Orthop.,* 194, 87, 1985.
13. **Williams, P. F.,** Arthrogryposis. Management of upper limb problems in arthrogryposis, *Clin. Orthop.,* 194, 60, 1985.

Chapter 15

SEATING THE HEAD INJURED

R. Mervyn Letts

TABLE OF CONTENTS

I. THE HEAD INJURY PROBLEM

The number of individuals with severe residual disability following head injury is increasing due to improved resuscitation techniques at the scene of the accident as well as subsequently in intensive care units. While many lives are saved, increasing numbers of head-injured persons with major musculoskeletal deformity are being salvaged. Many of these persons will be permanently nonambulatory and will require wheelchair support.[1,2,6,7]

In children, the incidence of significant head injury has been estimated to be 220 per 100,000 children. Fortunately, over 90% of these will recover with little residual disability.[14-16] Severe head injury often results in prolonged coma, during which time the immobility contributes to further deformity that may compromise future sitting stability. Spasticity, abnormal posturing, muscular imbalance, and ataxia frequently complicate the musculoskeletal deformity, resulting in major seating difficulties. Unrecognized and, hence, untreated injuries may accentuate these problems. As a result, head-injured persons are very prone to develop contractures, joint dislocations or subluxation, scoliosis, fracture malunion, and heterotopic ossification as a consequence of their cerebral injury.[2-6,19] Such deformities interfere with nursing and medical care, ambulation, seating, and activities of daily living, greatly prolonging the hospital stay. This is a cumulative population group which requires increasing support by seating clinics as well as ongoing requirements for wheelchair modifications and support systems.

II. ASSESSMENT OF THE HEAD INJURED

In the assessment of the seating needs of head-injured persons, it is essential that the seating team thoroughly understand the timing of the assessment and where the individual is in the rehabilitation process. During the first year after recovery from coma, there may be significant change and improvement in the status of the patient. Early seating is important and provides an opportunity for an improvement in tolerance for the upright position, environmental sensory stimulation, and mobility (Figure 1). Extensive customization of the wheelchair should be deferred until improvement has plateaued. At this time, residual deformities can be corrected, orthoses applied, a therapy program arranged, and the appropriate wheelchair choice decided upon.[9]

Other modalities which may influence the seating team in their choice of insert or customization of the wheelchair are

1. Medical status — Postural hypotension can be a problem in older head-injured individuals who may require a reclining feature for the chair so that a gradual gradation to upright sitting can be undertaken.
2. Musculoskeletal considerations — The presence of unrecognized injuries, such as fractures, dislocations, or contractures, may influence the course of action that needs to be taken. Some of these may require correction prior to the acquisition of a seating system.
3. Cognitive function — The residual cerebral function should be assessed to ascertain the need for special adaptive equipment to the wheelchair, such as environmental controls, communication systems, powered mobility, etc. These special adaptive aids can then be appropriately added to the wheelchair system.
4. Visual skills — Head-injured patients may be left with residual visual impairment which may influence their ability to utilize the wheelchair effectively. Assessment by an ophthalmologist, with input to the seating team, is essential with this type of patient.
5. Spasticity and motor control — An in-depth therapy review of the head-injured patient is essential to ascertain the potential for wheelchair usage and modifications, such as power adaptation, footplates, and wheeling rings.

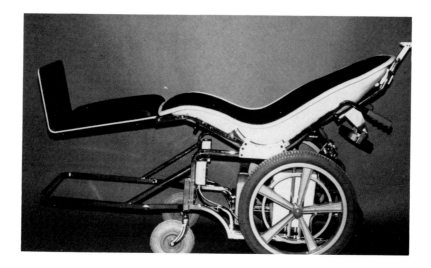

FIGURE 1. A tilting feature of the wheelchair is helpful in head-injured patients who experience severe hypotension in the upright sitting position. (Reproduced with permission from Letts, M., Rang, M., and Tredwell, S., Seating the disabled, in *American Academy of Orthopaedic Surgeons: Atlas of Orthotics,* 2nd ed., C. V. Mosby, St. Louis, 1985.)

6. Head and trunk posture — After head injury, some individuals' may require support to prevent the development of spinal curvature and to allow upright sitting (Figure 2). Such control may improve with experience and the maintenance of good sitting posture with a good wheelchair insert.[12]

III. SEQUELAE OF CEREBRAL INJURY CONTRIBUTING TO POOR SITTING

It must be emphasized that some head-injured patients will be so compromised following a head injury that it will be impossible or indeed impractical to seat them in a wheelchair. These unfortunate individuals are best managed in comfortable recumbent seats, and for those who would benefit from mobility, the bean bag stretcher is a practical device, especially for those who are institutionalized (Figure 3). Unfortunately, the seating team often has to face established contractures that have developed during the comatose period and that may be exaggerated or perpetuated by significant spasticity that often persists following significant head trauma. In a recent review of this subject in post-head-injury children, it was found that equinus deformities and hip adduction contractures were the most common residual contractures, followed by hamstring tightness and valgus deformities of the foot.[2] Ideally, it would be best to have the head-injured person assessed very early by the seating team so that some deformities may be avoided or aborted by physiotherapy, orthotic management, or early surgical correction. Few seating clinics have the luxury of this early consultation since the team is usually called in after the head-injured subject is able to sit upright. Established equinus deformities unresponsive to stretching and/or casting should be surgically lengthened in order to allow the feet to rest comfortably on the foot pedals (Figure 4). Hamstring shortening is usually not severe enough to compromise a good sitting posture, although in some head-injured persons the contractures may be well established and accentuated by spasticity, necessitating hamstring lengthening to avoid sacral sitting. Adductor contractures and gradual subluxation of the hips may occur over a period of time, often while the head-injured individual is in the process of rehabilitation. This may necessitate releasing the adductor contractures and ensuring good abduction seating through maintenance of hip reduction (Figure 5). In many instances, the spasticity that ensues as a result of head

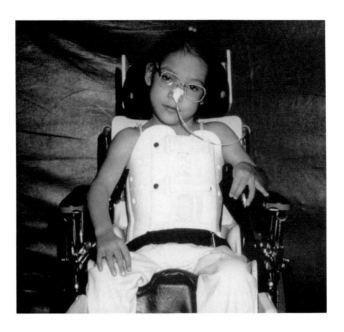

FIGURE 2.   Soft Aliplast spinal support is well tolerated and effective in controlling trunk instability and facilitating stable sitting post-head injury.

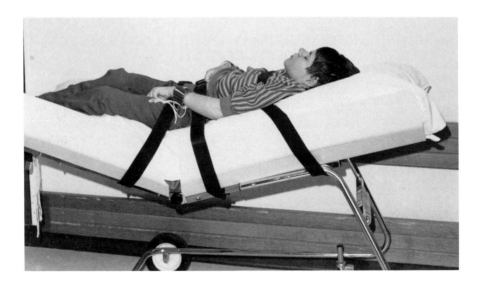

FIGURE 3.   Head-injured patients with continued cerebral irritation, irritability, and combativeness may be more effectively managed on a mobile, well-padded tilt stretcher. (Reproduced with permission from Letts, M., Rang, M., and Tredwell, S., Seating the disabled, in *American Academy of Orthopaedic Surgeons: Atlas of Orthotics,* 2nd ed., C. V. Mosby, St. Louis, 1985.)

injury results in progressive and recurrent deformities similar to those seen in cerebral palsy (Figure 6). Postoperative maintenance of correction utilizing ankle-foot orthoses following tendoachilles lengthenings and maintenance of abduction seating, especially after adductor tenotomies, is strongly recommended.[9-12]

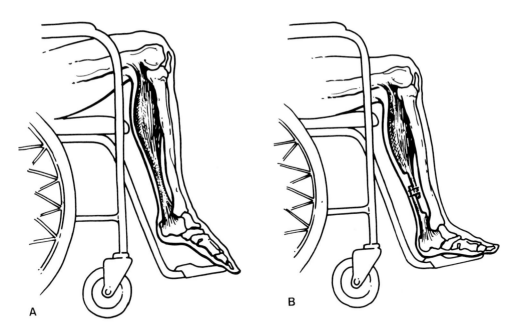

FIGURE 4.   Contracture of the tendoachilles (A) is the most common type of persistent deformity following severe head injury; (B) surgical lengthening may be necessary to facilitate shoe fitting and enhance wheelchair seating.

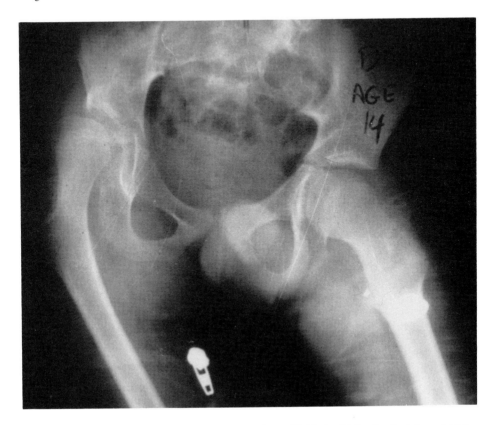

FIGURE 5.   Pelvic obliquity and windswept hips must be avoided in head-injured patients by maintaining abducted hips in the wheelchair and releasing contractures when necessary. (Reproduced with permission from Letts, M., Rang, M., and Tredwell, S., Seating the disabled, in *American Academy of Orthopaedic Surgeons: Atlas of Orthotics,* 2nd ed., C. V. Mosby, St. Louis, 1985.)

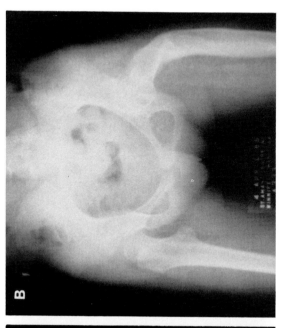

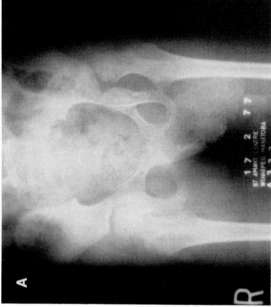

FIGURE 6.   Persistent subluxation or dislocation of the hip (A) after head injury in the child should be managed as in other spastic conditions with varus femoral osteotomy to maintain reduction and pelvic stability to facilitate seating (B). (Reproduced with permission from Letts, M., Rang, M., and Tredwell, S., Seating the disabled, in *American Academy of Orthopaedic Surgeons: Atlas of Orthotics*, 2nd ed., C. V. Mosby, St. Louis, 1985.)

IV. SPINAL DEFORMITY IN THE HEAD INJURED

Spinal curvature in the head-injured patient usually has an insidious onset that will lead to a rapid deterioration in seating if left untreated. The development of scoliosis in the head injured is similar to the onset in muscular dystrophy and coincides with the assumption of upright wheelchair seating.[8] There is frequently asymmetry in the paraspinal muscles, which contributes to the development of a long C-type curve or thoracic kyphosis or sometimes both (Figure 7). Other factors which can contribute to spinal deformity subsequent to head injury are unilateral head injury, pelvic obliquity secondary to intrapelvic causes, hip dislocation, poor trunk control, and asymmetric sitting posture.[13] It is frequently extremely difficult or indeed impossible to control these curvatures with wheelchair inserts in this type of individual as they usually are unable to tolerate passive bracing due to curve rigidity, resulting in skin irritation. The more forgiving Soft Boston type of orthosis is a temporizing compromise better tolerated by the head injured and may slow down curve progression to some extent. Head-injured children, especially those whose injury occurred prior to their adolescent growth spurt, have the potential to develop the greatest spinal deformity. Progressive curvatures over 40° should be surgically stabilized in order to prevent severe deformity and subsequent sitting instability. These curvatures should be dealt with in a manner similar to those in cerebral palsy, with instrumentation supplemented by sublaminar wire fixation and, in severe curves, circumferential fusions both anterior and posterior.

V. PREVENTION OF DEFORMITY SECONDARY TO HEAD INJURY

Established deformity subsequent to head injury is almost impossible to correct with physiotherapy, phenol blocks, or simple orthoses. Even in the immediate post-head-injury period, it is difficult to completely prevent the development of such deformities as equinus at the ankle or varus of the foot secondary to spasticity in the tendoachilles and/or posterior tibialis muscles. Therapy and orthoses may, however, slow the onset and prevent major fixed deformities and should always be attempted. However, when it is apparent that such modalities are not improving the particular deformity, the patient's sitting stability should not be compromised by a reticence to correct such deformities surgically. This frequently speeds up the rehabilitation of the patient and allows a much more functional sitting posture which allows the individual to utilize the full potential of any remaining cerebral function.

Early arrest of progressive hip contractures and scoliosis is necessary to control the onset of pelvic obliquity and the windswept hip deformity (see Figure 5). In late, established cases, accommodative seating may be all that is necessary since extensive surgery would be required when deformities become major and fixed for long periods of time.

Management of the musculoskeletal sequelae of head injury is similar to those of cerebral palsy, with a few distinct differences. While the typical patient with cerebral palsy experiences some degree of developmental delay, the head-injured person undergoes a true reversal of development, with variable recovery. The manifestations of cerebral palsy are the result of a stable neurologic lesion by definition, while the neurological signs following head injury may be variable, especially in the first year. For this reason, there may be a marked variance in the degree of spasticity, especially in the first year after head injury. Deformity secondary to spasticity in cerebral palsy is often much more responsive to physiotherapy and orthotic management than in the head injured.

The coexistence of musculoskeletal trauma at the time of injury may also have a considerable effect on later management, particularly if adequate management is precluded or delayed by the head injury. Unrecognized dislocations or fractures of the patella as well as malunions of femoral fractures treated in traction may compromise future seating. In children,

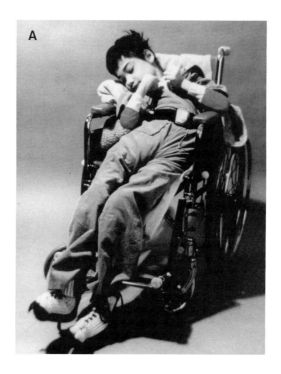

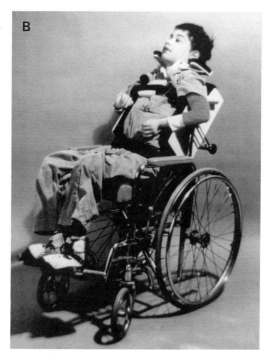

FIGURE 7. During rehabilitation from coma secondary to head injury, (A) avoid prolonged propping of the patient with pillows; (B) keep the hips abducted, the spine supported, and the feet at or near neutral position. (Reproduced with permission from Letts, M., Rang, M., and Tredwell, S., Seating the disabled, in *American Academy of Orthopaedic Surgeons: Atlas of Orthotics,* 2nd ed., C. V. Mosby, St. Louis, 1985.)

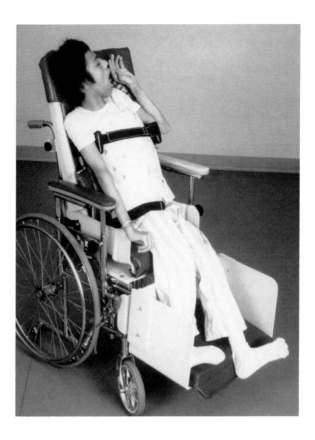

FIGURE 8. Extensor thrusting may be difficult to manage post-head injury, but tilting the insert, pelvic bars, and use of antithrust seat cushions may be helpful.

distal femoral growth-plate arrest may contribute to severe limitation of function as well as difficult seating due to limb-length inequality. Femoral fractures in both head-injured children and adults should usually be reduced and held with internal or external fixation to avoid major malunion problems later on.[18,19]

A particularly troublesome deformity that occurs secondary to head injury is the extension-abduction contracture of the hip which results in difficult seating as a consequence of the extended position of the hip.[17] This results in considerable difficulty for the seating team in maintaining a comfortable sitting posture, with the result that groin straps and pommels become necessary to try and maintain a partial sitting position (Figure 8). Unfortunately, these devices are usually insufficient and are not tolerated by the patient, resulting in poor sitting tolerance or seating which occurs in a semistanding position. This is often associated with considerable spasticity secondary to the head injury. Surgical release of the proximal hamstrings is necessary to improve hip flexion for proper sitting. In very severe and recalcitrant cases, the gluteus maximus insertion into the iliotibial band in the femur may also have to be released together with the external rotators and posterior hip capsule. The magnitude of the surgery will frequently depend upon the length of time the deformity has been present subsequent to the head injury. These releases should be followed up with regular physiotherapy to avoid hip stiffness, although the seated position usually maintains the correction fairly adequately. Occasionally, this deformity may occur after an extensive release of tight adductors and hip flexors. Seating teams must be vigilant in detecting the development of this type of deformity and must ensure that aggressive physiotherapy is embarked upon in the initial stages and that surgical correction in the established contracture is performed to maintain good stable sitting posture.

VI. SUMMARY

The head-injured population represents a significant and cumulative group with major disabilities for the seating team. The physical problems of the head injured are similar to those with cerebral palsy, but with some distinct differences. An aggressive surgical approach to the prevention and treatment of musculoskeletal deformity will facilitate good stable seating, with physiotherapy and appropriate orthotic management being used to maintain the correction and to prevent the development of future deformities that will compromise such seating.

REFERENCES

1. **Annegers, J. F.**, The epidemiology of head trauma in children, in *Pediatric Head Trauma*, Shapiro, K., Ed., Futura, Mt. Kisco, NY, 1983.
2. **Blasier, D. and Letts, M.**, The orthopedic manifestation of head injury in children, *Orthop. Rev.*, 28, 350, 1989.
3. **Brink, J. D. and Hoffer, M. M.**, Rehabilitation of brain injured children, *Orthop. Clin. North Am.*, 9, 451, 1978.
4. **Brink, J., Garret, A. L., Hale, W. R., et al.**, Recovery of motor and intellectual functions in children sustaining severe head injuries, *Dev. Med. Child Neurol.*, 12, 565, 1970.
5. **Brink, J. D., Imbus, C. and Woo-Sam, J.**, Physical recovery after severe closed head trauma in children and adolescents, *J. Pediatr.*, 97, 721, 1980.
6. **Bruce, D. A.**, Outcome following head trauma in childhood, in *Pediatric Head Trauma*, Shapiro, K., Ed., Futura, Mt. Kisco, NY, 1983.
7. **Bruce, D. A., Schut, L., Bruno, L. A., et al.**, Outcome following severe head injuries in children, *J. Neurosurg.*, 48, 679, 1978.
8. **Clark, P. R. and Hardy, J. H.**, Scoliosis following juvenile brain injury, *J. Bone Jt. Surg. Am. Vol.*, 56, 1767, 1974.
9. **Flach, J. and Malmros, R.**, A long-term follow up study of children with severe head injury, *Scand. J. Rehabil. Med.*, 4, 9, 1972.
10. **Hoffer, M. and Brink, J.**, Orthopedic management of acquired cerebrospasticity in childhood, *Clin. Orthop.*, 110, 144, 1975.
11. **Hoffer, M., Garrett, A., Brink, J., et al.**, Orthopedic management of brain injured children, *J. Bone Jt. Surg. Am. Vol.*, 53, 567, 1971.
12. **Letts, M., Rang, M., and Tredwell, S.**, Seaating the disabled, in *American Academy of Orthopaedic Surgeons: Atlas of Orthotics*, 2nd ed., C. V. Mosby, St. Louis, 1985.
13. **Letts, M., Shapiro, L., Mulder, K., and Klassen, O.**, The windblown hip syndrome in total body cerebral palsy, *J. Pediatr. Orthop.*, 4, 55, 1984.
14. **Mayer, T., Walker, M. L., Shasha, I., et al.**, Effects of multiple trauma on outcome of pediatric patients with neurological injuries, *Brain*, 8, 189, 1981.
15. **Molnar, G. E. and Perrin, J. C. S.**, Rehabilitation of the child with head injury, in *Pediatric Head Trauma*, Shapiro, K., Ed., Futura, Mt. Kisco, NY, 1983.
16. **Stover, S. and Zeiger, H. E.**, Head injury in children and teenagers — functional recovery correlated with the duration of coma, *Arch. Phys. Med. Rehabil.*, 57, 201, 1976.
17. **Szalay, E. A., Roach, J., Houkom, J., Wenzer, D., and Herring, J.**, Extension-abduction contracture of the spastic hip, *J. Pediatr. Orthop.*, 6, 1, 1986.
18. **Szuchan, L. A.**, Implications in the seating of head injured clients, in Proc. Seating the Disabled, Memphis, TN, February 1984.
19. **Zazbon, I., Najenson, T., and Tartakovsky, M.**, Widespread periarticular new bone formation in long term comatose patients, *J. Bone Jt. Surg. Br. Vol.*, 63, 120, 1981.

Chapter 16

SEATING AND THE SPINAL CORD INJURED

John E. Latter and Eric Dehoux

TABLE OF CONTENTS

I. INTRODUCTION

A continuous improvement of the survival and lifestyle of spinal cord-injured persons has been achieved over the second part of this century, but only in the last 15 years has proper attention been devoted to improvement in the design of wheelchairs and seating systems for this population.

The problem of pressure sores and its relationship to seating has always been (and still is) a major consideration when prescribing a wheelchair, but today more care is taken to also consider the comfort and the whole functionality of the patient in the sitting position.

In the last few years, technology has proliferated and can lead to confusion for the physician, who faces so many different systems, add-ons, and seating concepts.

The end result of any seating system for spinal cord-injured (SCI) persons should be to provide as upright a position as possible, reduce the risk of skin breakdown, and allow easy mobility, independence, and as much control of the environment as possible.

Depending on the level of the lesion, the prescription may be limited to a "standard" wheelchair plus a cushion or may entail a postural support system, including a back, a seat, and thoracic and lumbar supports.

II. CUSHION

Although we have chosen to discuss the cushion first, we must emphasize the importance of prescribing the whole system, including wheelchair, seat, and other components, at the same time, as one will influence the choice and measurements of the others.

The ideal cushion should be comfortable, provide stability, and act in some capacity to help prevent pressure sores.

Priority should be placed on the prevention of pressure sores. Maximal pressure occurs over bony prominences, and in the sitting position, pressure is exerted mostly on the ischial tuberosity region, followed by subtrochanteric and then coccygeal areas. The cushion should allow pressure distribution over as wide an area as possible.

Although ischial tuberosities are the most common area for pressure sores in the sitting position, Zacharkow has emphasized that subtrochanteric and coccygeal sores are also possible (up to 50% of coccygeal and 20% of trochanteric sores).[10]

Tissue tolerance to pressure is complex and still debated in the literature.[3] Both horizontal shear and vertical stresses are acting on loaded tissues. Some clinics use interface pressure-measuring devices, but caution should be exercised as they only measure vertical pressure and represent, at best, a relative indicator of deformations occurring deeper in the tissues.[3]

No currently available system is capable of reducing the tissue pressure below the capillary pressure level of 30 mmHg necessary for maintaining tissue perfusion. Therefore, ischemia always occurs in tissues loaded with body weight in the sitting position and must be periodically relieved by the individual, an assistant, or a mechanism included in the chair design.

Although different cushions allow variable tolerance time to sitting by distributing body weight over the largest possible area and by reducing shear forces, there is no good way of predicting how long individual patients can sit on different cushions without pressure relief. Individual resistance to tissue trauma by yet-unknown adaptive mechanisms to ischemia must surely play a role.[4]

Our experience is that the early months following SCI are a particularly risky period. Most clinicians use a trial-and-error approach with cushions, while frequently monitoring skin reaction until it is clear which cushion will be best for the patient in the long term.

The following should help identify high-risk individuals:

- Poor compliance with education and prevention measures
- Previous history of pressure sores

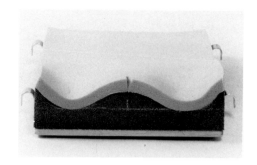

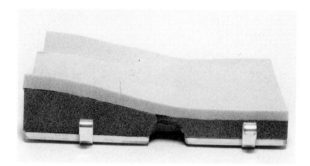

FIGURE 1.   Custom-made foam cushions (two views).

- Decreased tissue coverage over buttocks
- Bony deformities or asymmetry (e.g., previous ischiectomy)
- Heat and moisture accumulation
- Inability to perform pressure-relief maneuvers

Although a fair number of SCI patients have some preserved sensation, skin breakdown may still occur because of immobility, and it is recommended that the seating system be designed as if one were dealing with a complete lack of sensation below the level of injury.

In a large proportion of SCI individuals, the risk is moderate to low, and comfort, reliability, moderate cost, durability, and ease of replacement of the cushion should guide the choice. Excellent reviews of the components of cushions for SCI persons at moderate-to-low risk for skin breakdown are provided by Ferguson-Pell et al.[2,3] The basic materials and principles involved in custom cushion fabrication are also described[3] (Figure 1).

Our experience with adults has been that three types of cushions cover 95% of the needs: ROHO® (High- and Low-Profile or Enhancer models) (Figure 2), Jay® (Regular or Combi models) (Figure 3), and the foam cushion provided by the chair manufacturer. Over the last few years, the first two have been chosen more and more frequently by the patient and the seating team over the foam cushions.

The major disadvantage of foam cushions (commercial or custom fit) is their rapid deterioration with time, with the patient "bottoming out" after 6 to 12 months. Often, this may be the reason for an unexpected pressure sore. Frequent replacement offsets the initial, cheaper cost, and in the case of custom fabrication, patient compliance with follow-up by a seating clinic is essential. Ferguson-Pell recommends restricting the use of custom-fit foam cushions to cases where commercially available cushions fail to reduce interface pressure sufficiently.[3]

In children, the situation is different, as the need for frequent replacement is more often due to growth than to cushion breakdown.

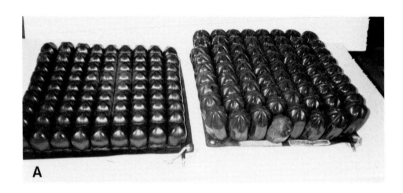

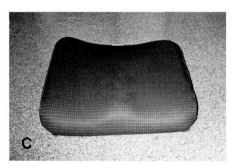

FIGURE 2.   ROHO® cushions. (A) Low- and High-Profile models; (B) Enhancer model.

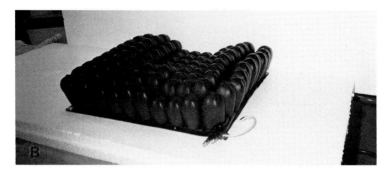

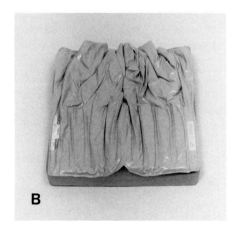

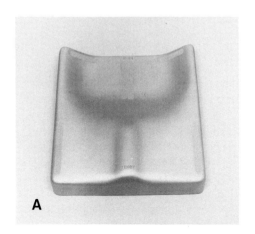

FIGURE 3.   Jay® cushions. (A) Regular model base; (B) gel pad added to cushion; (C) Combi model.

On the other hand, ROHO® cushions require care in monitoring air pressure (we recommend it once a week), and noncompliance with this may have the same results. ROHO® and other air-filled cushions tend to be more sensitive to underinflation than to overinflation, but the optimal range of internal air pressure (under load conditions) to achieve the lowest interface pressure possible is narrow (6 to 8 mmHg) and varies with the patient's body weight.[5]

Because of its contoured surface, the JAY® cushion may impair independent transfers in some quadriplegic patients with borderline ability to do so.

Paraplegics should be able to perform pressure-relief maneuvers (push-ups), and pressure sores are more often a problem of patient compliance than a true postural problem. In our experience with adults, sitting pressure sores are more common in paraplegics than quadriplegics, in spite of the better ability of the former with pressure-relief maneuvers. Quadriplegics depend more on caregivers for skin inspection during daily routine care and therefore problems tend to be detected earlier than with the often neglected self-inspection in some paraplegics.

This difference usually is not as common in children, as the role of skin inspection is assumed by the caregivers in both paraplegic and quadriplegic groups.

The literature has shown superior pressure reduction ability with the ROHO® cushion, compared to foam cushions.[3,4] In our experience, it has been sufficient to improve recurrent skin ulcers (in compliant individuals) at the expense of the some stability, and custom-fit cushions have rarely been necessary. We have occasionally used multiple-density, foam-"sculptured" cushions fabricated along the line of principles described elsewhere.[2,6,9]

The ROHO® cushion provides less trunk stability and a sense of flotation. The Jay® cushion allows a better posture, but in our experience, it does not offer the same amount of tissue protection as the ROHO® in patients with recurrent skin problems. In new, uncomplicated patients, the final choice between comfort, stability, and skin protection is often left to the individual.

III. POSITIONING

Most SCI persons, with the exception of quadriplegics at level C4 and above, retain sufficient mobility of their upper extremities and will not need or tolerate too much trunk restraint.

To provide good positioning (i.e., prescription of support devices), it is important to be aware of:

- Trunk support and balance
- Upper extremity function
- Skin tolerance to prolonged pressure
- Spasticity in trunk and legs
- Ability to transfer
- Scoliosis

Proper positioning should be conceived by starting with the pelvis as a base, then moving up. Two particularly important considerations are pelvic obliquity and the amount of posterior tilt of the pelvis in the seat.

Pelvic obliquity is often the result of the so-called "hammocking" effect from the wheelchair sling seat and results in asymmetrical pressure on the ischia and trochanters, as well as a scoliotic posture (Figure 4). Other consequences of the hammock seat are hip adduction, internal rotation of thighs, high trochanteric pressure, and reduction of the effective base for support, with consequent reduction in stability[8,10] (Figure 5). These effects can be prevented by a rigid base under the cushion.

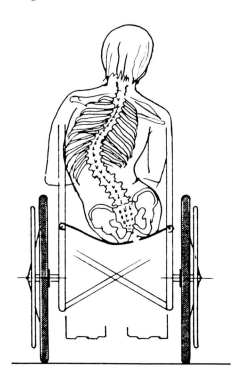

FIGURE 4. Scoliotic posture — ''hammocking'' effect of wheelchair sling seat.

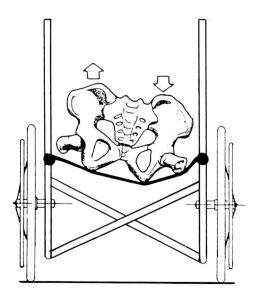

FIGURE 5. Pelvic obliquity.

Most SCI patients (except the lower paraplegics) lack trunk or pelvic muscles to maintain lumbar lordosis and will tend to sit on their coccyx (posterior pelvic tilt) (Figure 6). Restoration of some anterior pelvic tilt by a lumbar support is felt to be important in order to maintain a proper lumbar lordosis and improve trunk stability. Furthermore, the use of a

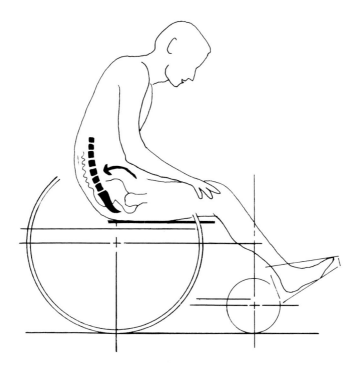

FIGURE 6.   Posterior tilt of pelvis.

lumbar support has been shown to decrease ischial pressure by allowing wider weight distribution on the posterior thighs and away from the coccygeal area.[7]

The lumbar support is not in itself a guarantee of better posture and is best combined with a 10° inclination of the seat to help prevent the pelvis from being pushed forward and remain posteriorly tilted. A tight pelvic belt is also important in that sense. Other factors maintaining a posterior tilt are hamstring tightness, excessive footrest height, and increased lumbar range of motion.[7]

Placement of the lumbar support pad is important: its lower part should be slightly below the iliac crest level. If too low, the pelvis will be pushed forward. If too high, the sacrum and pelvis will not be supported and may still be tilted posteriorly. An adequate recess should be left below the pad to accommodate the buttock tissues.[9,10] More recently, a new and interesting concept developed by Zacharkow[11] suggests placement of an inclined pad at the level of the posterior-superior iliac spines in order to support the anterior tilt of the pelvis. Another inclined pad between the T8 to T12 levels completes the postural system.

The trunk-to-thigh angle is usually kept at 90 to 100° between thighs and trunk, the knee angle at 80 to 90°, and the ankles/feet at 90°.

Recommendations for the seat angle to the floor varies from 3 to 10°. This should result in a trunk inclination of 10 to 15° from the vertical[7,9] (Figure 7).

Various methods are available to obtain that angle:

- Seat wedge
- Raising the front casters
- Rear axle adjustment (on new manual wheelchairs)
- Power tilt mechanism

Using a wedge board under the seat has the advantage of leaving the antero-posterior stability of the chair unchanged.

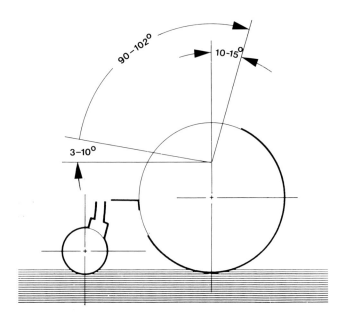

FIGURE 7.   Recommended seat angles.

The proper back height is 1 to 2 cm below the tip of scapulae for most patients. The backrest may also suffer from some hammocking effect after some time. Excessive concavity in the horizontal plane of forward inclination in the vertical plane pushes the upper limbs and shoulders forward and away from the backrest and results in difficulty maintaining contact with the lumbar support.[10]

Armrests are often not used by patients with sufficient lateral trunk stability. However, the fact that they also carry some upper body weight and help unload the buttocks is often overlooked.

Footrests are usually the ones provided with the chair and should offer a support area for the feet from the heel to at least the metatarsal heads, with appropriate foot/ankle restraints in spastic individuals.

IV. OTHER TECHNICAL COMPONENTS

Type of chair: manual or powered — Positioning in a powered wheelchair is not basically different from that in a manual one. Powered chairs are used by patients with less upper extremity function and probably less trunk control. They are usually unable to readjust their posture in the chair. The velocity of the ride as well as the use of chairs on bumpy terrain may result in subtle changes in position during the day. Contoured cushions such as the Jay® are usually preferable for trunk stability if skin tolerance is not a problem. There is usually no concern for transfers, as such patients are usually dependent. For manual chairs, the lightweight alloy-frame models with a seat angle of 5 to 10° to the floor (by adjusting the rear axle position) have become the standard today (for both paraplegics and lower quadriplegics) (Figure 8).

Rigid or folding frame — A rigid frame on manual chairs is usually beneficial at both ranges of functional abilities. For the quadriplegic with borderline upper extremity strength, it is usually lighter and easier to push; for the lower paraplegic involved in sports or with a very active outdoor lifestyle, sturdiness and durability are an advantage.

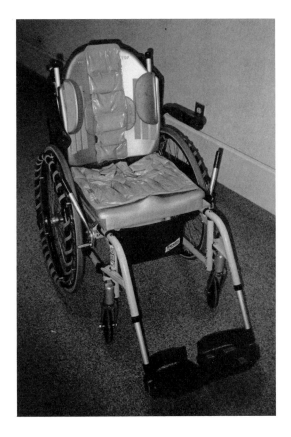

FIGURE 8. Lightweight manual wheelchair with Jay® cushion and Jay® back support.

V. QUADRIPLEGICS

For their postural needs, quadriplegics can be grouped into three levels:

- High-level quadriplegics (C1 to C4)
- C5 and C6 quadriplegics
- C7 and C8 quadriplegics

A. HIGH LEVELS (C1 TO C4)

Quadriplegics from C1 to C4 lack all upper extremity and trunk movements and require a powered chair. Problems include:

1. Total inability to adjust own position in chair
2. Decreased upright sitting tolerance (chronic orthostatic hypotension, usually more severe than lower quadriplegics)
3. Effect of upright position on respiration (Patients using a diaphragmatic pacemaker, C1 and C2 levels, show a decrease in vital capacity and usually cannot tolerate the same upright position as those with an intact diaphragm or a ventilator.)

More trunk support (contoured back) as well as a higher back (to the shoulder level) are indicated. It may be necessary to set the back at an angle of 25 to 30° to the vertical in

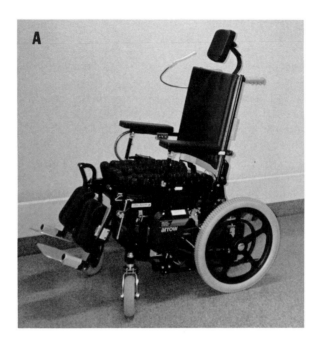

FIGURE 9.   Multisystem power wheelchair. (A) Upright position.

order to increase trunk stability by shifting the center of gravity of the head and trunk well behind the pelvis.

Head support is usually indicated in C1 to C3 patients, who may lack sufficient strength of neck muscles to maintain their head upright in the sitting position. It is also necessary if the back has to be reclined by more than 25 to 30°. "Sip and puff" or occipital controls are available for driving the chair and operating electronic environment control devices.

Armrests have to be wider and longer to accommodate forearms and hands in a trough.

The wheelchair base needs to allow for some reclining manually or, preferably, by a electric system controlled by the person. Two principles are available, i.e., "reclining" of back and elevation of legs vs. "tilting" the back-seat-legrest as a whole, thereby keeping the hip and knee angles unchanged (Figure 9).

Problems with the former system include shearing at the level of the sacrum and forward sliding on the seat. These problems have been reduced in recent designs which allow for a concomitant sliding motion of either the seat or the back (Figure 10).

We prefer the tilt-back system, which has the advantage of not changing the person's basic posture once he is installed, thus causing fewer problems in spastic individuals.

Chairs for respiratory-dependent quadriplegic persons will include a platform at the back of the chair for the ventilator.

B. C5 AND C6 LEVELS

At this level, a powered wheelchair can be controlled by a joystick activated by the person's hand. C5 quadriplegic persons will often use wrist splints that will require some adaptation of the control stick (Figure 11).

A back postural insert is rarely necessary and may simply consist of some slight lateral thoracic contouring and a lumbar support along principles described previously. Reclining chairs are not usually necessary.

Paralysis of trunk muscles most often results in quadriplegics sitting with a long thoracolumbar, C-shaped curve and leaning more to one side (scoliotic posture). It has been

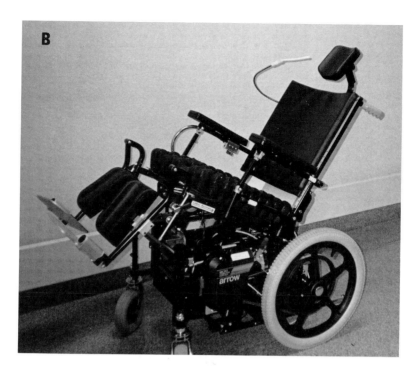

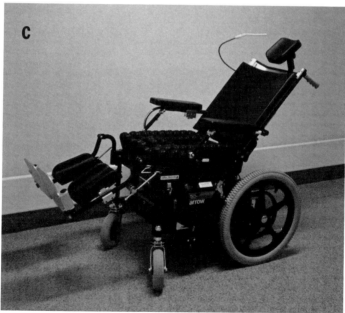

FIGURE 9 (continued).   (B) Electric tilt position; (C) electric reclining position.

postulated that reversal of lumbar lordosis ("unlocking" of facets) in sitting may be instrumental in developing the scoliotic posture and pelvic obliquity in paralyzed individuals.[7,9] In children and adolescents, this can result in permanent scoliosis, while in the adult, loss of sitting balance and discomfort are still a concern.

The back height should be at standard height in order to allow free backward shoulder movements. Individuals at that level can partially adjust their posture by extending their

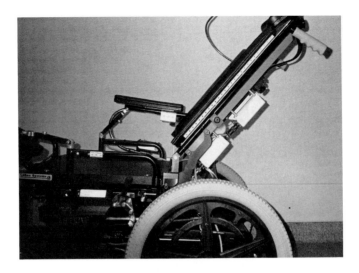

FIGURE 10.   Sliding back system to decrease shearing during reclining.

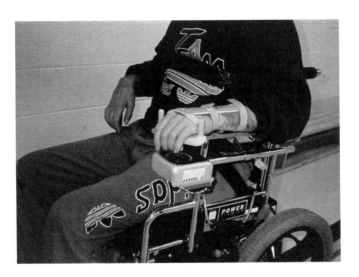

FIGURE 11.   C5 quadriplegia: wrist splint and joystick adaptation.

upper back with their trapezius and posterior deltoid muscles and hooking their arm around the wheelchair handle.

Individuals with serratus anterior weakness (C5) will have increased arm function if the scapula is supported against the backrest[10] and they may prefer a back raised to the level of the spine of the scapula.

A lap tray should be offered to help maintain an upright position by supporting the forearms and to provide a functional platform for those patients who cannot get sufficiently close to tables (Figure 12).

A standard pelvic strap should be pulling down and back at an angle of 45° over the iliac crest and not the upper abdomen. A chest strap helps maintain straight posture, especially during travel (Figure 13).

These individuals also require a manual wheelchair, and some will use it more than the electric one when indoors or for some exercise. It is essential when a van is not available

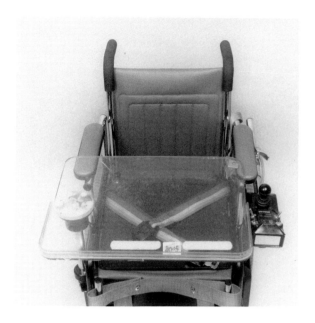

FIGURE 12. Lap tray.

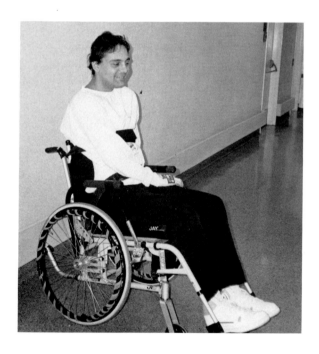

FIGURE 13. Properly positioned C6 quadriplegic. Note rubber tubing on hand rim to improve grip.

and the chair must be transported in a car trunk or when occasional visits to nonaccessible places (e.g., stairs) is likely (with help).

Other devices such as antibacking brakes (''grade-aid'') and brake extensions are also helpful. As these patients have no hand grip, rubber tubing wrapped around the hand rims helps manual propulsion by friction. This has almost completely replaced the projection

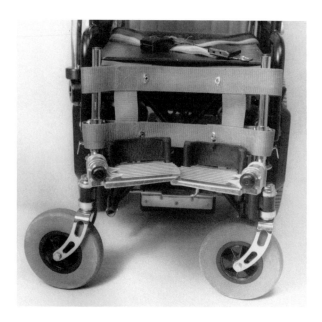

FIGURE 14.   H-strap calf restraints.

pegs on the rims formerly used for the same purpose. At the C6 level, similar principles apply, but wrist splints and lap trays are not required. Increasing trunk control by periscapular and shoulder muscles allows for some pressure-shift maneuvers.

C. C7 AND C8 LEVELS

These individuals often function without an electric wheelchair, except for long distances and inclines, and have the capacity to do "push-ups" for pressure relief. The wheelchair requirements are essentially the same as those for paraplegics, as described below.

VI. PARAPLEGICS

Most individuals can be accommodated with manual wheelchairs without custom-made modifications. Locking front casters are sometimes required for stability during sliding transfers. Folding chairs are a must for cars, and rigid frames are usually reserved for sport activities. Armrests and footrests come in a variety of models, and the latter may require slight custom modifications to offer sufficient contact to the sole of the foot.

The lower the level of paraplegia, the lower the chair back can be. We still recommend a standard below-scapula height for most. Chairs with very low backs are often chosen for increased mobility in sports by lower paraplegics. However, this is done at the expense of insufficient back support and may result in back pain if used continually. We tend to discourage their use on the patient's first chair.

A pelvic belt is still recommended in all but low, nonspastic paraplegics.

In very spastic persons, an abduction pummel in the base cushion is often not sufficient and extra straps may be necessary at distal thigh and foot levels.

Footrests may include heel-loop or H-strap calf restraints (Figure 14). Heel loops on the foot pedals are sufficient when involuntary spastic movements are not a problem. We prefer the H-strap which provides a larger area of calf support, but this might interfere with the use of swing-away footrests for transfers. However, many paraplegics do not bother swinging the footrests for transfers.

VII. CHILDREN

The same principles discussed above for adults pertain to the seating requirements of children.

A very important issue to take into account when dealing with children is their physical and psychological development. The seating system has to allow for normal growth and development in the areas of fine motor, gross motor, and communication ability.

Another difference is the invariable development of a structural scoliosis which will affect nearly all children with quadriplegia. Its management will require a spinal orthosis and thus could eliminate the need for thoracic lateral supports. Depending on the severity of the scoliosis, this could influence the development of pelvic obliquity and its inherent problems for seating. Surgical correction may be necessary to ensure sitting stability and will usually have a positive influence on the postural support system prescribed.

Also, in children, the issue of sphincter incontinence is an ongoing problem which is most often less controllable than in the adult. Thus, the cushion needs to be covered with a water-resistant layer of material and then an esthetically acceptable outer layer that reduces perspiration and is durable and washable.

With paraplegics under the age of 4 to 5 years, the mobility base is often not a wheelchair. It may be a stroller or caster cart (Figure 15). The caster cart allows the children to move easily and to be with their peers, who are "close to the ground" at that age. Modifications to the length of the cushion and contouring of the back cushion are usually needed to fit this mobility base.

Gibbus formation is rare in young SCI patients. If present, the back component needs to be cut out and padded to accommodate it or sufficient padding should be used to let the gibbus "sink in" so as to prevent skin breakdown. The first option is recommended, however, so as to reduce the chance of placing the child too far forward on the base. This would result in decreasing the support taken through the femurs and might also lead to inefficient self-propulsion because of the poor position of the hands.

A severe kyphosis may also require surgical stabilization to prevent future skin breakdown. This is more common in the spina bifida patient than in later-onset spinal cord injury.

In all cases of spinal instrumentation, care should be taken to use contoured rods as much as possible in order to preserve some lumbar lordosis.[1] Otherwise, excessive posterior tilting of the pelvis will occur in the sitting position. This results in a change in weight distribution between the ischial tuberosities, coccyx, and posterior thighs which can lead to tissue breakdown for the reasons explained earlier.

In the paraplegic 6 years of age and older, upper extremity strength is usually such that the child can easily do push-ups to relieve pressure on the buttocks and help reduce the risk of pressure sores.

The adolescent paraplegic has concerns similar to those of the adult.

VIII. SUMMARY

There probably is not perfect seating system for any individual, and compromises must always be achieved between stability, comfort, cost, ease of maintenance, and repair. One cannot overemphasize that appearance and acceptance by the person are essential and should never be ignored. Often, a little creativity with colors and choice of covering material is useful.

A team approach including physicians (physiatrist, orthopedic surgeon), occupational and physical therapists, orthotist, seating technician, and rehabilitation engineer is more likely to cover all aspects of complex cases.

As with other disabilities, the principles of proper seating for the SCI person will continue to evolve over the years. Rehabilitation engineering has allowed for a much better under-

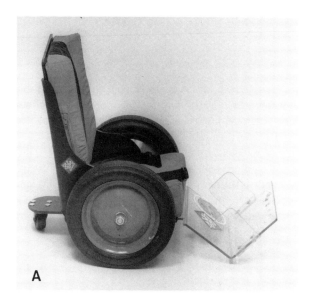

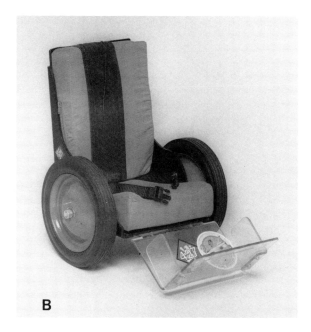

FIGURE 15.   Caster carts (A and B).

standing of the mechanics related to seating and tissue trauma. New technology and materials are constantly introduced and make it difficult to be aware of all possible systems commercially available.

The views represented in this chapter, especially with respect to cushions and the literature that we chose to present, are by no means the only ones considered valid. Each clinic should be familiar with the equipment it prescribes, rather than try to offer every choice available on the market.

REFERENCES

1. **Drummond, D., Narechania, R., Rosenthal, A., Breed, A., Lange, T., and Drummond, K.,** A study of pressure distributions measured during balanced and unbalanced sitting, *J. Bone Jt. Surg. Am. Vol.,* 64, 1034, 1982.

2. **Ferguson-Pell, M., Cochran, G. V., Palonieri, V. E., and Brunshi, J. B.,** Development of a modular wheelchair cushion for spinal cord injured persons, *J. Rehabil. Res. Dev.,* 23(3), 63, 1986.

3. **Ferguson-Pell, M.,** Seat cushion selection, *J. Rehabil. Res. Dev. Clin. Suppl.,* 2, 49, 1990.

4. **Fisher, S. V. and Patterson, P.,** Long term pressure recordings under the ischial tuberosities of tetraplegics, *Paraplegia,* 21, 99, 1983.

5. **Krouskop, T. A., Williams, R., Noble, P., and Brown, J.,** Inflation pressure effect on performance of air-filled wheelchair cushions, *Arch. Phys. Med. Rehabil.,* 67, 126, 1986.

6. **Nelham, R. L.,** Principles and practice in the manufacture of seating for the handicapped, *Physiotherapy,* 70, 54, 1984.

7. **Shields, R. K. and Cook, T. M.,** Effect of seat angle and lumbar support on seated buttock pressure, *Phys. Ther.,* 68, 1682, 1988.

8. **Vaughan, M.,** Seating for the disabled — positioning, *Australas. Phys. Eng. Sci. Med.,* 9(1), 45, 1986.

9. **Zacharkow, D.,** *Wheelchair Posture and Pressure Sores,* Charles C Thomas, Springfield, IL, 1984.

10. **Zacharkow, D.** *Posture. Sitting, Standing, Chair Design and Exercise,* Charles C Thomas, Springfield, IL, 1988.

11. **Zacharkow, D.,** personal communication.

Chapter 17

SEATING THE SELF-ABUSIVE

R. Mervyn Letts

TABLE OF CONTENTS

I. INTRODUCTION

The added disability of self-mutilation in a wheelchair sitter presents major problems to the seating team as well as to the caregivers for the unfortunate person. Such patients will injure themselves purposely on any exposed metallic or hard surface of the wheelchair or the seating system. Care must be taken to ensure that there are no hard edges available anywhere on the wheelchair insert and everything must be padded meticulously (Figure 1). In some children, the addition of a toy bar to secure toys on the wheelchair tray may provide enough distraction through play activity to greatly ameliorate self-injury (Figure 2).

II. LESCH-NYHAN SYNDROME

Although there are many types of patients who may be self-mutilating, the classic example for self-mutilation is the Lesch-Nyhan syndrome.[2,3,5,6,9] Patients suffering from this disorder realize that they should not injure themselves, but they have an uncontrollable urge to do so and will accomplish self-mutilation whenever possible[11-15] (Figure 3). Rather than restrict the extremities of these patients with straps to the chair, the wheelchair team should design a comfortable seating system with protective devices for the hands. The protective Plexiglass™ box shown in Figure 4 allowed this child with Lesch-Nyhan syndrome to lead a very comfortable existence without major injury to his extremities.[8] The child can be taught much more effectively with this protective attachment to the wheelchair tray since neither he nor the caregiver or instructor need worry about injury to the extremities (Figure 5).

III. OTHER HIGH-RISK, SELF-ABUSIVE GROUPS

Chronic head banging may have to be controlled with a protective helmet. This is sometimes encountered in severe mental retardation and subsequent to head injury.

In some severe cases of self-abuse, often associated with mental retardation, institutional care may be required. The mobile bean bag chair is safe and practical in these instances (Figure 6).

Several other conditions with congenital insensitivity to pain may pose some difficulty in seating due to associated musculoskeletal complications of the syndrome.[4,10] Children with familial dysautonomia or so-called Riley-Day syndrome are prone to develop spinal curvature and even neuropathic deformities of the spine.[1] This compounds the seating problem and may contribute to skin breakdown from attempts to provide adequate truncal support. Early stabilization of the spine surgically to prevent such progression is recommended. Congenital insensitivity to pain with associated self-mutilation is a disastrous situation, and keeping the hands occupied becomes a major objective of treatment. Behavior modification combined with innovative designs such as a Plexiglass™ box on the wheelchair tray may help to minimize this type of self-abuse. Deformities such as club feet can pose major problems for seating in children with congenital insensitivity to pain if the deformity has not been adequately corrected and the foot constantly rests in an abnormal position on the footrest of the wheelchair. Charcot joint formation in the lower extremities often occurs in individuals who are ambulatory prior to being relegated to a wheelchair existence. This may necessitate orthotic management of the ankles and feet in order to ensure functional and stable seating. Auto-amputation of digits in insensate wheelchair users will compromise independent use of the wheelchair as well as the activities of daily living.

In spite of innovative seating, individuals with the syndrome may still be able to mutilate themselves orally using their teeth, and, in some instances, teeth have had to be removed in order to prevent major mutilation to the lips.[1] Problems with pathological fracturing

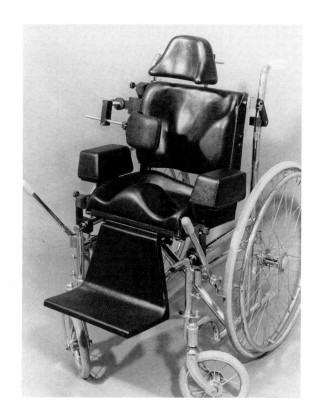

FIGURE 1. Complete padding of all contact surfaces of the wheelchair is often necessary to minimize intentional injury in self-abusive wheelchair users.

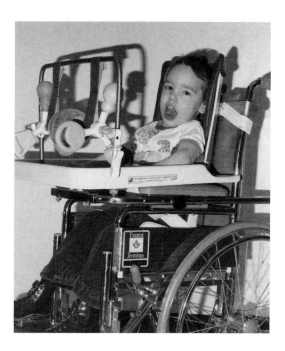

FIGURE 2. The addition of a toy bar and tray to the wheelchair may provide enough distraction to greatly lessen self-abusive tendencies in the same children.

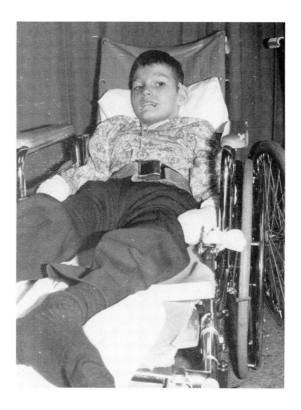

FIGURE 3.   A 14-year-old boy with Lesch-Nyhan syndrome as
seen initially by the seating team. Note hands tied down and
protected and poor attempts to improve seating with pillows and
foam. (From Letts, M. and Hobson, D., *Pediatrics*, 55, 852,
1975. With permission.)

secondary to the lack of sensation may occur in falls from the wheelchair. Such fractures
are usually metaphyseal, involving the distal femur or tibia. In the insensate individual,
these fractures are sometimes misinterpreted as infection since the first indication of any
underlying problem is the swelling and redness at the fracture site. Such an event in an
insensate wheelchair user should always be investigated for fracture before instituting treatment for possible infection.

IV. SELF-ABUSE IN THE BRAIN INJURED

Wheelchair sitting may be compromised by self-abusive behavior secondary to head
injury which is secondary to both trauma and hypoxia. In such instances, head banging may
be a difficult and annoying habit which requires helmeted protection for the patient. Helmeted
protection combined with a well-padded wheelchair may avoid serious injury. Self-abuse
through scratching and hitting can often be controlled by extension splints on the elbow
and, indeed, such patients are often more relaxed as a result of this type of immobilization.
The goal of the seating team should always be to provide the least amount of rigid immobilization necessary for good functional seating (Figure 7).

V. SUMMARY

Fortunately, the number of disorders that result in self-abuse are small, but the problems,
when they occur, can be immense for the family, caregivers, and the seating team.

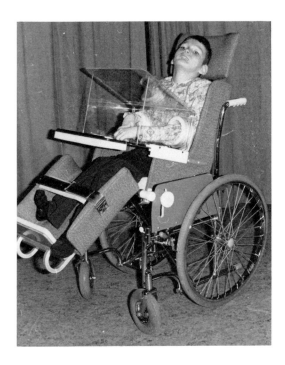

FIGURE 4.　Same child as in Figure 3 with custom insert and protective Plexiglass™ box to prevent self-mutilation of hands and fingers. (From Letts, M. and Hobson, D., *Pediatrics,* 55, 852, 1975. With permission.)

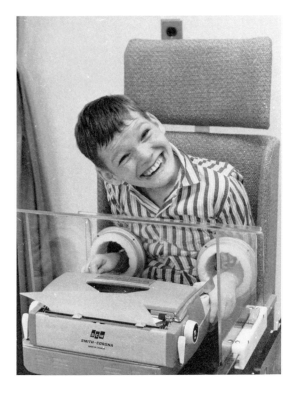

FIGURE 5.　The 9-year-old younger brother of the child shown in Figure 3 illustrating functional aspects of the protective Plexiglass™ box to facilitate learning and communication.

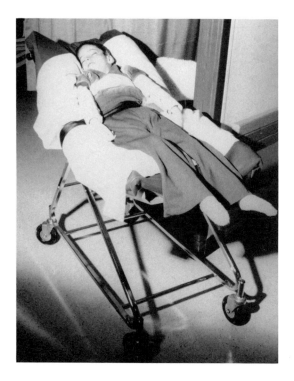

FIGURE 6.   Severely abusive patients with mental retardation may require institutional care. A mobile bean bag chair is often a safe and practical solution.

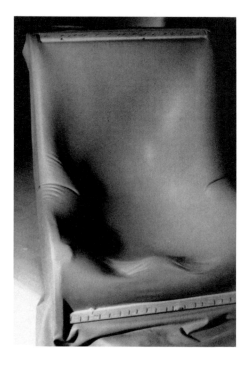

FIGURE 7.   Well-padded Foam-in-Place wheelchair insert being fabricated for self-abusive wheelchair user.

Recognizing the tendency to self-abuse at an early age is probably the best way to avoid major problems from established patterns of self-destruction in the future. Some element of behavior modification can be applied, and severe damage and deformity can often be avoided. Pressure sores secondary to skin breakdown must be identified early, and just as this is important in the spinal cord-injured seating program, so it is essential to educate families and caregivers in good skin care for those patients with congenital insensitivity to pain who may also have the added difficulty of noncompliance and self-mutilation. These families require extra support from the seating team, and a good seating program may make the difference between the child being managed in a home environment or requiring institutionalization because the family can't cope with the very demanding care of the child.

REFERENCES

1. **Albanese, S. A. and Bobechko, W. P.,** Spine deformities in familial dysautonomia (Riley-Day syndrome), *J. Pediatr. Orthop.,* 7, 179, 1987.
2. **Crawhill, J. D., Henderson, J. F., and Kelly, W. N.,** Diagnosis and treatment of the Lesch-Nyhan syndrome, *Pediatr. Res.,* 6, 504, 1972.
3. **Dizmanj, L. H. and Cheathman, C. F.,** The Lesch-Nyhan syndrome, *Am. J. Psychiatry,* 127, 671, 1990.
4. **Guidere, K. J., Multhopp, H., Ganey, T., and Ogden, J. A.,** Orthopedic manifestations in congenitally insensate patients, *J. Pediatr. Orthop.,* 10, 514, 1990.
5. **Hoefnagel, D.,** The syndrome of athetoid cerebral palsy, mental deficiency, self-mutilation, and hyperuricemia, *J. Ment. Defic. Res.,* 9, 69, 1965.
6. **Hoefnagel, D., Andrew, E. D., and Berndt, W. O.,** Hereditary choreoathetosis, self-mutilation and hyperuricemia, *N. Engl. J. Med.,* 273, 130, 1965.
7. **Janovic, J.,** Orificial and other self-mutilations, *Adv. Neurol.,* 49, 365, 1988.
8. **Letts, M. and Hobson, D.,** Special devices as aids in the management of child mutilation in the Lesch-Nyham syndrome, *Pediatrics,* 55, 852, 1975.
9. **Lesch, M. and Nyhan, W. L.,** A familial disorder to uric acid metabolism and central nervous system function, *Am. J. Med.,* 36, 561, 1964.
10. **MacEwan, G. D. and Floyd, G. C.,** Congenital insensitivity to pain and its orthopedic implications, *Clin. Orthop.,* 68, 100, 1970.
11. **McGreevy, P. and Arthur M.,** Effective behavioral treatment of self-biting for a child with Lesch-Nyham syndrome, *Dev. Med. Child Neurol.,* 29, 536, 1987.
12. **Partington, M. W. and Hennen, B. K.,** The Lesch-Nyhan syndrome: self-destructive biting, mental retardation, neurological disorder, and hyperuricemia, *Dev. Med. Child Neurol.,* 9, 563, 1967.
13. **Piazza, M. R., Bassett, G. S., and Gunnell, W. P.,** Neuropathic spinal arthropathy in congenital insensitivity to pain, *Clin. Orthop.,* 236, 175, 1988.
14. **Singh, S., Willers, J., Ulbrick, K., and Gustmann, H.,** A case of Lesch-Nyhan syndrome with delayed onset of self-mutilation, *Adv. Exp. Med. Biol.,* 195, 205, 1986.
15. **Winter, J. S. D.,** Metabolic effects of adenine therapy in Lesch-Nyhan syndrome, *J. Pediatr.,* 78, 1068, 1971.

Chapter 18

POWER WHEELCHAIRS AND OTHER MOBILITY AIDS

R. Mervyn Letts

TABLE OF CONTENTS

I. MOBILITY AIDS FOR THE WHEELCHAIR USER

Although much of this book is devoted to the provision of good stable and comfortable seating for the disabled population, we must not lose sight of the fact that mobility for these individuals is of paramount important to enhance their independence and in many instances pursue gainful employment and a higher education. This was brought home to me recently by a 10-year-old paraplegic girl with a bumper sticker on the back of her electric wheelchair which read "Mobility is Life."

II. IMPROVED PERCEPTIONS OF THE WHEELCHAIR

We are fortunate to be living in an era where the wheelchair population is "coming of age." Thanks to individuals such as Rick Hansen, who wheeled his chair around the world, as well as the growing interest in wheelchair sports, the manufacturing community is now addressing the problems of improving wheelchair mobility using the most up-to-date technology. Thus, there is no longer "a standard wheelchair". Lightweight chairs with various degrees of versatility are now available, depending on the needs of the particular wheelchair user. The lightweight sports wheelchair has been a boon to wheelchair users with muscle disabilities who have found it difficult or impossible to wheel the larger, more standard chairs of the 1960s and 1970s.[12] Out-flared wheels, balloon tires, improved gear ratios, unilateral wheeling rings, and improved wheeling grips have all enhanced the manual wheelchair and made it much more user friendly from a mobility standpoint (Figure 1).

III. POWERED WHEELCHAIRS

In spite of the advances that have been made over the past two decades in streamlining and upgrading manual wheelchairs to facilitate mobility, there are many wheelchair users who will be much more functional with an electric wheelchair.[1,12] Although using the manual chair will develop upper limb strength and endurance, there are many individuals with muscular dystrophy, quadriplegia, severe disability secondary to cerebral palsy, arthrogryposis, or poor upper limb development who will require the assistance of a powered device. Fortunately, a similar improvement has been occurring in powered wheelchairs as in manual chairs. Rechargeable batteries are lasting longer and the chairs are not so cumbersome or heavy. Although still relatively expensive, these chairs are often very cost effective. Many members of the wheelchair community will be much more functional in the school and workplace environment with a powered chair which can be used in school hallways, in shopping centers, on sidewalks, or in factories where the architectural barriers are minimal. Many wheelchair users find it advantageous to have both a manual and an electric wheelchair, either individually modified to meet their seating requirements or using a transferable wheelchair insert (Figure 2). The powered chair, for example, may be much more functional at work or at school, whereas the manual chair may be quite appropriate for the home environment.[4]

Every seating clinic should have an evaluation team to assess the suitability of a wheelchair user for a powered device. Some of the most handicapped individuals can be taught to use a powered chair very effectively and safely.[10] This, however, does require driver training and assessment by knowledgeable members of the seating team. Often the position of the joystick is pivotal as to whether or not the wheelchair can be safely driven. Depending on the physical limitations of the wheelchair user, the joystick may have to be centralized in front where someone with, for example, muscular dystrophy can rest and easily reach the control box. In other instances, such as children with arthrogryposis with good hand

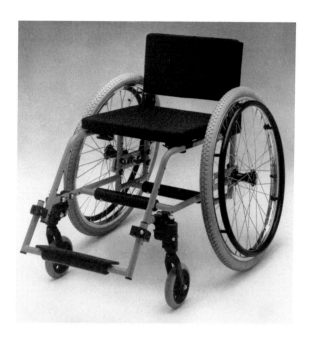

FIGURE 1. The sports wheelchair, built to be used in wheelchair athletics, but also used by many for everyday use (Enduro ''Bantam''; weight, 13 lb).

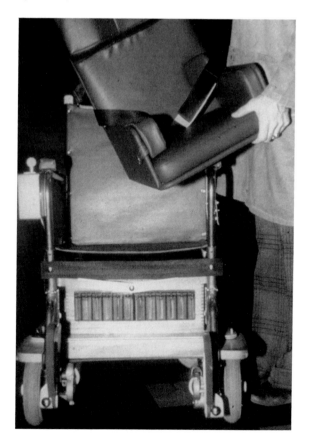

FIGURE 2. Transferable wheelchair inserts facilitate having a manual and a powered chair in different locations.

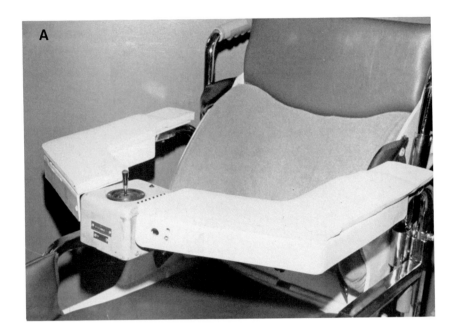

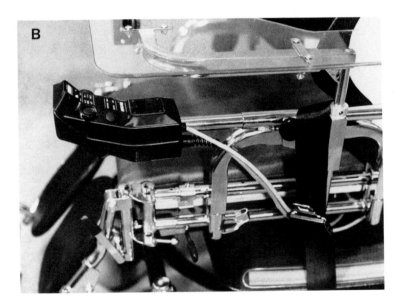

FIGURE 3.   Centralized power controls (A) to facilitate access in users with marked muscle weakness; (B) interface unit which permits easy control of many chair powered functions.

function but not elbow or shoulder motion, the control box may be much more appropriate lower down and to the side (Figure 3). Still others with severe spasticity may have to work the control box with their tongue. It is much more practical and effective to have a marginal manual wheelchair user converted to a powered device to increase independence and decrease the amount of time taken to get from one place to another than to continue to persist with the manual chair. Powered chairs can be virtually custom made to accommodate severe deformities and to compensate for certain types of terrain[13] (Figure 4). Modifications of

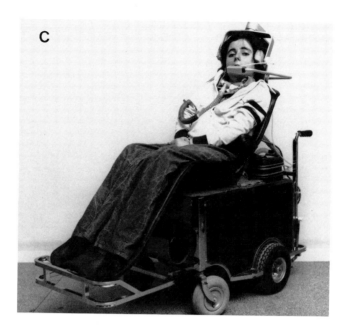

FIGURE 3 (continued).   (C) A 14-year-old boy with complete C2 quadriplegia uses a tongue control to direct his powered wheelchair with respirator. (Reproduced with permission from Letts, M., Rang, M., and Tredwell, S., Seating the disabled, in *American Academy of Orthopaedic Surgeons: Atlas of Orthotics,* 2nd ed., C. V. Mosby, St. Louis, 1985.)

such powered chairs may be required to accommodate respiratory equipment for the increasing number of wheelchair users who are quadriplegic and require ventilatory assistance (Figure 5). The commercially available group of powered wheelchairs such as the Pony™ or Amigo™ has provided a more avant garde type of mobility device and these powered chairs are frequently very adaptable to the school and workplace (Figure 6). Such units can also be used to do the grocery shopping and are frequently more adaptable to sidewalks and roads than the heavier, four-wheel powered chairs.

IV. INTERFACE UNIT

The wheelchair community is now demanding that the electronic industry address their needs and apply some of the advances of computerized technology to the requirements of wheelchair users. Results have been the development of "interface units" which allow the wheelchair user to control many of the functions of the wheelchair, as well as to interact with the environment and community through speech and communication and to interact with the home environment through environmental control modules, and which allow for user-controlled add-on air bladders or contours to assist proper posturing as well as chair tilting, reclining, and stand-up features when appropriate (see Figure 3B).

Controls can now be made to be very responsive so that a flicker of one finger or the tongue or hand can activate the control. Moreover, for individuals who do not have fine motor control, such as the very spastic, the controls can be made to be very durable so that they will stand up to rough use. The safety factors enters into prescriptions for more sophisticated types of mobility devices, and a training program together with an assessment, not only of the needs of the wheelchair user, but also of the ability of the user to safely apply the technology, is important. Each seating team should have a powered mobility assessment team capable of making these decisions. This may well have to include a home visit as well as a visit to the user's school or workplace.

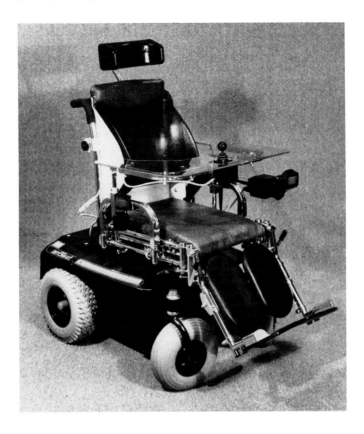

FIGURE 4.   Powered wheelchair with heavy-duty wheels for rough terrain.

V. POWER MOBILITY PRESCRIPTION

The seating team must be familiar with the various powered capabilities on the market, and within the seating team, a powered mobility assessment team must be developed. These individuals, usually consisting of a therapist, occupational therapist, and communication engineer, should be cognizant of all the electronic interfaces between the wheelchair and the environment. Ideally, it is best to have an example of each of these devices that can be used in the assessment of the individual being considered for a powered device. The reticence of ordering a powered wheelchair because of diminution in physical activity should no longer be a reason for deferring powered mobility. If a child or adult requires further therapy, this can be done on a regular and specific basis rather than relying on manual wheeling to provide the exercise. The basic requirements for the use of a powered device are an ability to use it safely and the physical ability to power the equipment switching. Independent mobility should be a *right* and not a *privilege* for both the child and the adult.

One of the major problems with accessing powered mobility is the cost of the device itself. Fortunately, these powered devices are now decreasing in price, but they are still a considerable financial outlay for families. In some areas, service clubs have contributed significantly to the acquisition of such powered mobility devices for those requiring them, but it is important that professionals in the field continue to communicate with insurance agencies, emphasizing the contribution to health care that powered mobility provides. It is often the difference between someone being gainfully employed or educated and obtaining the utmost of their potential in the wheelchair as opposed to sitting in the confines of their home environment. Patients in each geographical area should have access to a training assessment program whereby individuals being recommended for powered devices can be

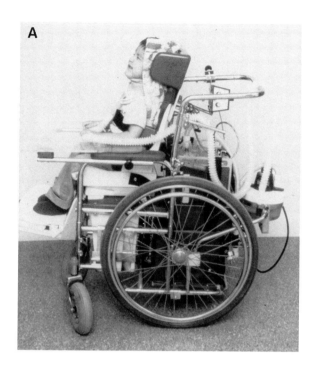

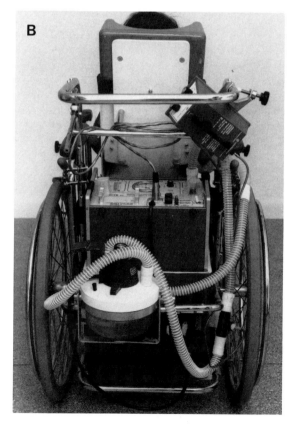

FIGURE 5. Wheelchair modified to incorporate equipment for respiratory support in a post-traumatic C3 paraplegic child (A and B).

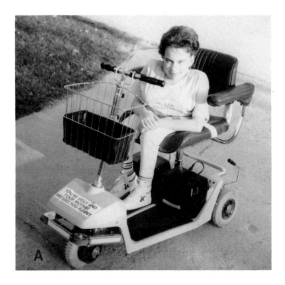

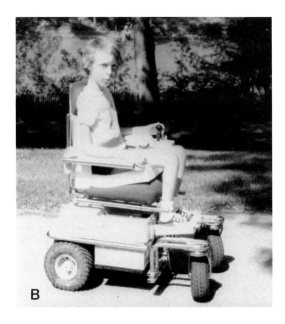

FIGURE 6.   The versatile Pony™ electric scooter (A) used here by a teenager with spina bifida who traveled miles in her neighborhood to visit friends and run errands; (B) powered base fitted with modular wheelchair insert interchangeable to a manual wheelchair.

assessed as to the safety of the equipment and be trained in proper use and maintenance of the powered device. A wheelchair simulator program is ideal and should be strived for by all seating teams.

VI. SAFETY IN TRANSPORT OF THE HANDICAPPED

Handicapped persons, both children and adults, need to be transported safely in their seating devices or wheelchairs in motor vehicles.[2,3] Better-designed car seats for handicapped

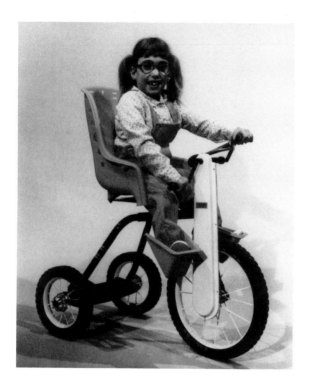

FIGURE 8. The "Tara Cycle" allows paraplegic children to ride tricycles with their friends. (Reproduced with permission from Letts, M., Rang, M., and Tredwell, S., The orthotics of myelomeningocele, *American Academy of Orthopaedic Surgeons: Atlas of Orthotics,* 2nd ed., C. V. Mosby, St. Louis, 1985.)

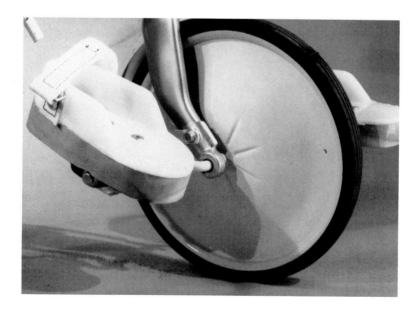

FIGURE 9. The attachment of a footpiece and strap to the pedals may allow a child with muscle weakness or spasticity to ride a tricycle.

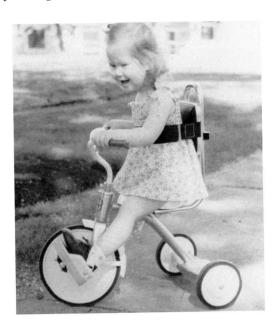

FIGURE 10.   A tricycle modified with a back support and seat belt to facilitate use by a child with athetotic cerebral palsy.

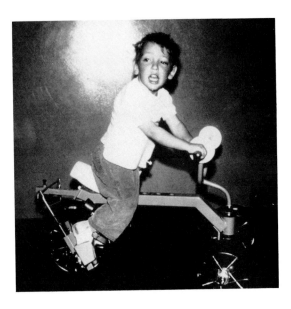

FIGURE 11.   The cerebral palsy tricycle can be a very effective mobility aid for the wheelchair user with spasticity.

X. MOBILITY ASSISTS IN CHILDHOOD

Many children who are wheelchair users will be quite capable of utilizing other mobility devices in a more effective manner than the wheelchair. Such devices often will place these children in more direct contact with their peer groups by allowing them to function at floor level and will avoid the barrier that the wheelchair sometimes imposes between wheelchair

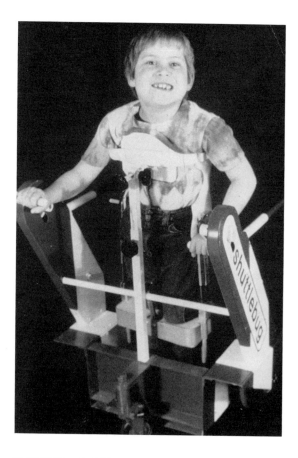

FIGURE 12. A child with paraplegia, but a good parapodium user, can use this mobility device in his parapodium to travel longer distances. (Reproduced with permission from Letts, M., Rang, M., and Tredwell, S., The orthotics of myelomeningocele, in *American Academy of Orthopaedic Surgeons: Atlas of Orthotics*, 2nd ed., C. V. Mosby, St. Louis, 1985.)

children and their ambulatory playmates. The energy cost of using such devices and propelling their light weights is also much less.

XI. CASTOR CARTS

The Castor Cart or spina bifida cart, first developed at the Ontario Crippled Centre in Toronto, is an effective alternative mobility device for children under 2 years of age (Figure 13). Although spina bifida children are the largest users of these devices, children with other disabilities also derive enjoyment from them. The use of the cart avoids skin abrasions from rug burns and allows the child to participate in games and activities at floor level (Figure 14). The use of the cart enhances upper extremity and trunk control and assists in the development of good sitting balance. The Castor Cart can be modified, depending on the seating needs of the child. Children with fixed deformities may require a specially molded seat which can be fabricated with the use of a Vacu-Form machine which enables the body of the Castor Cart to be molded directly to the child's contours (Figure 15). This is most frequently encountered in children who have poor head control or in those with marked scoliosis of the spine. Abduction can be built into the Castor Cart to ensure good hip stability. A removable handle at the back of the cart will allow it to be converted to a stroller type

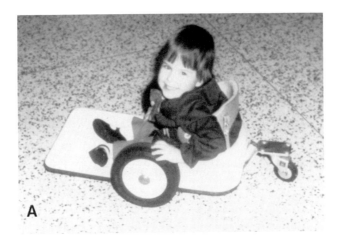

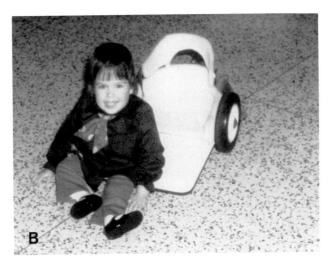

FIGURE 13. The Castor Cart (A) allows the nonambulatory child to propel the device easily; (B) mounting and dismounting are facilitated by the tilt feature.

of device in which the child can be pushed for longer distances. A castor wheel is sometimes built into the back of the cart, allowing multidirectional movement and making it easier for the child to propel and direct the cart by himself. Mounting and dismounting is facilitated by simply pressing down on the front of the cart which can be carefully balanced to tip forward and become a ramp so the child can disembark or access the cart without assistance.[7,8]

XII. STAND-UP WHEELCHAIRS

Various varieties of stand-up wheelchairs have appeared on the market from time to time (Figure 16). There are many advantages to the stand-up wheelchair for wheelchair users who are capable of bearing weight for short periods of time. Most are brought up to a vertical position by the use of a simple ratchet or hydraulic system. In the upright position, school activities can be participated in with greater ease (Figure 17) and activities of daily living such as standing at the sink, etc. can be accomplished with minimal difficulty (Figure 18). Care must be taken to educate the wheelchair user to avoid standing for long periods

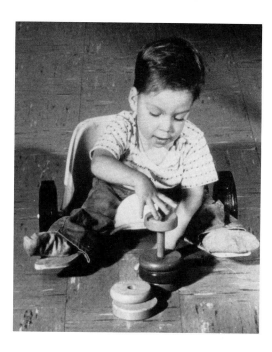

FIGURE 14. The Castor Cart avoids skin injury and floor burns in paraplegic children. Note leg abduction feature built into the cart to assist hip stability. (Reproduced with permission from Letts, M., Rang, M., and Tredwell, S., The orthotics of myelomeningocele, in *American Academy of Orthopaedic Surgeons: Atlas of Orthotics*, 2nd ed., C. V. Mosby, St. Louis, 1985.)

of time when the lower extremities are insensate, as pressure sores can develop. Children who have more serious handicaps and are unable to stand unaided may benefit from chairs that can be converted into supine standing devices (Figure 19).

XIII. STANDING AIDS

Even though most nonambulatory individuals will spend most of their time in the wheelchair, some may be able to function effectively for short periods of time in various forms of standing devices.[1-5] These standing devices provide respite from the wheelchair and allow children especially to participate more directly with their peer groups. Paraplegic children especially can utilize the parapodium,[9] the A-frame, and standing frames to increase their mobility. Prone and supine standers can be utilized by less coordinated wheelchair users (Figure 20). A more aggressive orthotic approach may be necessary if upright standing is to be instituted, with an ankle-foot orthosis often being necessary.[9] More research is needed in this area as well as in the continued improvement in wheelchair design[9] (Figures 21 to 23).

XIV. SUMMARY

Mobility is essential for all of us and is greatly appreciated by the wheelchair user since it contributes immensely to independence as well as to the ability to compete in an environment which often compromises wheelchair function and accessibility (Figure 24). The accessibility of such devices should be discussed by the seating team with the families of

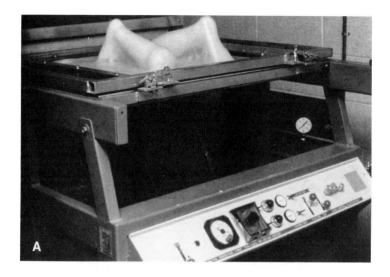

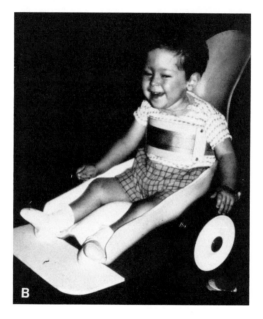

FIGURE 15. The Vacu-Form machine facilitates the fabrication of custom-made wheelchair inserts as well as modular systems from predesigned molds (A); (B) back support can be fabricated with the Vacu-Form machine to accurately provide molded total contact support for children with poor torso stability.

wheelchair users who might benefit from such mobility aids. Ideally, the seating team should have access to a number of these mobility aids to allow wheelchair users to try them out and be assessed on their ability to adapt to the particular device recommended. Specialized training teams should be set up to evaluate the feasibility of powered chair use as well as a training protocol for teaching these individuals safe and effective methods of using powered devices. The cost factor is a definite consideration with many of the more sophisticated types of mobility aids, and assistance may have to be obtained from service clubs, corporations, and government agencies in order to facilitate the purchase of the appropriate mobility assistance.

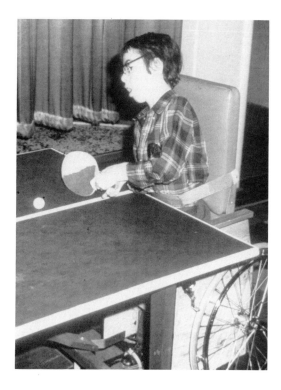

FIGURE 16. The stand-up wheelchair allows upright stance and stretches hamstrings and hip flexors as well as permits participation in upright activities including sports.

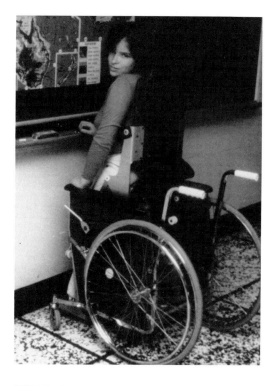

FIGURE 17. The stand-up wheelchair facilitates school activities such as board work.

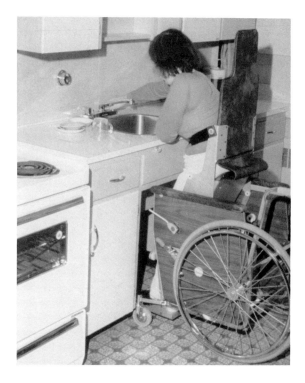

FIGURE 18.   The stand-up wheelchair facilitates activities of daily living.

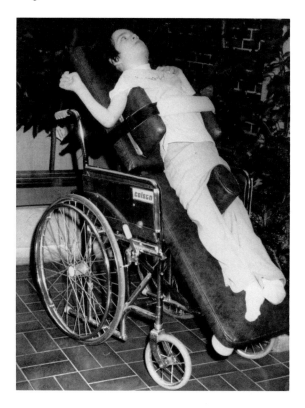

FIGURE 19.   A passive stand-up wheelchair feature that functions like a tilt board.

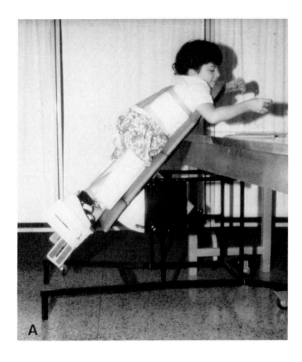

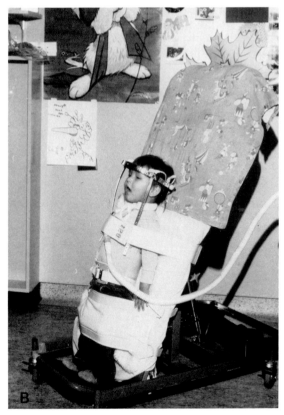

FIGURE 20. Prone stander (A) allows respite from the wheel-chair; (B) supine stander used by quadriplegic child.

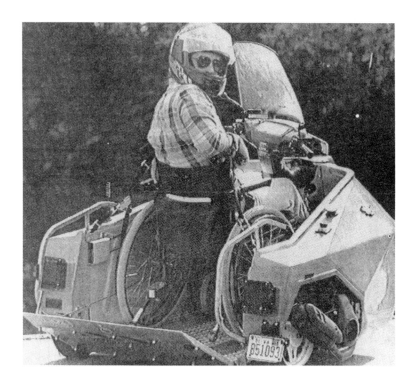

FIGURE 21.   The wheelchair chariot designed by Rick Balloon, a disabled Vietnam veteran, to give wheelchair users a practical and more exciting type of mobility.

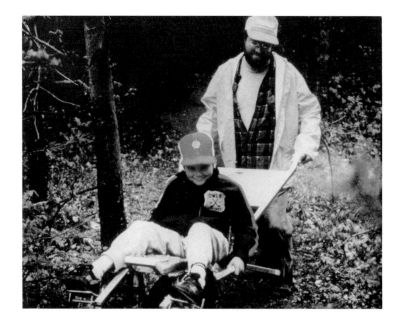

FIGURE 22.   The wheelbarrow chair designed for use on narrow forest paths in the woods.

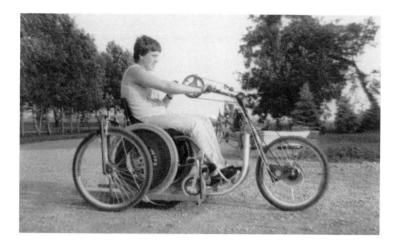

FIGURE 23.   The "Libre Trike" allows the wheelchair to roll onto platform with 18 speed gears for hand pedaling, allowing rapid transport over long distances. (Courtesy of Juan Neufeld, Cycling Future Co., Winkler, Manitoba, Canada.)

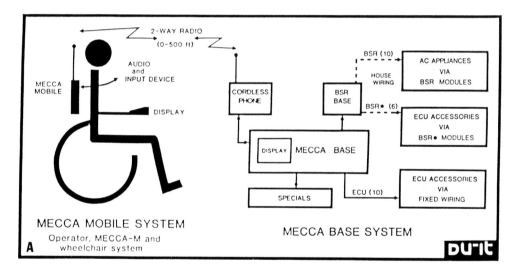

FIGURE 24.   Environmental control unit (ECU) utilizing cordless telephone technology (A). The MECCA system fully integrates into Du-it wheelchair systems. This approach permits nearly all functions of the system to be located anywhere in the household. It places the selection and control processes as well as all of the telephone functions with the user in his wheelchair; (B) wheelchair control system. By positioning a switch or sensing device at some anatomical location, signals can be derived which might be employed to operate a wheelchair. This listing represents potential control sources; controllers have been implemented to use many of these sites: A, chin control; B, headrest control — By pushing straight back against the headrest, a forward signal is produced. By rocking the head to the left or right against the headrest, turn signals are generated. A separate switch needs to be activated to reverse the sense for backward motion; C, joystick; D, arm/elbow control; E, head control — Direct use of forward/backward and left/right movement of the head is employed; F, shoulder position — Elevation and depression (or slump) provide forward/backward signals, while protraction/retraction of the shoulder provide the left/right signals; G1, pneumatic (puff/sip) control — This system uses hard puffs and sips to control forward and backward velocities, while soft puffs and sips introduce proportional turns; G2, spoken control — A computer can analyze the words spoken and use them to "drive" the wheelchair; G3, mouth, tongue, lip control — A head-mounted chin-controller element can make use of small movements to provide proportional control; H, foot control; I, knee control. (Courtesy of Du-it Control Systems Group, Inc., Shreve, OH 44476.)

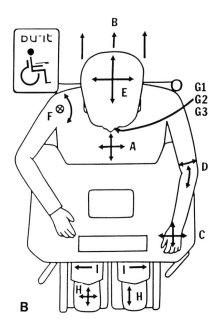

FIGURE 24 (continued).   (B) Wheelchair control system.

REFERENCES

1. **Balfour, L.,** Current trends in power mobility, in Proc. Seating the Disabled, Vancouver, British Columbia, February 1990.
2. **Bull, M. J. and Stroup, K. B.,** Premature infants in car seats, *Pediatrics,* 75, 336, 1985.
3. **Bull, M. J., Weber K., and Stroup, K. B.,** Safety seat use for children with hip dislocation, *Pediatrics,* 77, 873, 1986.
4. **Breed, A. L.,** The motorized wheelchair; new freedom, new responsibility, and new problems, *Dev. Med. Child Neurol.,* 24, 366, 1982.
5. **Feller, N., Gunnip, A., Stout, J., and Bull, M. J.,** A multidisciplinary approach to developing safe transportation for children with special needs, *Orthop. Nurs.,* 5, 24, 1986.
6. **Letts, R. M., Fulford, R., and Hobson, D. A.,** Mobility aids for the paraplegic child, *J. Bone Jt. Surg. Am. Vol.,* 58, 38, 1976.
7. **Letts, R. M., Hobson, D. A., Trefler, E., and Fulford, R. E.,** The role of special devices in the management of the handicapped child, *Can. Med. Assoc. J.,* 110, 925, 1974.
8. **Letts, M., Rang, M., and Treadwell, S.,** Seating the disabled, in *American Academy of Orthopaedic Surgeons: Atlas of Orthotics,* 2nd ed., C. V. Mosby, St. Louis, 1985.
9. **Schneider, L. W.,** Protection for the severely disabled: a new challenge in occupant restraint, in *Proc. Int. Symp. Occupant Restraint,* American Association of Automotive Medicine, 1981, 217.
10. **Scott-Taplin, C., Smith, M., McLaughlin, J., and Matthews, T.,** The wheelchair culmulator: powered wheelchair assessment and training, *Can. J. Rehabil.,* 3, 1, 1989.
11. **Shaw, G.,** Vehicular transport safety for the child with disabilities, *Am. J. Occup. Ther.,* 41, 35, 1987.
12. **Warren, G. G.,** Powered mobility and its implications, in *Proc. Wheelchair IV,* Brubaker, C., Ed., RESNA, Washington, D.C., 1990.
13. **Warren, C. G., Ko, M., Smith, C., and Imre, J. V.,** Reducing back displacement in the powered reclining wheelchair, *Am. Phys. Med. Rehabil.,* 63, 447, 1982.
14. **Wisbeach, A. and Holt, K. S.,** Children in wheelchairs, *Br. Med. J.,* 281, 199, 1980.

Chapter 19

ALTERNATE SEATING

R. Mervyn Letts and Erica von Kampen

TABLE OF CONTENTS

I. INTRODUCTION

Sitting for prolonged periods of time in one seating device is frequently not well tolerated, especially by children. In some situations, there may not be any alternative form of seating system that is appropriate, but in those instances where respite seating can be offered, the seating team should discuss this with the family and/or caregivers. Many disabled persons will have a need for at least two wheelchairs, often one being motorized and the other being manual. For the more severely handicapped, the wheelchair insert can often be transferred from one wheelchair to another, and even in custom-designed chairs, the change offers slightly different seating mechanics and provides some respite for the individual (Figure 1). It is important that alternative seating include the basic important concepts of seating required for the particular disability for which the person is being treated. For example, in children with cerebral palsy, the hips should be in abduction, whether the child is in a regular wheelchair or in an alternative seating device, to ensure proper development of the acetabulum from a well-reduced femoral head. Alternatively, in insensate disabled individuals, good skin care must be ensured to avoid pressure sores, no matter what type of seating device the person is using. This chapter will cover a number of alternative seating and positioning devices which are frequently used to provide respite for the wheelchair sitter and assist in both occupational and physiotherapy for the enhancement of wheelchair sitting.

II. ALTERNATIVE SEATING DEVICES

A. FLOOR SEAT
This seating device is primarily used for preschool-age children, ensuring safe sitting on the floor for play as well as instruction (Figure 2). The floor seat has the therapeutic benefit of stretching the hamstrings, and in children requiring abduction seating, abducting wings can be inserted to keep the hips abducted. Such a seat is often referred to as a CP floor seat (Figure 3). Floor seats are usually more effective when combined with working tables for playing or reading. Some sitting balance is needed to effectively use the floor seat, although some trunk support can be built into the backrest.

B. POMMEL SEAT
The pommel seat is a comfortable and practical type of sitting device, providing trunk support for the child to enable hands-free sitting (Figure 4). The size of the pommel allows the legs to be kept in abduction which is particularly important in children with spasticity to stretch the adductors and allow the femoral head to be nicely seated within the acetabulum of the hip joint. Play activities are facilitated by a table in front of the pommel seat, and the pommel itself is capable of being adjusted forward or backward, or to a 30° forward slope.

C. CORNER SEAT
The corner seat can be used by children from ages 2 to 10 years and promotes symmetrical upright positioning with hip abduction (Figure 5). Depending on the size of the child, the back support can be elongated, and the seatbelt provides further support. Headrests can be attached to the corner seat for children with poor head control. The pommel ensures good abduction with stretching of the adductor, ensuring good seating of the femoral head (Figure 6).

D. COZY SEAT
The Cozy Seat is a multipurpose seat made to support small children approximately 1 to 3 years of age. It can be used as an insert in strollers, highchairs, car seats, toboggans,

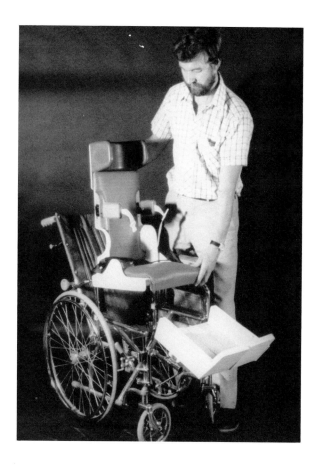

FIGURE 1. Wheelchair inserts can be designed and are available in modular seating systems (Gillette, Otto Bock, or Winnipeg) to be transferred from wheelchair to highchair, to car seat etc. (Reproduced with permission from Letts, M., Rang, M., and Tredwell, S., Seating the disabled, in *American Academy of Orthopaedic Surgeons: Atlas of Orthotics,* 2nd ed., C. V. Mosby, St. Louis, 1985.)

and other commercial bases as well as a free-standing unit on the floor (Figure 7). It is easily transferred from one base to another and therefore can support the child in most daily activities (Figure 8). It is particularly useful in children with difficult feeding problems since it is reclinable and will fit into most highchairs (Figure 9). It can be adapted with head supports and trunk bolsters as well as foot supports, thus providing good supportive seating for those children who have very poor balance.

E. ADAPTED SCHOOL OR OFFICE CHAIRS

Many disabled people can sit in standard chairs if they are modified somewhat to provide just a little more sitting support (Figure 10). This has the advantage of allowing the individual to participate in class activities and not be apt to rely on the wheelchair exclusively for all learning and work-related tasks. The modifications required may be minimal and only require some adjustments to seat height and some foot support for very short children, as in Figure 11. Minor modifications to the chair to provide some trunk support to avoid falling out of the chair may be all that's required (Figure 12). In some instances, a more elaborate support system may have to be added to the chair; however, this may well be more appropriate than wheeling in a wheelchair into a particular environment. The exact requirements of each

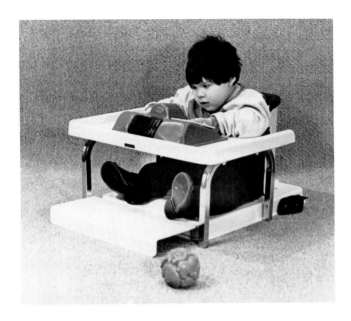

FIGURE 2.   The floor seat provides sitting support to allow floor play activities.

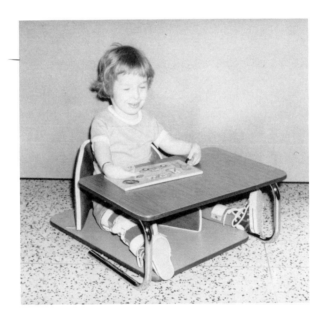

FIGURE 3.   The cerebral palsy floor seat with abduction wings to ensure abduction seating.

patient must be obtained through a good discussion with the individual as well as with the family and teacher and may require a site visit to the school or workplace.

F. BEAN BAG

The bean bag is a very forgiving type of seating support system which provides respite for people of all ages (Figure 13). For some, this will be a fun type of respite seating,

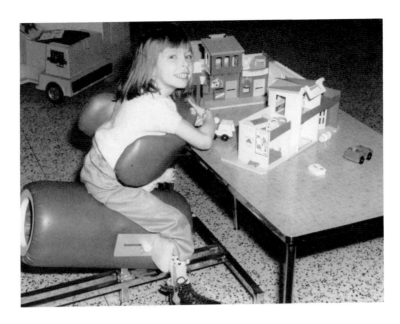

FIGURE 4. The pommel seat provides respite from the wheelchair and ensures abduction seating during play activities.

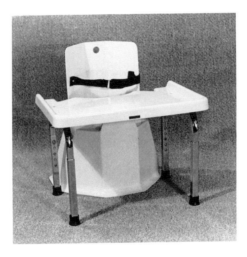

FIGURE 5. The corner seat resembles a corner table, but is a very comfortable and functional chair for seating handicapped children.

whereas in other instances where there are many deformities that almost defy proper seating in conventional devices, the bean bag may well be the most comfortable alternative that can be obtained. These may be mounted on wheels (Figure 14) and used very effectively, especially in institutional environments (Figure 15).

G. EDU-CUBES

Commercially made seating devices such as the Edu-Cube may answer a particular need for the child with mild-to-poor seating balance (Figure 16). Many other commercially available seating devices may well be found on the market from time to time which will answer

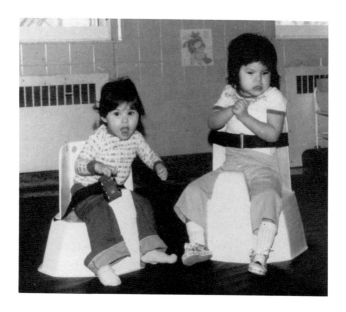

FIGURE 6.   Corner seats ensure abduction seating and can be fitted with higher backs or headrests. (Reproduced with permission from Letts, M., Rang, M., and Tredwell, S., Seating the disabled, in *American Academy of Orthopaedic Surgeons: Atlas of Orthotics,* 2nd ed., C. V. Mosby, St. Louis, 1985.)

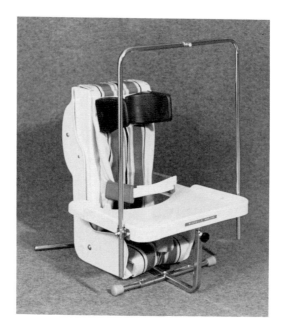

FIGURE 7.   The Cozy Seat fitted with a tray and toy bar.

a particular sitting problem and be more economical than trying to fabricate a special type of seat to address a unique problem for a particular child (Figure 17).

H. SLEEK SEAT

The Sleek Seat was designed to provide relaxation for children with spasticity (Figure 18). The child in this seat assumes the comfortable fetal position which relaxes most of the

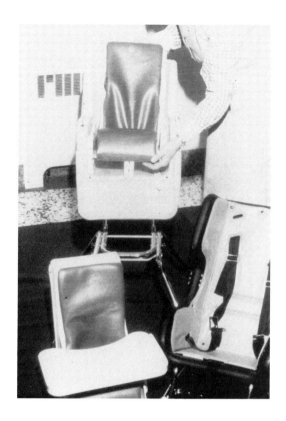

FIGURE 8. The Cozy Seat is easily transferable to high chair, car seat, or stroller.

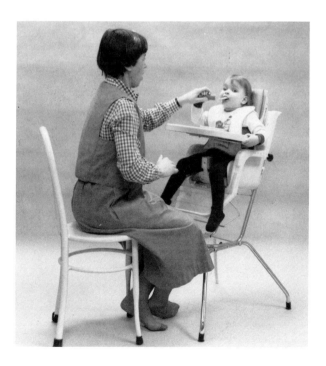

FIGURE 9. The Cozy Seat facilitates feeding especially in children with cerebral palsy.

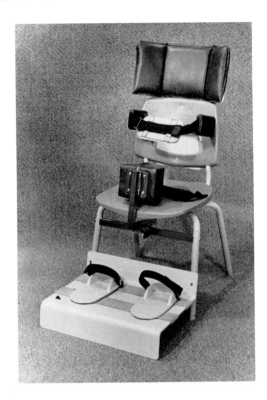

FIGURE 10.   Modified standard chair to enable teenager with cerebral palsy to sit in class.

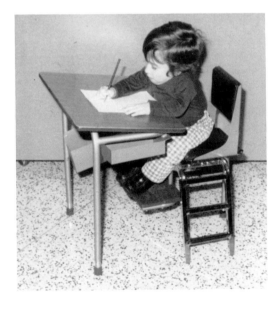

FIGURE 11.   A teenage boy with short stature secondary to spondyloepiphyseal dysplasia able to sit normally at classroom desk with seat elevation and foot support.

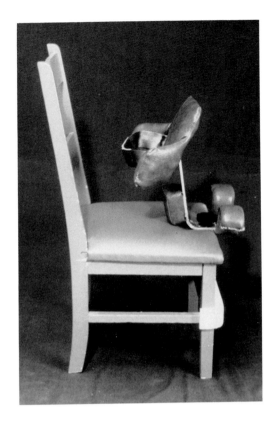

FIGURE 12. Anterior trunk support attached to standard chair.

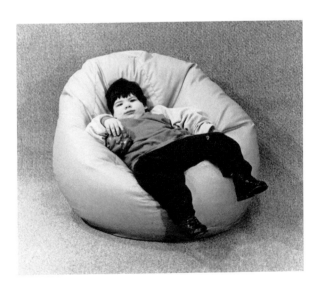

FIGURE 13. The bean bag seating device.

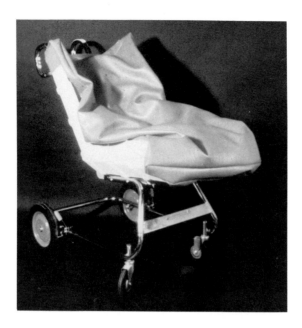

FIGURE 14.   The bean bag mobile seating system.

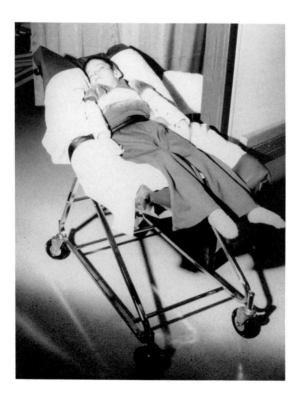

FIGURE 15.   The bean bag chair is applicable to individuals with severe deformity who cannot be seated appropriately in any seating system.

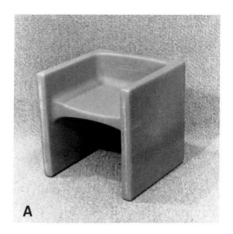

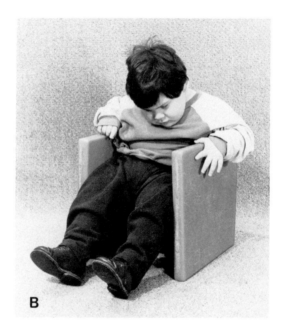

FIGURE 16.   The Edu-Cube seat (A) may be a useful, alternate seating device for some handicapped children (B).

spastic muscle groups. Children with spastic cerebral palsy especially are quite comfortable
in this type of seat, and although one would not wish them to sit for long periods of time
in this position, it does offer a comfortable respite from the wheelchair insert. The seat is
attached to a base with a handle and rear wheel so that it can be easily moved from one site
to another by the caregiver (Figure 19).

I. ADAPTED COMMODES

Toileting children with handicaps is a major problem, especially when cooperation may
be minimal or the type of disability is such that good support is essential to both allay anxiety
and decrease injury, as in osteogenesis imperfecta (OI) children. Commodes can be fabricated
to build in good head support as well as trunk support to facilitate this activity of daily
living (Figure 20).

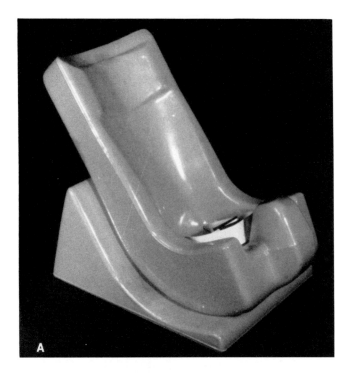

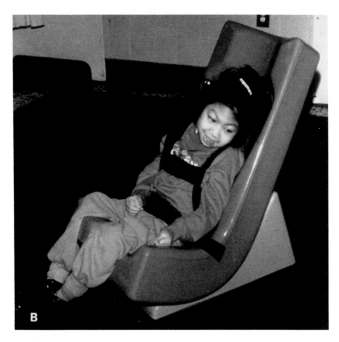

FIGURE 17.   The Tumbleform℠ seat (A) is another example of commercially available alternative respite seating especially for hand-dependent sitters (B). (Reproduced with permission from Letts, M., Rang, M., and Tredwell, S., Seating the disabled, in *American Academy of Orthopaedic Surgeons: Atlas of Orthotics,* 2nd ed., C. V. Mosby, St. Louis, 1985.)

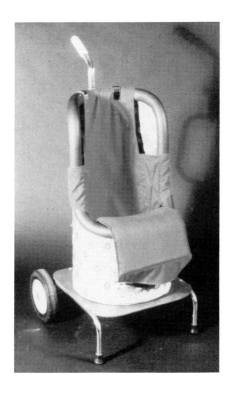

FIGURE 18.   The Sleek Seat.

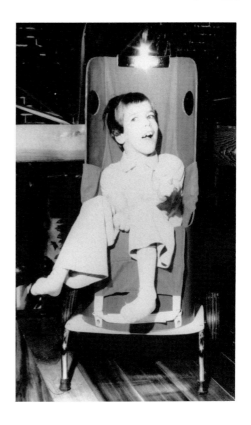

FIGURE 19.   The Sleek Seat allows a return to fetal positioning, one of comfort for children with spasticity.

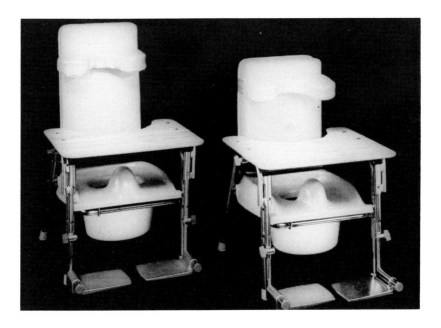

FIGURE 20.   Modified commodes provide supportive toileting for severely handicapped osteogenesis imperfecta (OI) children.

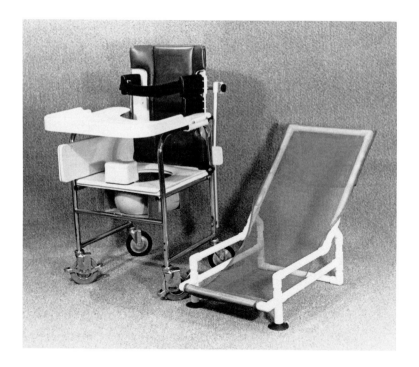

FIGURE 21. Reclining bath seat (right) to assist bathing handicapped wheelchair users; portable commode with trunk bolster and tray (left) to provide seating support during toileting.

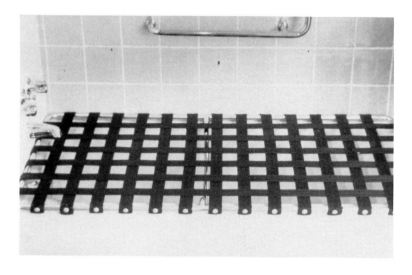

FIGURE 22. Bath frame facilitates bathing of the older handicapped wheelchair user.

J. BATH SEAT

Bathing a handicapped child can be a harrowing experience which doesn't improve as the child gets older. Lightweight but sturdy bath seats can be used to immerse the child in a bath if the child is under good control and support in the bath seat (Figure 21). A bath frame to go over the bathtub is also available or can be fabricated to allow the child to lie on the frame quite comfortably while being showered or washed (Figure 22).

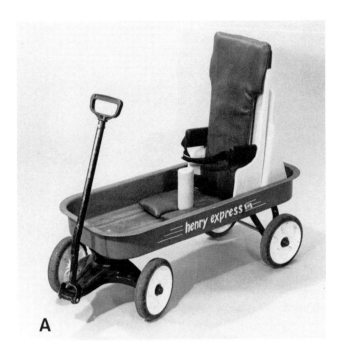

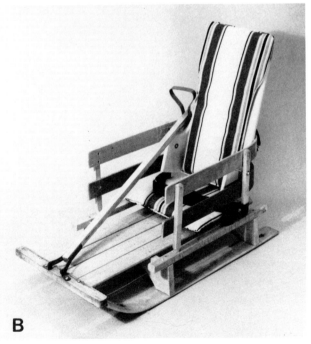

FIGURE 23.   Modular wheelchair inserts can be transferred to other seating devices to enhance seating stability as in (A) wagon and (B) sleigh.

K. TOY MODIFICATION

Children relegated to a wheelchair existence enjoy the same play activities as their ambulatory peers. Modifications to wagons, toboggans, bicycles, and even saddles will allow them to enjoy these activities and obtain some respite from the wheelchair. (Figures 23 and 24). Even rocking horses can have seating support added to allow the handicapped child to participate (Figure 25).

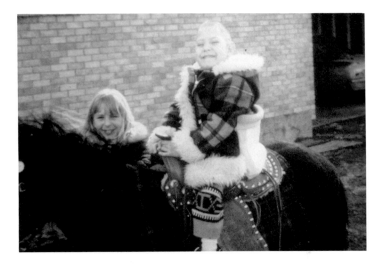

FIGURE 24.   Saddle modified to provide seating support in a child with paraplegia, enabling her to participate in a riding program.

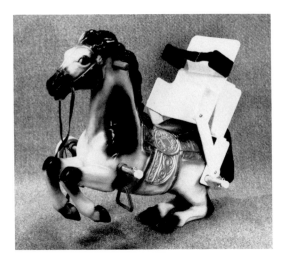

FIGURE 25.   Rocking horse with customized supportive seat for a child with cerebral palsy.

III. SUMMARY

Alternative seating provides respite for the disabled wheelchair user and, in many instances, this is therapeutic and assists in the learning or work experience. The above descriptions of various alternative methods of seating are by no means exhaustive, and each seating team will probably find similar devices in their area which can be purchased or fabricated at minimal cost to provide alternative seating for the handicapped.

Chapter 20

COMMUNICATION IN THE WHEELCHAIR

Arthur Quanbury and Julie Huish

TABLE OF CONTENTS

I. INTRODUCTION

Many individuals who require a wheelchair or other special seating also require alternate and/or augmentative methods of communication to improve their ability to interact with those around them. Some typical examples are the nonverbal cerebral palsy child or adult, stroke patients who have not yet regained their speech, some amyotrophic lateral sclerosis (ALS) patients, head-injured patients whose speech and/or verbal skills have been affected, some spinal cord-injured patients, and some developmentally delayed individuals. In fact, any individual whose interactive communication ability is limited by his/her physical disability is a candidate for some form of communication enhancement.

II. ALTERNATIVE/AUGMENTATIVE COMMUNICATION (AAC) SYSTEMS

Verbal communication is enhanced in a number of ways. Hand gestures, facial expressions, and other subtle or not-so-subtle body cues are used to emphasize the message content of the words we speak.[4] The individual with a physical disability may lack not only the function of clear, intelligible speech, but also these other enhancements that require a high level of physical control. An AAC system must attempt to substitute for as many of these natural abilities as possible as well as to provide an alternative to speech. A picture or Bliss Symbol pointing board used by a cerebral palsy child, a writing board or pencil and paper used by a person with temporary loss of speech, or a computer with voice output to speak messages used by a head-injured person are all examples of AAC communication systems.

III. FACE-TO-FACE VS. WRITTEN COMMUNICATION

People communicate by two primary methods: face-to-face communication, which includes speech and all the body language components associated with it, and written communication for educational purposes, permanent messages, or communication at a distance such as letter writing. An individual in a wheelchair may require an alternative/augmentative method for either or both of these communication types.

IV. ALTERNATE ACCESS TO A COMPUTER

With the current widespread use of computers, the ability to operate a computer is essential for the broadest range of communication function. Operation of a computer can provide not only the ability to use the computer for educational, vocational, and recreational purposes, but also for augmentative/alternative forms of communication (face-to-face or written).

For the individual who cannot use the regular computer keyboard effectively, there are a number of options and alternate access methods available.

Positioning — Position the regular keyboard in a particular way to make it easier to use, such as placing it to one side or the other, resting it on an easel or sloping base, etc. The detached computer keyboards of the Apple IIGS and the IBM and IBM-compatible computers are easier to position than ones integral to the computer body (Figure 1).

Special physical aids — A keyguard can often improve keyboard use with a finger or with a mouth stick or head stick by preventing errors in pushing the incorrect key. A keyguard is a metal or plastic cover that fits over the keyboard keys with a hole for each of the keys (Figure 2). A keylock can be used to hold down more than one key at a time, e.g., the shift and letter keys, when only one finger or a pointer is used.

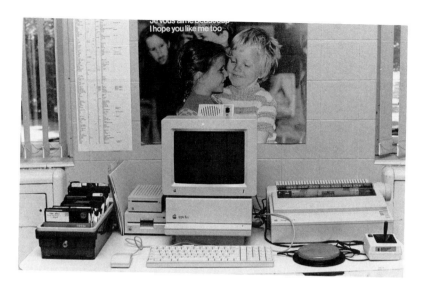

FIGURE 1. Typical setup of a multiaccess computer system with mouse, detached keyboard, single switch, and joystick.

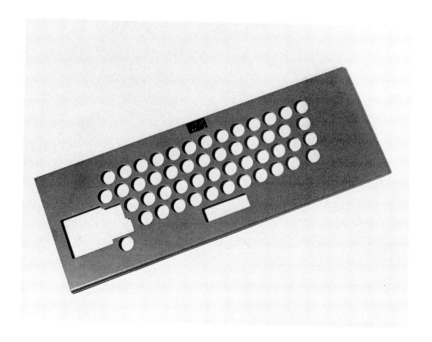

FIGURE 2. Keyguard to improve access to the regular computer keyboard.

Special software — Computers with an MS-DOS or IBM operating system can use special software to improve standard keyboard use by individuals with disabilities. These programs can provide a locking feature for the shift, alt, and control keys for single-finger typing, can slow down or disable the auto repeat function of the keyboard, and can provide abbreviation/expansion facilities and word prediction capabilities to speed up the typing of frequently used words (Figure 3).

Special hardware/software combinations — For individuals who cannot use the standard computer keyboard, special hardware/software systems can be used to provide alternate

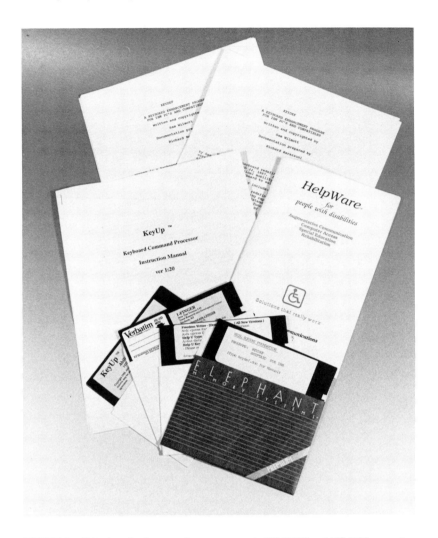

FIGURE 3.   Selection of software to improve access to IBM-DOS and MS-DOS computer.

forms of computer access. The Adaptive Firmware Card for the Apple Computer (Figure 4) allows use of the computer with special keyboards (Figure 5), single-switch scanning methods (Figure 6), or by Morse code input. The PC Serial A.I.D. allows the same range of input methods for IBM and IBM-compatible computers (Figure 7).

V. AIDED VS. NONAIDED SYSTEMS

AAC systems can cover the whole spectrum, from those that require no equipment (nonaided), such as a signing or gesturing system, to those that utilize complex electronic equipment (aided)[1] (Figure 8). In addition, they may be portable or nonportable, may have a permanent form of output (print on paper) or a temporary form of output (light scanning, finger pointing), and may have auditory and/or visual output. The proper selection of an appropriate system will depend on many factors, such as use requirements (functions and locations) as well as on the physical, perceptual, and cognitive abilities of the user.

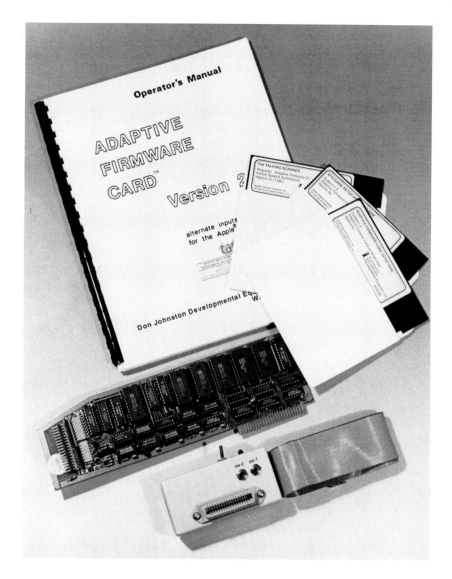

FIGURE 4.   Adaptive Firmware Card to provide alternative access to Apple II family of computers.

VI. COMPONENTS OF AN AAC SYSTEM

An AAC system must replace the functions of speech for face-to-face communication and provide writing ability for written communication. To accomplish this, it must have a vocabulary of message elements, a means of selecting and presenting them, and a set of rules (syntax, grammar) giving a string of message elements meaningful content. In addition, the AAC user must have the necessary discourse strategy skills to use the AAC system effectively in a variety of settings and for a variety of communication purposes (i.e., getting attention, requesting objects/information, clarifying, expanding on a topic, etc.).

VII. VOCABULARY/SYMBOL SYSTEMS

A symbol system is a set of pictures/symbols/words/characters that have a specific meaning associated with them. In order of degree of increasing cognitive requirements,

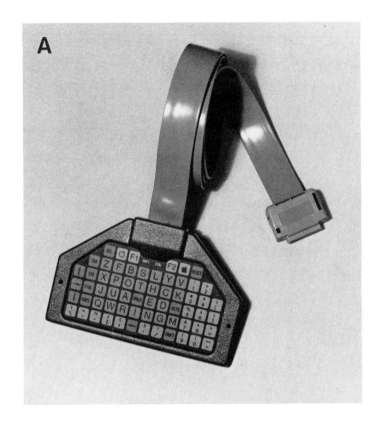

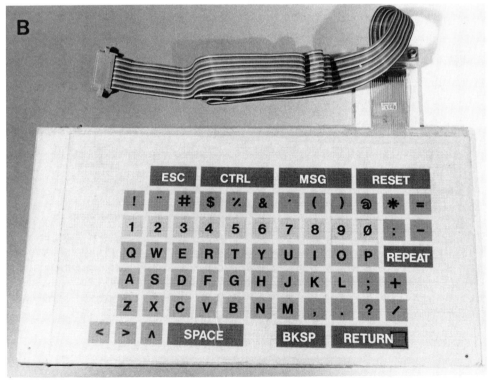

FIGURE 5. Miniature keyboard for alternate keyboard access to computer (A); (B) enlarged keyboard for alternate keyboard access to computer.

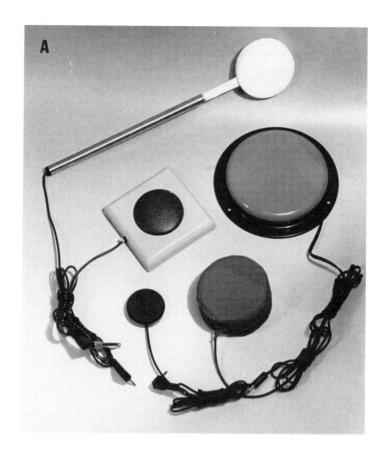

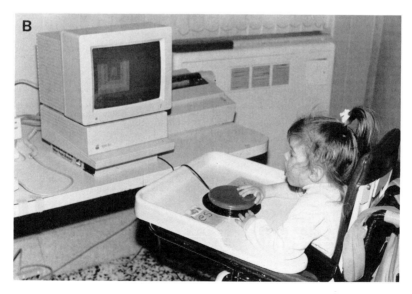

FIGURE 6. Array of switches for single-switch access to computer or other electronic aids (A); (B) using a single switch with a computer program to reinforce cause-and-effect relationship.

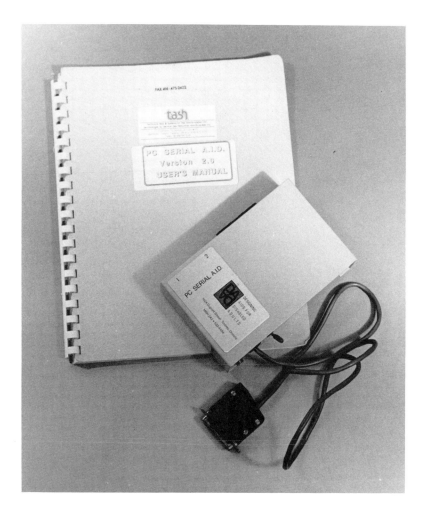

FIGURE 7.   PC Serial A.I.D. to provide alternate access to IBM-DOS and MS-DOS computer systems.

symbols systems would include objects, photographs of objects, line drawings, symbolic drawings (e.g., pictogram ideogram communication, PIC), Bliss symbols, and words (Figure 9). A variety of hand signs, including American Sign Language (ASL), Signing Exact English (SEE), and Amerind, are also options for a nonverbal individual with suitable hand skills. The particular symbol system used with a particular individual will depend on the mental, cognitive, and perceptual ability of the individual as well as the requirements of the AAC system. The vocabulary includes all the symbols/message elements that are needed to satisfy the communication requirements of the individual. Vocabularies are dynamic, growing, and changing as the individual changes, develops, and moves from one environment to another. Vocabulary selection is a complex task.

VIII. A MEANS OF SELECTING/INDICATING

An individual using an AAC system must be able to operate the system in as efficient a manner as possible. Unaided systems generally require only a yes/no response or a means of physically indicating a choice. Aided systems have some form of interface (switch/keyboard) that must be operated by the user in order to control the device.[3] Determining the

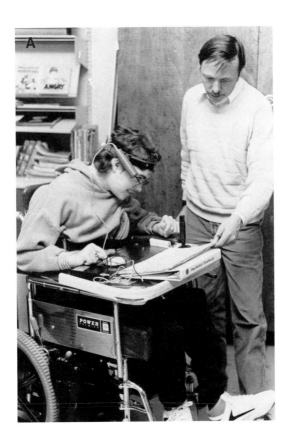

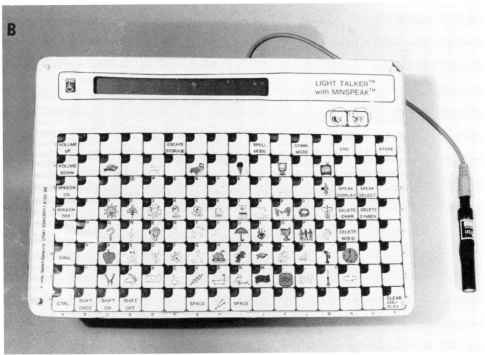

FIGURE 8. Communication with a light-beam head pointer (A); (B) portable, electronic, multiple access communication aid with voice output.

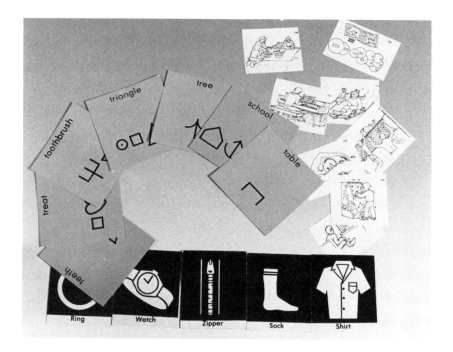

FIGURE 9. Variety of symbol and picture sets for alternate communication.

most appropriate interface, its position, and the part of the body that will be used to operate it requires a very thorough assessment procedure.

The interface used must direct and control the electronic equipment to display the desired message elements. There are three basic methods of achieving this.

Direct Selection — If there is one interface or switch for each message element, that element can be selected directly by pushing the appropriate key/switch. A typewriter or computer keyboard is an example of direct selection because there is a key for each letter of the alphabet (Figure 10). Direct selection is, potentially, the fastest method of selection, but requires the greatest amount of physical control.

Scanning — If the number of interfaces/switches is fewer than the number of message elements, a scanning method can be used to select items. Scanning can be rotary (Figure 11), linear, or row-column (Figure 12). The number of switches used in the scanning approach is typically one, two, or four (see Figure 6).

Encoding — A more abstract method of selection using a small number of switches is encoding. Operating the switches in a particular pattern or code will result in the selection of a particular message item. For example, two switches could be used to produce a Morse code pattern, one switch being used for the ''dits'' and the other for the ''dahs''. Tapping out the appropriate code pattern would produce the corresponding letter of the alphabet. Eye movements can often be used effectively in conjunction with an encoding technique by individuals without reliable limb or head control. An ETRAN Board is a popular method of using eye movements (Figure 13). A coding technique is used to make letter selections from the board by gazing to the group containing the desired letter and then to the corner of the board corresponding to the letter's position in the group.

IX. DISCOURSE SKILLS AND STRATEGIES

The physical components of an AAC system are of little use to an individual who has either no desire or no skills to use them.[4] Unfortunately nonverbal communicators do not

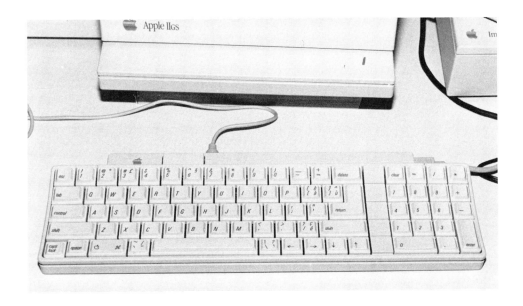

FIGURE 10. Computer keyboard as an example of a direct selection input device.

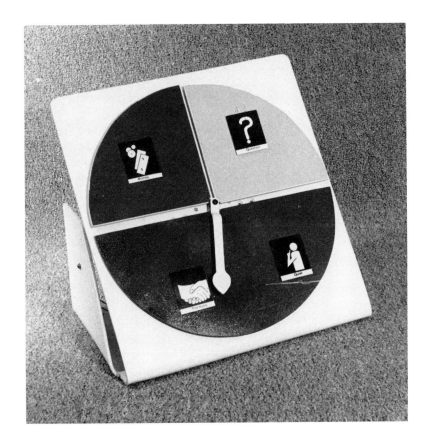

FIGURE 11. A rotary scanning message selector.

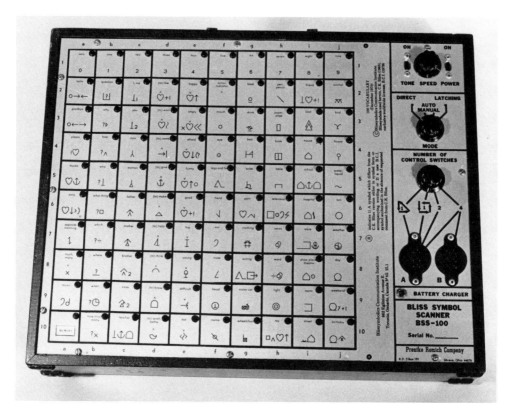

FIGURE 12.   A row-column scanning communication aid.

"automatically" learn discourse skills like verbal individuals do when they are learning to speak. The verbal individual learns discourse skills hand-in-hand with the development of verbal skills, primarily by copying the actions of verbal individuals with already developed skills. The nonverbal individual has no role model to follow. The techniques of getting someone's attention, requesting information, clarifying a point, etc. must all be taught using the AAC system appropriate for the individual. This is particularly true for children who have never had any speech, but is also a factor for adults who have lost their verbal ability and are using a nonverbal method of communication.

X. ASSESSMENT, GOAL SETTING, AND INTERVENTION

Assessment for an AAC system is a multidisciplinary team effort. The team may consist of the client, parents/partners/caregivers, teachers, occupational therapists, engineers, and speech-language pathologists, among others. In assessing for a communication system, a detailed look at the individual's capabilities as well as the requirements of the system and constraints of the environment is necessary. Critical to the development of an AAC system is an understanding of the client's expressive and receptive language skills, cognitive and perceptual abilities, vision, sensation, and hearing. Also to be considered are the age and development potential of the client.

The individual should be properly positioned in a wheelchair before beginning any physical assessment. At least one voluntary behavior is needed to produce alternate communication. When the best behavior(s) have been established, the range which can be accessed (with limb, head pointer, mouthstick, light pointer, etc.) needs to be determined. The accuracy within this range will dictate the size of the symbols/digits/switches which

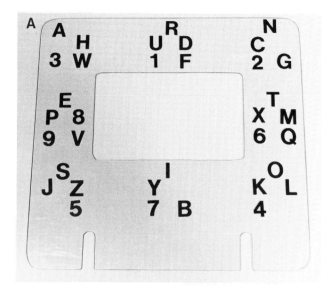

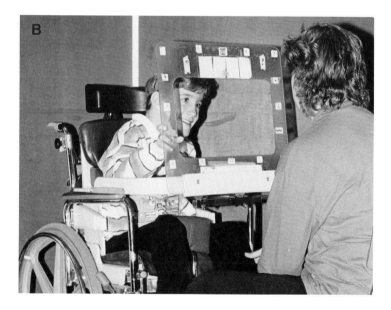

FIGURE 13. ETRAN board to allow communication using eye gazing (A); (B) communication by eye gaze and ETRAN communication board.

can be used. A small range or poor accuracy may preclude direct selection. Other physical considerations may be activation force (affects which input device can be used), reaction time, reliability, and fatigue.

Requirements of the system which need to be considered are when, where, and how often the system will be used, who the communication partners are likely to be, how portable, durable, and cleanable the system is, how it will be mounted on the wheelchair, and how compatible it will be with other systems which may be used. The output requirements (voice, visual display, and written copy), the amount and type of feedback necessary, and the room for expansion will influence the choice of system.

Individuals must be trained in the use of AAC systems, and those close to the user must be trained to be effective communication partners. The most meaningful systems should be usable and used throughout the individual's daily routine and in all environments.[2]

There is an ever-growing number of excellent books and references addressing the many areas of augmentative communication and the delivery of AAC service. The following references contain a number of the more current ones.

REFERENCES

1. **Bengston, D., Bradenburg, S., and Vanderheiden, G. C.,** *Non-Vocal Communication Resource Book,* Trace Research and Development Center, Madison, WI, 1985.
2. **Blackson, S. W., Cassatt-James, E. L., and Bruskin, D. M.,** Teaching effective use of communication aids and techniques, in *Augmentative Communication — Implementing Strategies,* Blackstone, S. W., Cassatt-James, E. L., and Bruskin, D. M., Eds., American Speech-Language-Hearing Association, Rockville, MD, 1988, chap. 5.
3. **Fishman, I.,** *Electronic Communication Aids and Techniques: Selection and Use,* College Hill Press, San Diego, 1987.
4. **Vanerheiden, G. C. and Yoder, D. E.,** Overview, in *Augmentative Communication, An Introduction,* Blackstone, S. W. and Bruskin, D. M., Eds., American Speech-Language-Hearing Association, Rockville, MD, 1986, chap. 1.

Chapter 21

SEATING AND SPORTS

R. Mervyn Letts

TABLE OF CONTENTS

I. INTRODUCTION

Following World War II, there was a tremendous increase in the number of young, previously active individuals who were relegated to a wheelchair existence because of a spinal cord injury sustained during conflict. To provide recreation as well as rehabilitation therapy for this group of active individuals, Sir Ludwig Guttmann, then Director of the National Spine Injury Centre in England, introduced a program of wheelchair sports primarily for paraplegic war veterans.[11] This was shown to have superb physical and psychological value in the rehabilitation process for the paraplegic population. In North America, this trend also developed under the auspices of the Paralyzed Veterans of America and in Canada it developed through the Canadian Paraplegic Association. Basketball was one of the first sports to be played and organized by the wheelchair athletic community. In 1949, the National Wheelchair Basketball Association was formed, with teams competing from all over the U.S. and, ultimately, internationally. Once the concept of wheelchair athletics was shown to be of great value and, indeed, of interest to the nondisabled spectator population as well, other sports were entered into by the wheelchair athletic population. The National Wheelchair Athletic Association was formed in 1958, governing competition in archery, swimming, track and field events, and weight lifting.[3]

It was a great achievement for wheelchair sports that in 1976 the first Olympiad for the physically disabled was held in Toronto, Ontario.[12] At that time, more than 1500 disabled athletes, many in wheelchairs, competed from 38 countries. These competitions have continued, and in October 1988, over 3000 athletes competed in 19 events at the Eighth Para Olympics in Seoul, South Korea.

II. LEVELS OF PARTICIPATION FOR WHEELCHAIR ATHLETES

Since there are many reasons why an individual must use a wheelchair, the degree of disability must be classified to provide fair and equal competition. To avoid athletes with generalized impairments such as quadriplegia or muscular dystrophy having to compete against a paraplegic with normal upper extremity function, a classification system has been devised by both the National Wheelchair Association and the National Wheelchair Basketball Association to allow individuals with similar disabilities to compete against each other (Table 1).

These competitions are now much more advanced than simply a form of rehabilitation, although they still function very much as an important rehabilitation medium and really are an outlet for wheelchair users to test their skills and develop a maximum level of physical performance.[10] Associated with this are improved self-image, a greater degree of independence, and increased physical fitness.[1,2,4]

III. SPORTS WHEELCHAIRS

Just as the wheelchair athlete has become a participant in almost every athletic endeavor, the wheelchair manufacturing community also had to strive to keep up to the technology required to enable these athletes to compete to the maximum of their abilities. Many of the innovative designs and suggestions have actually come from participating wheelchair athletes (Figure 1). It is beyond the scope of this chapter to deal with all of the various lightweight sports wheelchairs which have, indeed, revolutionized the wheelchair industry, since many ''nonathletic wheelchair users'' prefer to have lightweight chairs simply because they are easier to propel and transport and have a certain image about them that is psychologically pleasing to users, regardless of whether they are athletes! There are over 30 companies in

TABLE 1
Classification Systems for Wheelchair Athletes

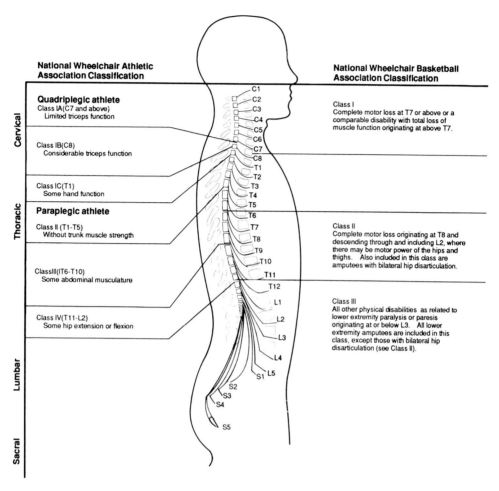

National Wheelchair Athletic Association Classification	National Wheelchair Basketball Association Classification
Quadriplegic athlete Class IA(C7 and above) Limited triceps function	**Class I** Complete motor loss at T7 or above or a comparable disability with total loss of muscle function originating at above T7.
Class IB(C8) Considerable triceps function	
Class IC(T1) Some hand function	
Paraplegic athlete	
Class II (T1-T5) Without trunk muscle strength	**Class II** Complete motor loss originating at T8 and descending through and including L2, where there may be motor power of the hips and thighs. Also included in this class are amputees with bilateral hip disarticulation.
ClassIII(IT6-T10) Some abdominal musculature	
Class IV(T11-L2) Some hip extension or flexion	**Class III** All other physical disabilities as related to lower extremity paralysis or paresis originating at or below L3. All lower extremity amputees are included in this class, except those with bilateral hip disarticulation (see Class II).

Modified from Schaefer, R. S. and Proffer, D. S., *Am. Fam. Physician*, 39, 239, 1989.

North America that produce lightweight sports-type wheelchairs, with many designs for specific athletic endeavors, such as racing, basketball, tennis, etc. (Figure 2). Most of these chairs now have standard components, quick-release wheels, modular construction, and adjustable axle positions and are very lightweight, on the order of 20 to 30 lb, with some ultralightweights weighing only 14 to 17 lb.[3,7] Many are adjustable, and some companies will even manufacture the wheelchair directly to the specifications of the individual athlete (Figure 3). With improvement in the design and innovative mechanical features of the chair have come improvements in the quality of the chairs, and many lightweight wheelchairs come in a variety of colors and designs, with competition coloring available for team sports. The improved design of athletic chairs has been a great asset to the overall wheelchair user population since a number of the features used in these chairs are now standard for all wheelchairs (Figure 4). The aluminum construction has been found to be very durable and has led to a marked decrease in the weight of most wheelchairs. The modular construction utilized for athletic chairs, primarily to allow the athletes to change back heights and seat widths, has now been applied to standard wheelchair models. The ability to adjust the widths

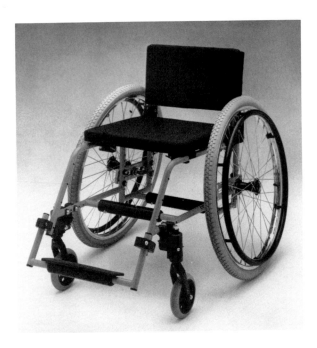

FIGURE 1.   The Enduro "Bantam". A sports wheelchair for children constructed of lightweight titanium and weighing only 13 lb. Seat height is adjustable. Note cambered wheels and adjustable one-piece footrest. (Courtesy of Wheel Ring, Inc., Manchester, CT.)

of the wheelchairs has also been a great advantage, allowing wheelchair users to get through narrow doorways and passageways. Improved balancing of the wheels for responsive, easy rolling and the popularity of pneumatic tires together with improved balance between the front and rear axels has enhanced the responsiveness of the chair for all wheelchair users. The names that have been given to various manufacturers' designs for various models of the sports wheelchair also reflect the dynamic development that is occurring and has occurred in this field, e.g., Eagle IV, Hurricane II, Ultralight Lightening, Champion 2000, Shadow One, Glove Rover, and Quickie, to name a few.

A testimony to the athletic endurance of the wheelchair athlete was exemplified by Mr. Rick Hansen, who in 1987 wheeled his chair around the world in a tremendous feat of stamina and endurance and in the process raised millions of dollars for spinal cord research in Canada (Figure 5).

A. ADVANTAGES

Many of the advantages of the sports wheelchair have been alluded to in the previous discussion; however, it often is not recognized that the wheelchair becomes part of the body image of the wheelchair owner. Because of this, the chair becomes a reflection of the user and therefore must be acceptable to the owner and project the image the user wishes to project. The sports wheelchair is capable of all these requirements. A major advantage is that they do not look as if they had been designed for a handicapped person, as many of the older, standard wheelchairs often did. For the younger wheelchair user who is still physically active, the sports chair is a welcome alternative to a more standard seating device (Figure 6).

The role of sports in rehabilitation is self-evident, but at the same time, sports activities assist the individual to feel self-confident and to leave what is sometimes an isolated environment (Figure 7). It also provides an opportunity to participate in sports activities with the able-bodied, such as table tennis and wheelchair tennis.

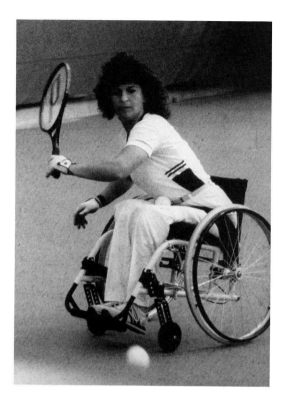

FIGURE 2. The tennis wheelchair with low back to allow freedom of trunk movement, large hand rims for rapid acceleration, and low hip position for increased stability. The rules of wheelchair tennis are identical to those of standard tennis except two bounces are allowed the wheelchair player.

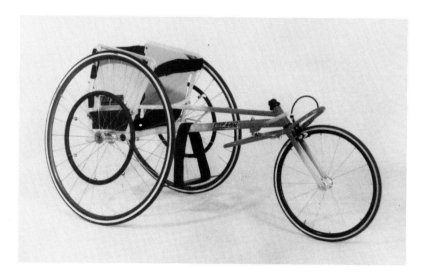

FIGURE 3. Top End Racer. A three-wheeled racing sports wheelchair illustrating many innovative design features to enhance speed and competitiveness such as large, cambered drive wheels, low-slung seat, and small hand rims. (Courtesy of Top End, Inc., Pinellas Park, FL.)

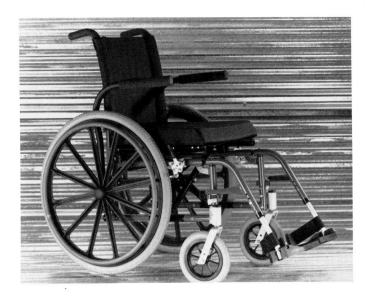

FIGURE 4. The "Quickie". An example of sports wheelchair technology applied to chairs for regular, everyday usage. This chair is lightweight and designed for the active child user. It has many of the features of a sports chair incorporated into its construction. (Courtesy of Quickie Designs, Inc., Fresno, CA.)

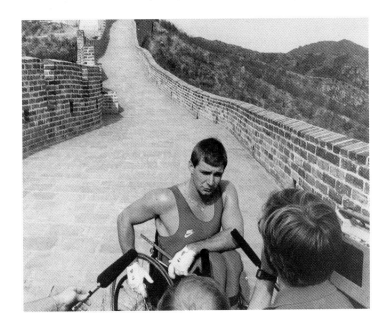

FIGURE 5. Rick Hansen on the Great Wall of China during his wheelchair marathon around the world in his lightweight sports wheelchair.

The direct interaction between disabled athletes and the manufacturing community has resulted in a better understanding of the needs of the wheelchair community, with the result that engineering innovations are being discovered and applied to solve many problems that plagued the more standard designs in the past. For example, the center of gravity of the chair can now be changed, depending upon the particular sports activity that is being carried

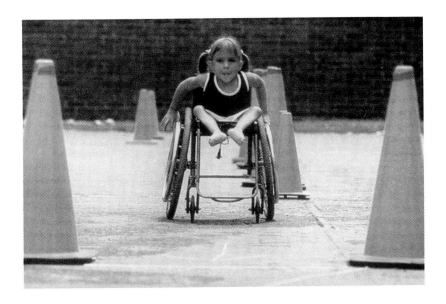

FIGURE 6. Ultralightweight sports wheelchairs may be appropriate for everyday use for users such as this little girl with paraplegia, but with normal upper extremities and good trunk stability.

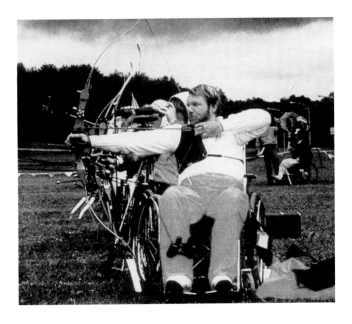

FIGURE 7. The wheelchair serves as a stable platform for such sport activities as archery or bowling.

on or on the size and ability of the wheelchair user.[6] This can only aid in the future development of a more efficient and supportive chair. New materials such as titanium, graphite tubes, and aircraft aluminum have all decreased the weight of the chair. It remains for industry to design an adjustable wheelchair seat and to provide good torso support similar to the adjustability of automobile seats (Figure 8). Through the medium of sports, wheelchair users themselves are directing the design and development of their own vehicles, and this

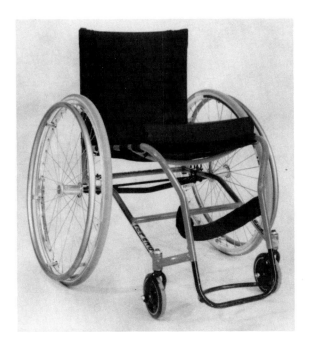

FIGURE 8. Basketball sports wheelchair with high-set seat, solid
front casters, large hand rims for rapid acceleration, and removable
seatback to allow change to low back during actual participation.
(Courtesy of Top End, Inc., Pinellas Park, FL.)

is exactly what needs to happen, rather than the able-bodied attempting to identify all the
problems and needs and rectifying them in a unilateral manner.[19]

There is now development of a series of wheelchairs that fall between the sports wheelchair and the ''standard wheelchair''. Many of the innovations and advantages of sports
wheelchairs have now been put into wheelchairs for regular use such as negative wheelchair
camber and adjustable centers of gravity. These features combined with the very pleasing
appearance of the wheelchair are much more acceptable to both the athletic and nonathletic
wheelchair populations.[15]

B. DISADVANTAGES

The popularity of the design of sports wheelchairs and the positive image that they
portray for the wheelchair user have made such chairs very attractive, especially to the
younger wheelchair user. Unfortunately, the sports wheelchair, unless modified, does not
provide much upper body support because of the low backrest and, in some instances, an
absence of sturdy armrests. Such chairs have to be carefully prescribed in order to avoid
problems with the progression of scoliosis and increase in kyphosis or marked fatigue from
no support in the upper body. It is possible to provide some modification to the seats of
sports wheelchairs, but this is at the expense of the appearance and image of these chairs.
A compromise has to be reached between the needs of the wheelchair user and their desire
to have the sporty, low-profile, speedy type of chair. This is one of the modern roles of the
seating clinic and may require tact, time, and a careful explanation of the goals required
for good stable sitting for the particular individual.

IV. NONWHEELCHAIR SPORTS

The seating team may be asked to address modifications to standard sports equipment
such as toboggans or sleighs in order to allow participation in sports activities that do not

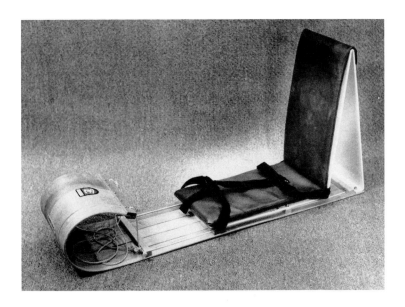

FIGURE 9.   Custom-made back support for toboggan to facilitate sitting for child with poor trunk control. (Courtesy of Erika von Kampen, Rehabilitation Centre for Children, Winnipeg, Manitoba.)

require wheelchair use (Figure 9). In most instances, this basically will be the provision of trunk support to prevent the individual from falling to the side and out of the device, be it a toboggan, sleigh, snowmobile, or saddle! This requires some innovation on the part of the seating clinic, but is usually achievable. A new sport that is becoming very popular is sledge hockey, which is played on sleighs with small runners, with rules similar to those in regular hockey (Figure 10). Back support may be required for some players. This sport is one started primarily for the nonambulatory, however, the ambulatory population now participates and is becoming interested in it as a sport for the able-bodied as well!

V. POWERED RECREATIONAL EQUIPMENT

Powered-wheelchair competitive events are increasing in acceptability and frequency. Hopefully, as more powered sports activities occur, the design and development that has occurred with manual wheelchairs will also take place with powered wheelchairs.

The power capability allows the disabled individual to participate in a number of sports activities, such as hunting, fishing, or hikes through the woods, over terrain only accessible by powered vehicles such as snowmobiles or all-terrain vehicles. The concept that the powered wheelchair is a symbol of greater disability must be erased in the minds of both the disabled themselves and the health care professionals. For many disabled persons, the powered chair saves an immense amount of time and effort and results in a remarkable improvement in the quality of life. Powered mobility will probably never be as popular in the sports arena as in manual sports wheelchair athletics; however, for those individuals who require powered chairs or who prefer them over manual chairs, it is hoped that a similar availability of sports activities will develop.

VI. INJURY PREVENTION IN WHEELCHAIR SPORTS

Injuries to wheelchair athletes can occur from entanglement within their own chair and from falls due to tipping of the chair and direct contact with other wheelchairs.

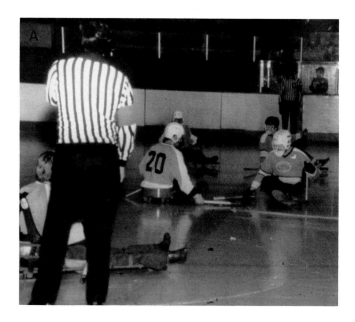

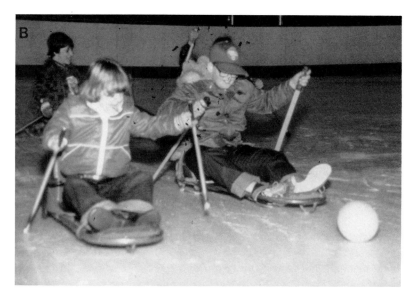

FIGURE 10.   Sledge hockey can be played by (A) adults or (B) children; the player is strapped into a sledge and propelled by ice pick poles. The poles are used to propel the ball.

Stability of the chair is of utmost importance to prevent tipping and outright falls out of the chair. To enhance stability, the wheels of the sports chair are cambered (angled in at the top) to provide a wider base for the chair and also an improved mechanical advantage for wheeling the chair. Spoke protectors can be applied to the drive wheels to prevent breakage by footrests of opposing players as well as to prevent feet from becoming entangled. There is now an international agreement that, in an attempt to minimize leg injuries, sports wheelchairs must have a standard footrest height of 10 cm above the ground, with the seat no higher than 50 cm above the ground. Leg straps around the legrests and behind the legs keep the feet from sliding off the foot supports and becoming entangled in the wheelchair or sustaining burns from the floor.[5,17,18]

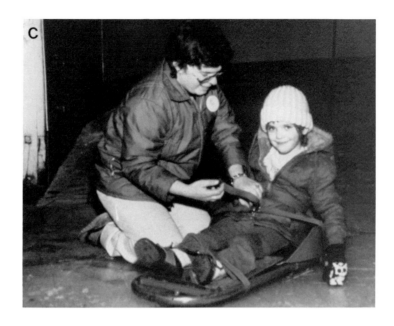

FIGURE 10 (continued).   (C) The player is strapped into a sledge.

VII. WHEELCHAIR SPORTS INJURIES

Data concerning the incidence of injury to the wheelchair athlete are sparse. Curtis and Dillon,[8] in a survey of wheelchair athletic injuries which occurred in 1200 wheelchair athletes, found that 72% of the respondents reported at least one injury. These usually occurred in track, basketball, and road racing. Most injuries were to soft tissue, consisting of upper extremity strains, sprains, bursitis, and tendonitis, with an unusually high incidence of shoulder pain and rotator cuff injury. It is well known that there is a high incidence of shoulder injury in paraplegics who use wheelchairs.[20] The typical overuse syndromes seen in many athletes also occur in the wheelchair athlete, with tenosynovitis and soft tissue strains about the wrist, elbow, and shoulder being the most common.[14,18]

Trauma to the fingers as a result of contact with the chair's push rim or tire as well as recurrent sprain of the metacarpal phalangeal joint of the thumb because of contact with the push rim is not uncommon. Taping of the hands and fingers and protective gloves help to minimize these injuries in track athletes.[16]

Blistering of the hands is the second most frequent injury seen in the wheelchair athlete. The constant friction and contact with the wheelchair push rim results in blistering if protective gloves are not worn. Those wheelchair athletes with impaired sensation also may develop pressure sores over the sacral and ischial tuberosities during training and competition. This is accentuated due to the sweating and shear pressure that occurs during the athletic endeavor. If the wheelchair design results in the knees being higher than the buttocks, pressure will be increased over the sacral and ischial tuberosities, thus accentuating pressure in these vulnerable areas. This type of chair should be avoided for those athletes prone to pressure sores.

The spinal-injured wheelchair athlete will be particularly susceptible to hyperthermia and hypothermia due to the loss of normal sympathetic nervous control of body temperature and sweating below the level of the lesion. The combination of dehydration and intense athletic endeavor such as in a marathon race may result in the development of hyperthermia.[13] These athletes need to ensure an adequate fluid intake during the competition to minimize the development of hyperthermia. Hypothermia may occur after the athletic endeavor has

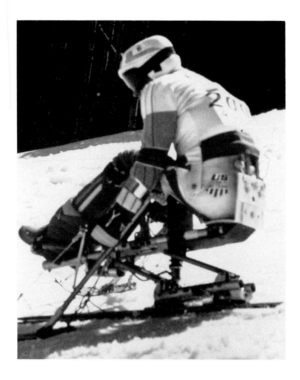

FIGURE 11. Seated skiing illustrating the innovation and technical possibilities allowing the nonambulatory to participate in virtually any sport! (From Michael, J. W., Gailey, R. S., and Bowker, J. H., *Clin. Orthop.*, 256, 64, 1990. With permission.)

been completed, especially in colder environments. Additional layers of clothing for protection against the loss of body heat are essential.

VIII. SUMMARY

Wheelchair sports have now obtained a very prominent place in the lifestyle of the wheelchair user. The advantages to both the wheelchair athlete and the entire wheelchair community through the improvement of wheelchair technology have been immense. The seating team must ensure that they are knowledgeable in this field so that appropriate prescriptions for wheelchairs and appropriate advice regarding the amount of support required for these athletic endeavors can be given. In some instances, these chairs will have to be modified to allow a disabled athlete to participate safely. Some guidance will also have to be given for those individuals who become so attached to their sports chair that they would prefer to use them as their permanent chair. In some instances, this may be appropriate; in others, an analogy must be developed for the athlete so that he/she will think of the sports wheelchair in the same way that the able-bodied individual relates to specialized running shoes for specialized sports! A sports wheelchair may be very appropriate for an evening basketball game, but will not provide the user with enough support during school activities or at the workplace. Attention must be paid to the prevention of injury through provision of appropriate protection for the athlete and a good stable, functional sports wheelchair. This is an exciting area of development for the wheelchair disabled and one that is still evolving and improving (Figure 11).

APPENDIX
MANUFACTURERS OF LIGHTWEIGHT SPORTS CHAIRS

Active Life Wheelchairs, Inc., P. O. Box 3926, Pinedale, CA 93650

Alt Design, South Third Street, P. O. Box 128, Wood Lake, MN 56297

CBS Custom Chairs, 1014 Main Street, Vancouver, British Columbia, Canada V6A 2WI

Cycling Future Co., 239 13th Street, Winnipeg, Manitoba, Canada

E & G Sportschairs, 2351 Parkwood Road, Snellville, GA 30278

Everest & Jennings, Inc., 3233 East Mission Oaks Boulevard, Camarillo, CA 93010

Hand Crafted Metals, Inc., 13710 49th Street North, Clearwater, FL 33520-3735

Invacare Corporation, 899 Cleveland Street, P. O. Box 4028, Elyria, OH 44036-2125

Magnium Poirier, Inc., One Madison Street, East Rutherford, NJ 07073

Motion Designs Inc., Marketing Department, 2842 Business Park Avenue, Fresno, CA 93727

Ortho-Kinetics, Inc., W220 N507 Springdale Road, P. O. Box 436, Waukesha, WI 53187

Quadra Medical Corporation, P. O. Box 7719, Thousand Oaks, CA 91360

Top End, Inc., 6551 44th Street North, 5002 Enterprise Business Park, Pinellas Park, FL 33565

Wheel Ring, Inc., East Coast 199 Forest Street, Manchester, CT 06040

REFERENCES

1. *Sports and Recreational Programs for the Child and Young Adult with Physical Disabilities,* AAOS Doc. No. 993-883, American Academy of Orthopedic Surgeons, Chicago, 1983.
2. **Beaver, D. P., Jackson, R. W., McCann, C., Messmard, G., and Ryan, A. J.,** Sports and recreation for the handicapped, *Physician Sports Med.,* 6, 44, 1978.
3. **Bernt, J.,** Wheelchairs designed for activity in sports, *J. Rehabil. Res.,* 10, 4, 1987.
4. **Bowker, J. H., Edwards, C., and Smeltzer, J. S.,** Orthotic and adaptive devices for recreation and driving, *American Academy of Orthopaedic Surgeons: Atlas of Orthotics,* 2nd ed., C. V. Mosby, St. Louis, 1985, 487.
5. **Corcoren, P. J., Goldman, R. F., and Hoernar, E. F.,** Sports medicine and the physiology of wheelchair marathon racing, *Orthop. Clin. North Am.,* 11, 697, 1980.
6. **Coutes, K. D.,** Kinomatics of sport wheelchair propulsion, *J. Rehabil. Res. Dev.,* 27, 21, 1990.
7. **Crase, N., Robins, S., and Schmid, R.,** Fifth annual survey of the lightweights, *Sports Spokes,* 12, 17, 1987.
8. **Curtis, K. A. and Dillon, D. A.,** Survey of wheelchair athletic injuries; common patterns and prevention, *Paraplegia,* 23, 170, 1985.
9. **Davis, G. M., Jackson, R. W., and Sheppard, R. J.,** Sports and recreation for the physically disabled, in *Sports Medicine,* Strauss, R. H., Ed., W. B. Saunders, Philadelphia, 1984, 286.
10. **Gairdner, J.,** *Fitness for the Disabled; Wheelchair Users,* Fitzhenry and Whitside, Toronto, 1983.
11. **Guttmann, L.,** Development of sports for the disabled, in *Sport in the Modern World; Problems and Chances,* Grupe, O., Ed., Springer-Verlag, Berlin, 1973, 254.
12. **Jackson, R. W. and Fredrickson, A.,** Sports for the physically disabled. The 1976 Olympiad, Toronto, *Am. J. Sports Med.,* 7, 293, 1979.
13. **Labanowichs, J.,** The physically disabled in sports, *Sports Spokes,* 12, 33, 1987.
14. **Madorsky, J. G. and Curtis, K. A.,** Wheelchair sports medicine, *Am. J. Sports Med.,* 12, 128, 1984.
15. **Michael, J. W., Gailey, R. S., and Bowker, J. H.,** New developments in recreational prosthesis and adaptive devices for the amputee, *Clin. Orthop. Rel. Res.,* 256, 64, 1990.
16. **Ragnarsson, K. T.,** Prescription considerations and a comparison of conventional and lightweight wheelchairs, *J. Rehabil. Res. Dev. Clin. Suppl.,* 2, 8, 1989.
17. **Schaefer, R. S. and Proffer, E. S.,** Sports medicine for wheelchair athletes, *Am. Fam. Physician,* 39, 239, 1989.
18. **Sheppard, R. J.,** Sports medicine in the wheelchair athlete, *Sports Med.,* 4, 226, 1988.
19. **Walsh, C. M., Marchiori, C. E., and Steadward, R. D.,** Effect of seat position on maximal linear velocity in wheelchair sprinting, *Can. J. Appl. Sports Sci.,* 11, 186, 1986.
20. **Wing, P. C. and Tredwell, S. J.,** The weight bearing shoulder, *Paraplegia,* 21, 107, 1983.

Chapter 22

THE HISTORY OF WHEELCHAIRS

Richard A. F. Perry

For man to sit has been a natural act from the beginning of time. With the passage of time, man has gone from sitting or squatting on the ground to sitting on carpets, mats, and cushions and then to chairs. The earliest chairs possibly were of ancient Egyptian origin, and these closely resembled the modern "camp stool" of today. The National Museum of Athens has a statue of a figure seated in a chair dating to about 2900 BC.

Evidence suggests that the wheel is older than the chair. Two- or four-wheeled carts were known in Sumeria and Assyria as early as 3500 BC. Putting the horse and cart together to serve man probably occurred in the second or third millennium BC in Mesopotamia, spreading quickly to Syria and then to Egypt. Chariots were certainly in widespread use in the area of the Holy Lands about 2000 BC. These used spoked wheels. However, the chair and the wheel were not formally introduced to carry the sick and infirm until the fifth century AD. Until that time, family members, servants, or slaves were the choice of transportation over the bad and bumpy roads of that era. A Chinese sarcophagus, now housed in Kansas City, MO, is decorated with many scenes. Among them is one of a gentleman seated upon a three-wheeled cart. This is dated about 525 AD[2,9] (Figure 1).

During the Middle Ages and Renaissance periods, a simple and versatile vehicle, the wheelbarrow, became quite appreciated. The invention has been attributed to Jugo Lyang (or Chu-Ko-Liang), a Chinese, in the third century AD. It found its way to Europe by way of the Crusades around the 12th century. It was soon adapted to the transport of the sick and dead. The painting, "The Fountain of Youth", by Lucas Cranach, dated 1546, depicts sick and lame individuals arriving on litters and in wheelbarrows and then led away under their own power after bathing in the mystical waters.[9] From litters to wheelbarrows, the return to litters for the gentry came about due to the lack of dignity the efficient and comfortable wheelbarrow provided.[2]

Applying wheels to chairs seemed popular around the 15th century. As time passed, these "comfort chairs" or "invalid chairs" became more elaborate, with armrests, recliners, and head wings. King Philip of Spain (1527 to 1598) was a long-standing gout sufferer. His "invalid chair", made for him by Flemish nobleman Johen Lhermite, featured reclining armrests and elevating legrests with footboard, all covered with a horsehair mattress. His Majesty was well pleased.[9]

Most invalid chairs of this era basically were rollers on heavily padded armchairs. For ease of transportation and not ease of the patient, wheels were applied to only one pair of legs. Also, the chairs were only for indoor use since the small wheels could not function on the poor roads of medieval Europe. Responsibility for outdoor excursions reverted to family members, servants, or slaves with strong backs to carry slings, litters, or sedan chairs.

Rolling chairs of the 17th century required able-bodied individuals to push them since they were quite heavy and cumbersome. Self-propelled wheelchairs, which featured hand cranks for paraplegics, were devised by Johann Hautsch of Nuremberg. Again, these were indoor chairs. Near the end of the 17th century, comfort became an important goal of chairmakers for the healthy as well as the wealthy. So comfortable were they that Louis XIV of France used them after his "Grande Operation" (closure of an anal fistula) in 1686. Entire days were spent in his "roulette". In 1700, the palace at Versailles contained 20 such chairs.[9]

Comfort, it was found, was important in the 17th century, and in the 18th century this concept was expanded. Adaptation to contours of the human body was as esthetic as it was

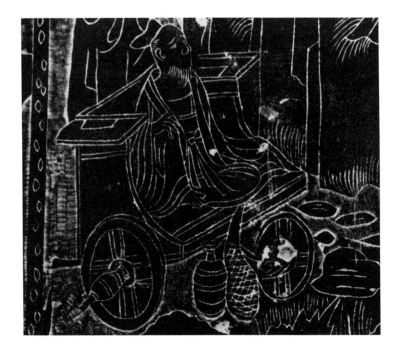

FIGURE 1.   Chinese sarcophagus ca. 525 AD. (From Kamenetz, H. L., *The Wheel-chair Book,* Charles C Thomas, Springfield, IL, 1969. With permission.)

practical. Wheels also were modified to enable self-propulsion. It was in the first half of the 1700s that two wheels large enough for the occupant to turn and a smaller pivoting rear wheel became a true precursor to the modern wheelchair. One noble manufacturer devised a leather belt suspension system that changed the center of gravity of the chair according to the plane in which the chair moved. For propulsion, the inside wheel moved, with power provided by the individual in the chair via crank and cog. Prior to this chair, all others were for indoor use.

During the 19th century, the Bath chair dominated the scene. It was developed in Bath, England at the site of the famous spas. The Bath chair was invented by John Dawson in 1798. The innovations he wrought earned him the title of ''Wheelchair Maker'' before anyone else. The Bath chair (Figure 2) consisted of two large wheels in the rear, on either side of the seat, and a single, smaller wheel in front. An attendant could push the chair from behind while the passenger steered by way of a steering handle, or the attendant could turn the handle and wheel 180° and pull the chair. The seat resembled that of a buggy of the era. Wheels and framework were of iron. A canvas hood could be raised or lowered and a hinged flap in front protected the rider's legs.[5,8,9]

The Bath chair was not only appreciated by invalids, but persons of position and influence found them fashionable, so much so that by 1840, sedan chairs had virtually disappeared from the streets and squares of Bath.

Another drawing, dated 1798, displays more modest chairs employing two large rear wheels and one smaller, forward-pivoting wheel, to be pushed by an attendant. This can be said to be the nearest ancestor to the 20th century wheelchair.

The 19th century wheelchair was initially constructed of wood, followed by wicker, and then back to wood. One footboard soon became two. The two large wheels were changed from back to front and vice versa. Hoods were added, then dropped. Wooden wheels were replaced by bicycle wheels, complete with cranks to be turned by the occupant to effect propulsion. Later, hand rims were added. Overall, the chairs were made smaller and lighter, more versatile, self-propelling, and practical enough for commercial production.

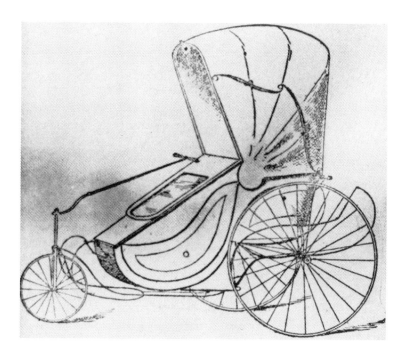

FIGURE 2. Bath chair. (From Kamenetz, H. L., *The Wheelchair Book,* Charles C Thomas, Springfield, IL, 1969. With permission.)

Prior to 1860, there are apparently no major records of the production or use of wheelchairs in North America, although they were obviously used. Everest and Jennings, Inc., long a wheelchair manufacturer, has in their archives a wooden New England chair made during the 1850s (Figure 3). During the American Civil War, there was the opportunity for major use of wheelchairs during the convalescing of untold thousands of wounded. The chairs were made of wood and were heavy, with two large (wooden) wheels forward with outside rims for propulsion and two smaller wheels at back (Figure 4). A Connecticut wheelchair in 1871 boasted a wood frame and a cane wicker seat, back, and legrest. This was considerably lighter than previous chairs (Figure 5).

In the 20th century, wheelchair developments followed industrial developments as a whole. Some of the evolutionary developments included wire-spoked wheels with inflatable tires as a result of the bicycle craze of the 1890s. A gentleman named A. O. Denly reported a cycle pioneer attaching a 1.75-horse power engine to an invalid tricycle in 1912.[3] This was probably the first motorized wheelchair. Carter of London began commercial manufacture of motorized chairs in 1916. An electrically driven chair was showing promise in 1903. In 1915, it was used during the San Francisco, San Diego, and Panama Pacific Expositions to shuttle hundreds of visitors to and fro. The chair consisted of a ten-cell, 12-V battery powering a three eighths-hp motor. Speeds could reach a mind-boggling 4.5 to 5 miles per hour.[5,9] Its four wheels and wicker body construction resembled a golf cart more than a wheelchair. Acceleration was accomplished by one of the two passengers depressing a pedal on the floor. Releasing the pedal would stop the conveyance within 24 inches.[5]

In post-World War I, the British Ministry of Pensions furnished hand-propelled tricycles to paraplegics and bilateral leg amputees. The British Red Cross provided motorized chairs to those who went farther than 3 miles to work.[6,7]

The first folding wheelchair was reported in a 1914 volume of *Scientific American.* The father of an invalid daughter collaborated with the superintendent of a wheelchair company who also had an invalid daughter. The result was a wheelchair that, when folded, measured

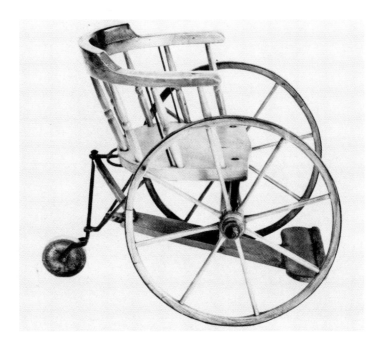

FIGURE 3. New England chair. (From *Wheelchair Selection: More Than Choosing a Chair with Wheels: Revised Edition,* Publ. No. 713, Sister Kenny Institute, Minneapolis, MN, 1977. With permission.

13 inches in height, 30 inches in length, and 20 inches in width. Made of seamless tubular steel and wood veneer, it weighed about 70 pounds, no more than the noncollapsing chairs of the era.[1,5] In 1933, Herbert A. Everest, a paraplegic, and Harry C. Jennings, a mechanical engineer, produced a lightweight, folding metal wheelchair which remained the standard for many years.

In 1950, a standing, self-propelled "chair" was demonstrated. It was propelled by hand cranks and chains turning the larger front wheels. In 1954, New York University constructed a curb-climbing chair under the sponsorship of the National Foundation For Infantile Paralysis. Via rotating handles, it allowed a person to get over curbs using the same force as on level ground.[11] The stair-climbing wheelchair was not a new idea. The first idea was patented in 1892, but of hundreds proposed, few have ever reached the market. Their size, weight, instability, and high price made them impractical. In 1960, the National Inventor's Council of the Department of Commerce, in cooperation with the President's Committee on Employment of the Handicapped (U.S.), offered a $5000 prize for the best design of a stair-climbing chair. The National Bureau of Standards selected, in 1965, a Canadian design from more than 500 entries. It featured battery-powered caterpillar tracks that could both ascend and descend (Figure 6). It has yet to reach major markets.[10]

Within the last 30 years, the availability of lighter, stronger metallic alloys plus the astute minds of disabled individuals not willing to vegetate have come together to produce wheelchairs that are lighter, more maneuverable, and more compact than any of the early fathers could have dreamed possible. Moreover, ambitious people like Kenneth Ginsterblum of Osage, Iowa, have added accessories such as a radio, head- and taillights, storage boxes, etc.[4] Also, current emphasis on wheelchair sports has resulted in the seat, frame, and wheels being moved, experimentally, to any and all positions in the quest for more speed and versatility.

Man's desire to move from one place to another, even if handicapped, has produced inventions over the years to reach this goal. The need for further improvement brings us

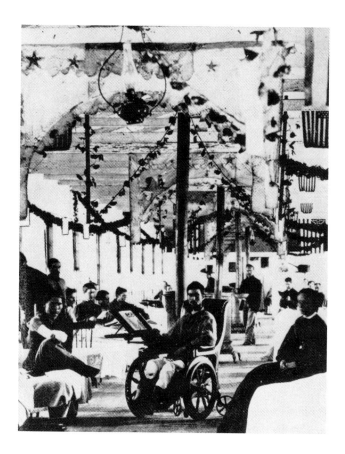

FIGURE 4. Union Convalescent Hospital ca. 1864. Illustration of heavy wooden, front-wheeled chair. (From Kamenetz, H. L., *The Wheelchair Book*, Charles C Thomas, Springfield, IL, 1969. With permission.)

closer to self-sufficiency. Development of the wheelchair from "wheeled cart" to modern sport chairs has had to proceed at a pace set by society as a whole, but society's attitudes toward the handicapped had to change as well. The "well-being" population had to realize the mental and physical needs of the "invalid". Once met and addressed, not shunted into a corner and ignored, the changed attitudes allowed others to take over and almost eliminate the word "handicapped" from a pitying vocabulary.

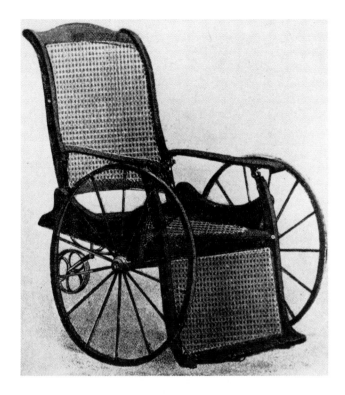

FIGURE 5. Wooden Connecticut chair ca. 1871. (From Kamenetz, H. L., *The Wheelchair Book,* Charles C Thomas, Springfield, IL, 1969. With permission.)

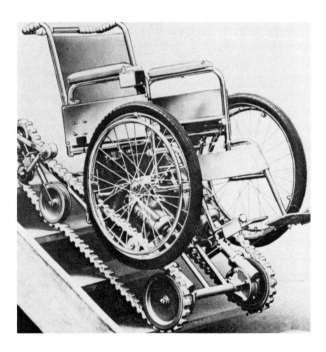

FIGURE 6. Stair-climbing wheelchair. (From Kamenetz, H. L., *The Wheelchair Book,* Charles C Thomas, Springfield, IL, 1969. With permission.)

REFERENCES

1. **Bond, A. R.,** A folding wheelchair, *Sci. Am.,* 110, 67, 1914.
2. **Conine, T. A. and Fuchs, E.,** Evolution of the wheelchair, *J. Am. Phys. Ther. Assoc.,* 45, 995, 1965.
3. **Denly, A. O.,** The user's viewpoint, *Paraplegia,* 2, 42, 1964.
4. **Anon.,** Electric wheelchair has radio and lights, *Pop. Mech.,* 88, 85, 1947.
5. **Anon.,** Evolution of the wheelchair, *Sci. Am.,* 112, 497, 502, 1915.
6. **Guttmann, L. (Chairman),** Symposium on the wheelchair (London 1963), *Paraplegia,* 2(1), 1964.
7. **Jolly, D. W.,** Symposium on the wheelchair, Ministry Practice (London 1963), *Paraplegia,* 2, 20, 1964.
8. **Kamenetz, H. L.,** A brief history of the wheelchair, *J. Hist. Med.,* 24, 205, 1969.
9. **Kamenetz, H. L.,** *The Wheelchair Book,* Charles C Thomas, Springfield, IL, 1969.
10. **Anon.,** Stair climbing wheelchair wins contest, *Bull. Prosthet. Res.,* 10, 212, 1965.
11. **Anon.,** Wheelchair that mounts curb to help patients travel unaided, *Paraplegia News,* 8, 1, 7, 1954.

Chapter 23

SEATING PROBLEMS AND SOLUTIONS

Stephen Tredwell and Lori Roxborough

TABLE OF CONTENTS

I. SEATING PROBLEMS AND SOLUTIONS

Although there is no "cookbook" approach to seating problems that can be used to solve all seating difficulties, certain seating scenarios, if identified, will respond to specific corrective measures. These may include modifications to the seating insert and the wheelchair and, in some instances, corrective surgery to the seated individual to improve an impediment to stable seating.

Problem solving in the quest for stable, comfortable, and functional seating requires the participation of all members of the seating team. Changes in one area may impact adversely in another, hence, it is essential in difficult seating situations that the problem be presented and discussed by the team at a seating clinic or rounds.

This section deals with commonly occurring postural problems, their possible causes, and suggested technical solutions. While not intended to be an extensive analysis, the following will serve as a quick reference for understanding and dealing with some of the common situations confronted when seating cerebral palsy children.

A. PELVIS

Problem: Posterior pelvic tilt (Figure 1)
Causes: 1. Hypertonicity of hip extensors or inability to silence hip extensor following active contraction
        2. Hamstring contracture
        3. Low tone or weakness of lumbar extensors
        4. Iatrogenic
          • Seat too long
          • Hammock seat
          • Legrest too extended
Solutions: 1. Firm back and seat of correct length
        2. Seat-to-back angle of <90° to inhibit hip extensor spasticity
        3. Hip belt — 45° in mild cases and bifurcating (Y-shaped) over anterior superior iliac spine in more severe cases (Figure 2)
        4. Antithrust seat — Provides a block to anterior movement of the ischial tuberosities (Figure 3)
        5. Pelvic stabilizer — Provides a block to anterior movement of the pubic symphysis (Figure 4)
        6. Pelvic bar — Rigid restraint positioned immediately inferior to the anterior superior iliac spines (Figure 5)
        7. Sacral pad and knee block (must be used with close attention to intervening joints when pelvic control is being attempted from a distant point, i.e., hip and knee joints) (Figure 6)

Problem: Anterior pelvic tilt
Causes: 1. Hypertonicity of hip flexors or inability to silence hip flexors following active contraction
        2. Hip flexion contracture
        3. Hypertonicity of lumbar extensors
        4. Hypotonia or weakness of abdominals
Solutions: 1. Inhibition of hip flexor tone through use of a flat seat (to increase hip extension)
        2. Accommodation of hip flexion contracture by wedging
        3. Hip belt positioned over the anterior superior iliac spines to prevent anterior movement of the upper pelvis

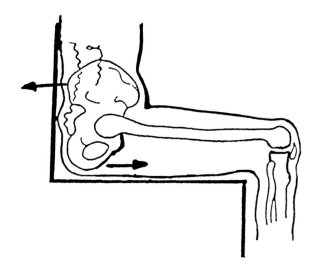

FIGURE 1.   Posterior pelvic tilt.

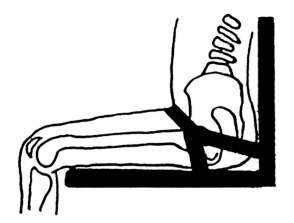

FIGURE 2.   ''Y''-belt.

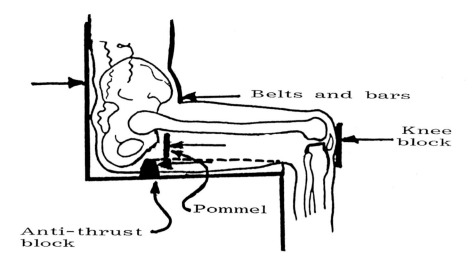

FIGURE 3.   Antithrust seat provides a block to anterior movement of the ischial tuberosities.

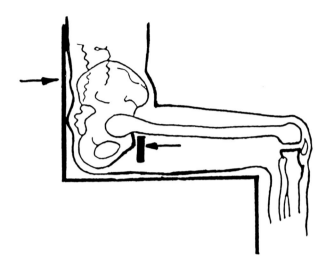

FIGURE 4.   Pommel pelvic stabilizers.

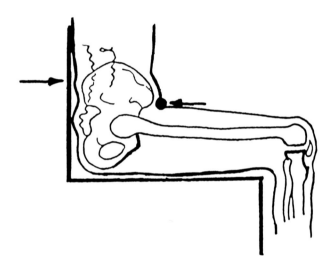

FIGURE 5.   Rigid sub-ASIS bar.

Problem: Pelvic obliquity
Causes: 1. Spasticity of trunk side flexors
2. Unilateral hip extensor spasticity
3. Iatrogenic — hammock seat
Solutions: 1. Firm seat
2. Lateral pelvic supports
3. Bifurcate hip belt
4. Pelvic positioners
5. Pelvic bar (Figure 7)
6. Accommodation through seat molding for fixed deformities

Problem: Pelvic rotation
Causes: 1. Asymmetrical tone in hip adductor or abductors
2. Asymmetrical tone in trunk rotators

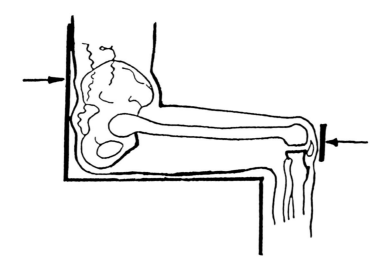

FIGURE 6.   Sacral pad and knee block for control of posterior pelvic tilt.

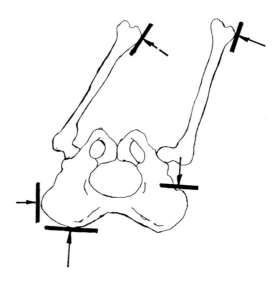

FIGURE 7.   Pelvic control of rotation with pelvic positioners or a pelvic bar for windswept hips.

3. Iatrogenic
   ● Failure to accommodate a true leg length discrepancy in the seating sys-
     tem
   ● Failure to accommodate a hip adduction or abduction contracture in the
     seating system

Solutions: 1. Bifurcate hip belt in mild cases
          2. Pelvic positioners placed below the anterior superior iliac spine on the side
             of the pelvis which is rotated forward (used in combination with a firm back
             board) (Figure 8)
          3. Appropriate accommodation of leg length discrepancy or hip abduction/ad-
             duction contracture

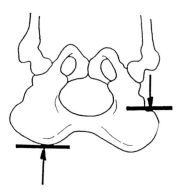

FIGURE 8.   Pelvic positioners placed below the anterior superior iliac spine with firm backboard to correct pelvic rotation.

B. TRUNK

Problem: Forward flexion
Causes: 1. Compensation for posterior pelvic tilt
                 2. Abdominal muscle hypertonicity
                 3. Weight of the arms pulling the trunk into flexion
                 4. Iatrogenic — sling back
Solutions: 1. Support the pelvis
                 2. Firm backboard
                 3. Use of arm supports (armrests, tray)
                 4. In severe cases, use of three-point sagittal plane control consisting of anterior pelvic control, firm backboard, and anterior trunk supports such as a chest panel or rigid shoulder pads
                 5. Use of a spinal orthosis if total contact required
                 6. Accommodate through custom contouring if a fixed kyphosis present
                 7. Alter the orientation in space to decrease the influence of gravity

Problem: Trunk side flexion
Causes: 1. Poor feedback
                 2. Poor sustained control of trunk muscles
                 3. Muscle tone imbalance in trunk side flexors
                 4. Compensation for pelvic obliquity
Solutions: 1. Firm seat board with lateral pelvic support
                 2. Use of a standard precontoured lateral trunk molding to provide midline feedback for individuals who are able to self-correct, but lack position sense
                 3. Lateral trunk supports
                 4. Three-point coronal plane control in severe cases, i.e., lateral pelvic support, trunk support over the apex of the curve, and a trunk support on the opposite side in the axillary region (Figure 9) (Swing-away trunk supports are required for a closer fit)
                 5. Use of thoraco-lumbar-sacral orthosis when total contact required

Problem: Trunk rotation
Causes: 1. Asymmetrical muscle tone
                 2. Asymmetrical trunk control

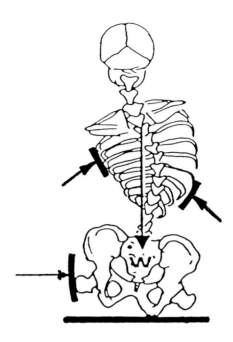

FIGURE 9. Three-point coronal plane control in scoliosis.

Solutions: 1. Use of curved trunk supports to provide anterior control on the side which is rotated forward (must be used in combination with a firm back)
2. Chest straps and panels
3. Anterior shoulder pads

C. HIPS

Problem: Extension
Causes: 1. Spasticity of hip extensors
2. Difficulty silencing extensors following active contraction
3. Hamstring contracture
4. Iatrogenic — sling seat
Solutions: 1. Firm seat and back
2. Seat wedging to decrease extensor tone
3. Accommodation of hamstring contracture by allowing sufficient knee flexion
4. Pelvic support

Problem: Flexion
Causes: 1. Spasticity of hip flexors
2. Hip flexion contracture
3. Difficulty silencing flexors following active contraction
4. Iatrogenic — footplates too high
Solutions: 1. Inhibition of flexor tone using a flat or anteriorly tipped seat
2. Footplates at appropriate height
3. Accommodation through wedging if fixed contractures present
4. Good pelvic control required to prevent anterior pelvic tilt during flexor spasms

Problem: Adduction
Causes: 1. Adductor spasticity
2. Adductor contracture
3. Inability to silence adductors following active contraction
4. Abduction of the opposite hip, inducing pelvic rotation and passive adduction of the observed hip
5. Dislocated hip
6. Iatrogenic
   - Sling seat
   - Footplates too high, resulting in loss of thigh contract with the support surface and consequent adduction and internal rotation of the hips to stabilize
Solutions: 1. Firm seat board with good thigh contact
2. Use of medial thigh support (abductor) as part of the seat contour in mild cases, as a separate component in more severe cases (The abductor should be constructed of rigid materials to prevent stimulation of the stretch reflex.)
3. Control pelvic rotation
4. Accommodation of fixed contracture through construction of an asymmetrical seat and placement of the abductor off-center

Problem: Abduction
Causes: 1. Abductor spasticity
2. Inability to silence the abductors following active contraction
3. Abduction contracture
4. Adduction of the opposite hip, inducing pelvic rotation and passive abduction of observed limb in the seating system
Solutions: 1. Use of lateral thigh supports (adductor)
2. Control pelvic rotation
3. Accommodate a fixed contracture through construction of an asymmetrical seat (if unilateral) or wide anterior seat surface (if bilateral)

Problem: Windswept hips
Causes: 1. Asymmetrical muscle tone above and/or below the hip
2. Different motor synergies present in each limb
3. Unilateral abductor or adductor spasticity or contracture inducing pelvic rotation and windswept positioning
Solutions: 1. Good pelvic control of rotation with pelvic positioners or a pelvic bar
2. Correction of abduction/adduction posture of hips if range is available
3. Accommodation of fixed hip deformities using an asymmetrical seat

Problem: Leg length discrepancy
Causes: True
1. Hip dislocation
2. Surgical shortening (varus osteotomy)
3. Unequal skeletal development

Apparent
1. Abduction or adduction contracture
2. Pelvic rotation

Solutions: 1. Accommodation is required in the case of a true leg length discrepancy through construction of a seat with a cutout at the anterior aspect for the shorter thigh.
2. Correction of an apparent leg length discrepancy through control of pelvic rotation and hip position

D. SCAPULAE POSITION
Shoulder girdle postural abnormalities are frequently compensatory in nature and therefore should be closely examined in relation to the posture of other segments.

Problem: Retraction
Causes: 1. Spasticity in scapular retractors
2. Fixing of the shoulders to compensate for poor trunk control
Solutions: 1. Provision of appropriate pelvic and trunk support
2. Provision of sternal pressure using a chest panel or anterior shoulder supports angled inward to facilitate active protraction
3. Use of a tray to support the upper limbs in forward flexion
4. Shoulder wedges (protractors) (Shoulder wedges should be used with good anterior trunk supports to prevent the trunk from being levered forward as the scapulae retract against the supports.)

Problem: Protraction
Causes: 1. Spasticity in scapular protractors
2. Weight of the arms when the trunk is forward flexed
Solutions: 1. Good pelvic and trunk supports
2. Armrests or a tray for arm support
3. Shoulder straps over the lateral aspect of the shoulders
4. Shoulder pads angled outward in more severe cases

Problem: Elevation
Causes: 1. Upward pull on the scapula by the upper fibers of trapezius and levator scapulae when the neck is side flexed
2. Inability to stabilize scapulae during attempted, active head movements
Solutions: 1. Shoulder straps with a slightly downward angle of pull over the shoulder
2. Rigid shoulder pads

E. HEAD/NECK
As with scapulae position, many abnormal head and neck postures are compensatory in nature.

Problem: Flexion
Causes: 1. Spasticity of neck flexors
2. Lack of stable origin for the neck extensors
3. Inability to actively extend against gravity
Solutions: 1. Appropriate support of the pelvis, trunk, and shoulder girdle
2. Good upper limb support on a tray
3. "Halo" to prevent neck flexion beyond the point of active recovery
4. Headband of elastic material to provide increasing resistance to flexion
5. Alter the orientation of the seating system in space to decrease the influence of gravity

Problem: Extension
Causes: 1. Spasticity of neck extensors
2. Compensatory for forward trunk flexion
Solutions: 1. Appropriate control of the pelvis, trunk, and shoulder girdle
2. Use of a neckrest (avoid occipital pressure)

Problem: Cervical flexion with atlanto-occipital extension (gooseneck posture)
Causes: 1. Compensatory for trunk flexion and scapular protraction
2. Compensatory posture when head control is poor
Solutions: 1. Appropriate control of the pelvis, trunk, and shoulder girdle
2. Neckrest contoured in two places (cup shaped)

II. SEATING SYSTEM SELECTION

Selecting the appropriate seating system for each child is a process of matching needs with available technology. For the child with mild seating problems, modular seating systems consisting of standard components are often selected. Multiadjustable seating systems are generally prescribed for individuals with moderate to severe motor disorders in the absence of severe deformities. Custom-contoured systems are generally prescribed for individuals with severe structural deformities. A number of commercial manufacturers produce seating systems within each of aforementioned categories. The ever-changing range of components available precludes an exhaustive list in a text of this nature.

In seating the cerebral palsy child, several factors must be considered:

1. The seat (i.e., the chair) is the primary treatment mode for these patients.
2. To understand handicapped seating, normal seating must be understood.
3. The chair seat must first be fitted; then the angle between the seat and back must be determined along with modifications, such as medial and lateral thigh bolsters being applied to the seat as needed; and, finally, the chair back should be fixed.
4. While surgery can be a powerful adjunct in the management of seating problems, nonoperative management is usually preferable in treating the cerebral palsy child.
5. The decision to operate cannot be made in isolation. Knowledge of the patient's current functional ability, including his/her sitting tolerances and communication skills as well as other environmental control needs, a survey of the patient's change in function over the past several years, and attendants' reports are essential parts of an appropriate evaluation.

ACKNOWLEDGMENT

The authors gratefully acknowledge the editorial assistance provided by Lawrence A. Davis, M.A.

SUGGESTED READINGS

Bergen, A. F. and Colangelo, C., *Positioning the Client with Central Nervous Systems Deficits,* Valhalla Rehabilitation Publications, Valhalla, NY, 1982.

Bobath, B. and Bobath, K., *Motor Development in Different Types of Cerebral Palsy,* White Friars Press, London, 1975.

Carr, J. H., Shephard, R. B., Gordon, J., Gentile, A. M., and Held, J. M., *Movement Science: Foundation for Physical Therapy in Rehabilitation,* Aspen Publishers, Rockville, MD, 1987.

Connolly, B. H. and Montgomery, P. C., Eds., *Therapeutic Exercise in Developmental Disabilities,* Chattanooga Corporation, Chattanooga, TN, 1987.

Henderson, B. (Compiler), *Seating in Review: Current Trends for the Disabled,* Otto Bock Orthopedic Industries, Winnipeg, Manitoba, 1989.

McDonald, E. T., *Treating Cerebral Palsy: For Clinicians by Clinicians,* PRO-ED, Austin, TX, 1987.

Nashner, L. M., *A Functional Approach to Understanding Spasticity, Electomyography and Evoked Potentials,* Struppler, A. and Weindle, A., Eds., Springer-Verlag, Berlin, 1985.

Nashner, L. M., Shumway-Cook, A., and Marin, O., Stance posture control in select groups of children with cerebral palsy: deficits in sensory organization and muscular coordination, *Exp. Brain Res.,* 49, 393, 1983.

Trefler, E., Ed., *Seating for Children with Cerebral Palsy: A Resource Manual,* University of Tennessee, Memphis, 1984.

Ward, D. E., *Positioning the Handicapped Child for Function,* 2nd ed. rev., Phoenix Press, Chicago, 1984.

Zacharkow, D., *Posture: Sitting, Standing Chair Design and Exercise,* Charles C Thomas, Springfield, IL, 1988.

APPENDIX
SEATING SYSTEMS

Mulholland Seating System

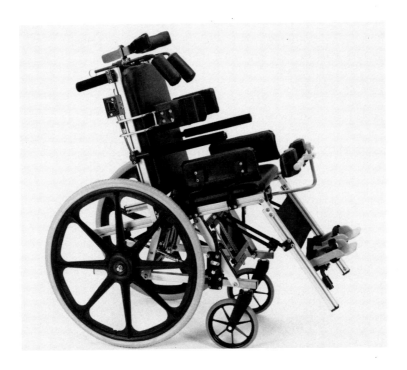

FIGURE 1. The Mulholland System. The Mulholland adjustable chair, developed in the early 1970s by Nancy Mulholland, a physiotherapist, and her husband, an engineer, provided a very versatile and adjustable seating unit. Optimum positioning of the child or junior adult in space is facilitated by variable geometric features. It is a modular unit and the insert has been crash tested to verify its suitability as a car seat.

Gillette Modular Seating System

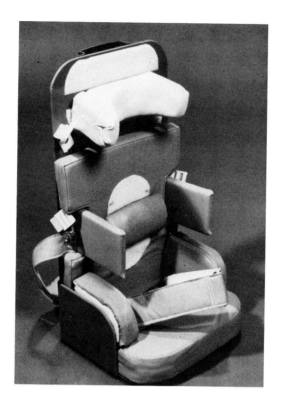

FIGURE 2. The Gillette seating support orthosis (SSO) System. The Gillette SSO, using premanufactured plastic shells, is a modular type of seating system that has greatly lowered the unit cost of the insert. A mobile seating service in Minnesota allows the delivery of seating services to more remote areas of the state.

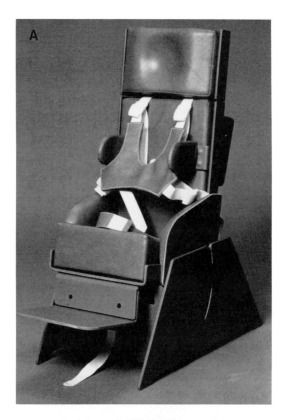

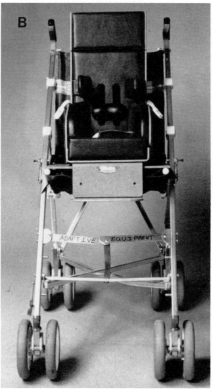

FIGURE 3.   The Gillette Upholstered Seating Support Orthosis. (A) Plastic frame with modular seating components; (B) modular insert which can be transferred to stroller.

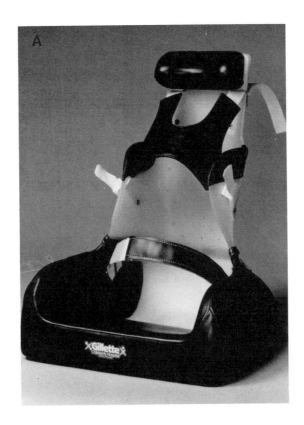

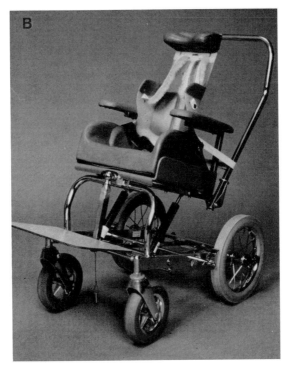

FIGURE 4. The Gillette molded seating support orthosis (SSO) (A and B). (Courtesy of David Wilkie, Gillette Children's Hospital, St. Paul, MN.)

Winnipeg Modular Seating System

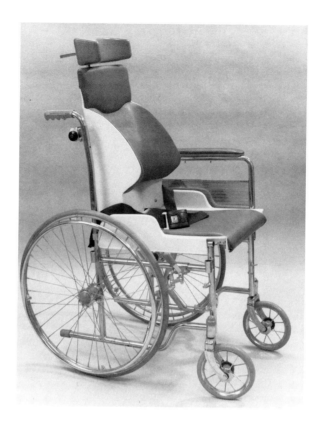

FIGURE 5.   The Winnipeg Modular Seating System. A modular seating system involving many separate components of the seat was developed at the Rehabilitation Centre for Children in Winnipeg. These were of various sizes and allowed a seating system to be fabricated from the component parts at much lower cost with functionality being maintained. This system has been further refined and marketed by the Canadian Posture and Seating Centre in Kitchener, Ontario.

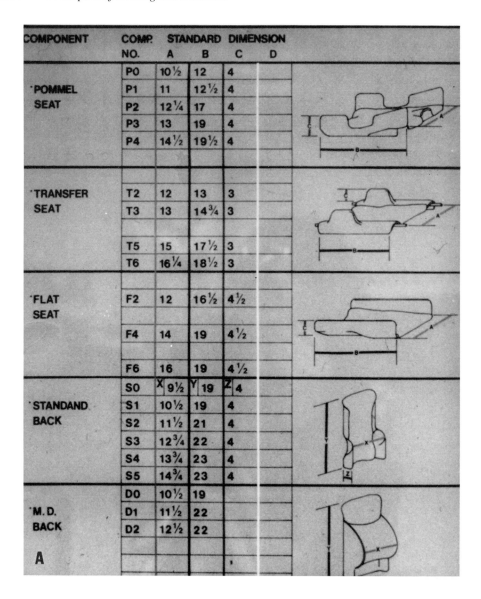

COMPONENT	COMP. NO.	STANDARD DIMENSION			
		A	B	C	D
POMMEL SEAT	P0	10½	12	4	
	P1	11	12½	4	
	P2	12¼	17	4	
	P3	13	19	4	
	P4	14½	19½	4	
TRANSFER SEAT	T2	12	13	3	
	T3	13	14¾	3	
	T5	15	17½	3	
	T6	16¼	18½	3	
FLAT SEAT	F2	12	16½	4½	
	F4	14	19	4½	
	F6	16	19	4½	
	S0	X 9½	Y 19	Z 4	
STANDARD BACK	S1	10½	19	4	
	S2	11½	21	4	
	S3	12¾	22	4	
	S4	13¾	23	4	
	S5	14¾	23	4	
M.D. BACK	D0	10½	19		
	D1	11½	22		
	D2	12½	22		
				•	

FIGURE 6. The Winnipeg Modular Seating System. (A) Examples of modular components available.

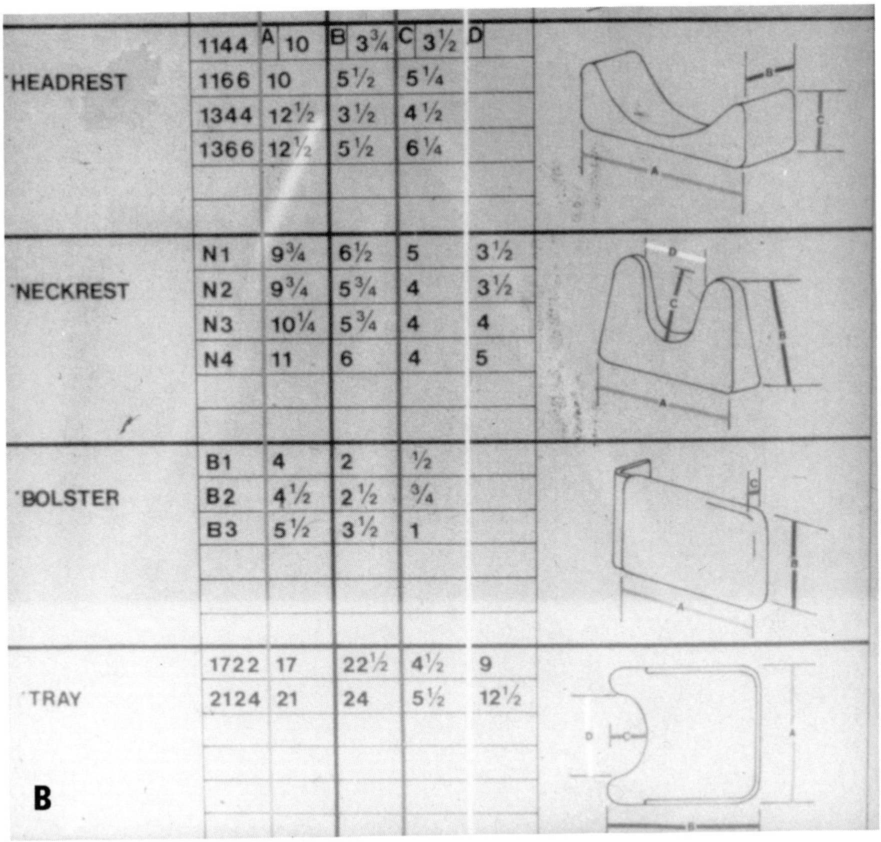

		A	B	C	D
HEADREST	1144	10	3¾	3½	
	1166	10	5½	5¼	
	1344	12½	3½	4½	
	1366	12½	5½	6¼	
NECKREST	N1	9¾	6½	5	3½
	N2	9¾	5¾	4	3½
	N3	10¼	5¾	4	4
	N4	11	6	4	5
BOLSTER	B1	4	2	½	
	B2	4½	2½	¾	
	B3	5½	3½	1	
TRAY	1722	17	22½	4½	9
	2124	21	24	5½	12½

B

FIGURE 6 (continued).   (B) Examples of modular components available.

Canadian Posture and Seating System

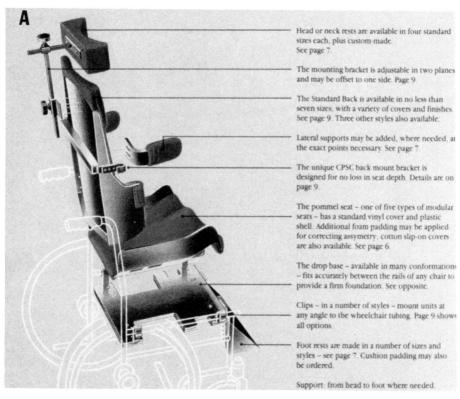

A

Head or neck rests are available in four standard sizes each, plus custom-made. See page 7.

The mounting bracket is adjustable in two planes and may be offset to one side. Page 9.

The Standard Back is available in no less than seven sizes, with a variety of covers and finishes. See page 9. Three other styles also available.

Lateral supports may be added, where needed, at the exact points necessary. See page 7.

The unique CPSC back mount bracket is designed for no loss in seat depth. Details are on page 9.

The pommel seat – one of five types of modular seats – has a standard vinyl cover and plastic shell. Additional foam padding may be applied for correcting assymetry; cotton slip-on covers are also available. See page 6.

The drop base – available in many conformations – fits accurately between the rails of any chair to provide a firm foundation. See opposite.

Clips – in a number of styles – mount units at any angle to the wheelchair tubing. Page 9 shows all options.

Foot rests are made in a number of sizes and styles – see page 7. Cushion padding may also be ordered.

Support: from head to foot where needed.

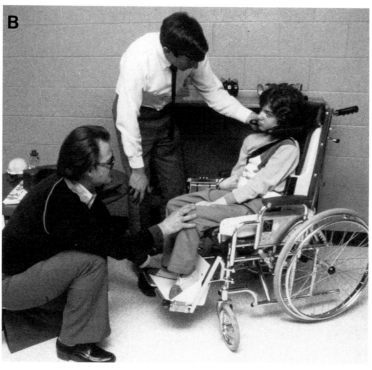

B

FIGURE 7.   The Canadian Posture and Seating Centre System. (A) Modular wheelchair insert system; (B) in use.

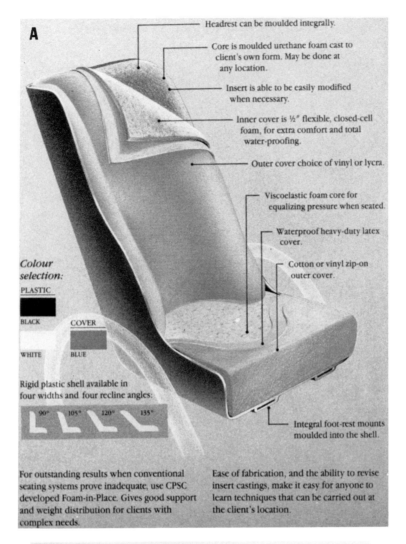

A

Headrest can be moulded integrally.

Core is moulded urethane foam cast to client's own form. May be done at any location.

Insert is able to be easily modified when necessary.

Inner cover is ½" flexible, closed-cell foam, for extra comfort and total water-proofing.

Outer cover choice of vinyl or lycra.

Viscoelastic foam core for equalizing pressure when seated.

Waterproof heavy-duty latex cover.

Cotton or vinyl zip-on outer cover.

Integral foot-rest mounts moulded into the shell.

Colour selection:

PLASTIC

BLACK   COVER

WHITE   BLUE

Rigid plastic shell available in four widths and four recline angles:

90°   105°   120°   135°

For outstanding results when conventional seating systems prove inadequate, use CPSC developed Foam-in-Place. Gives good support and weight distribution for clients with complex needs.

Ease of fabrication, and the ability to revise insert castings, make it easy for anyone to learn techniques that can be carried out at the client's location.

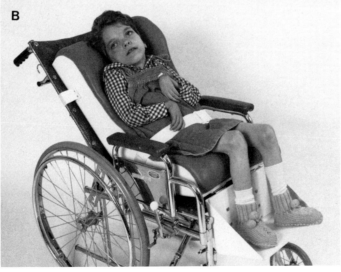

B

FIGURE 8. The Canadian Posture and Seating Centre (CPSC) System. (A) The CPSC Foam-in-Place (FIP) wheelchair insert; (B) in use.

Otto Bock Seating Systems

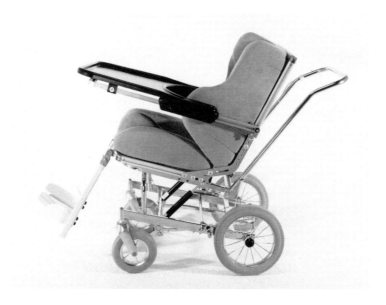

FIGURE 9. The Otto Bock Seating System. Customized wheelchair insert for the severely incapacitated.

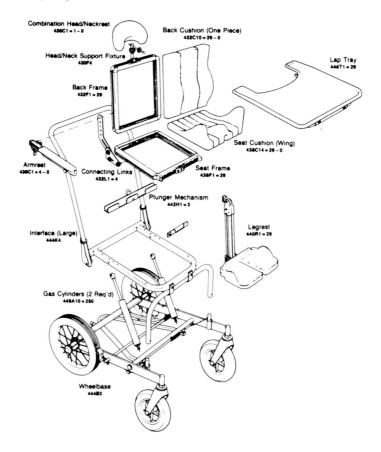

FIGURE 10. The Otto Bock Modular Orthotic Seating System.

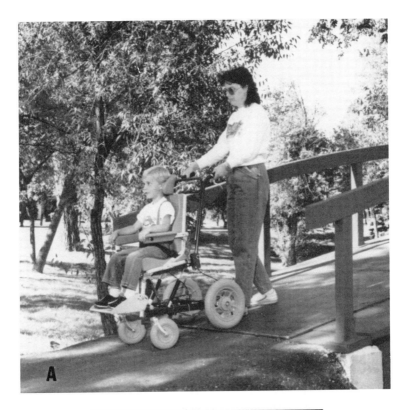

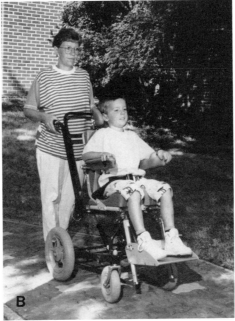

FIGURE 11. The Otto Bock Juvenile Modular Seating System. (A and B) Examples of two versions.

Bead Matrix Seating System

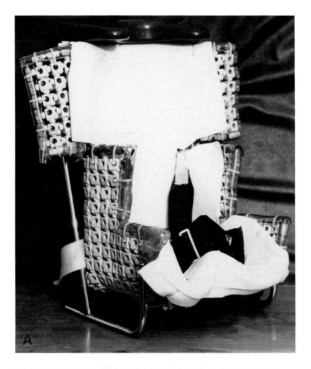

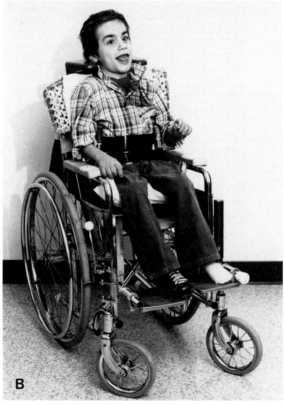

FIGURE 12.   The Bead Matrix System. (A) Component; (B) in use.

Foam-in-Place/Foam-in-Box Seating Systems

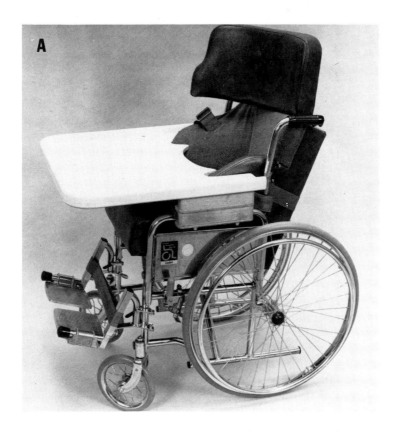

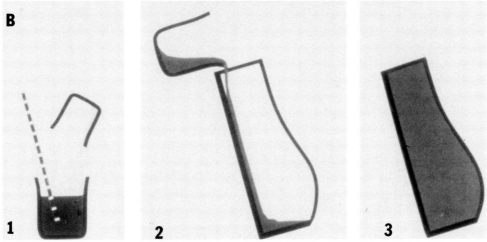

FIGURE 13.   The Foam-in-Place/Foam-in-Box Systems. (A) The Foam-in-Place system of seating was initially popularized by the seating team at the Rehabilitation Centre for Children, Winnipeg, Canada, and was further developed at the University of Tennessee, Memphis, by Hobson and Associates; (B) The Foam-in-Box system is a particularly useful technique for difficult deformities which are not amenable to surgical correction: (1) mix and stir liquid foam components, (2) pour into mold, and (3) foam rises, fills mold, and sets.

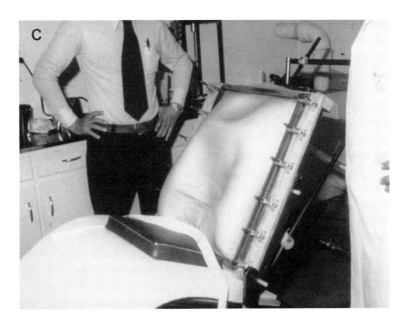

FIGURE 13 (continued).   (C) The seat is formed around the seated individual, resulting in a comfortable total contract unit that is both cosmetically and functionally very acceptable.

INDEX

A

Abduction seating
  alternative seating devices, 288
  castor carts, 277, 279
  infants, 9, 46
  juvenile seating goals, 69
  pelvic obliquity and, 133
Abduction wings, 68, 288, 290
Acetabular development, 46
Acrylonitrile-butadiene-styrene (ABS), 29—30
Active posture control, 5
Adaptive Firmware Card, 306
Adductor contracture, 346
  head-injured patient, 229
  hip dislocation and, 162
  pelvic obliquity and, 132
Adductor myotomy, 162
Adductor release, 62—63
Adductor tenotomy
  head-injured patient, 230
  hip pain relief, 84
  infant abduction seating and, 46
  pelvic obliquity prevention and, 135
Adolescent seating, 15—17, 80—94
  deformity severity, 80
  hip pain, 84—85
  powered chairs, 85—87
  spinal curvature, 82—84
  weight problems, 80—82
A-frame, 11, 279
Aging, physiological changes of, 98
Air-filled cushions, 28
Aliplast orthosis, 86
Allergic sensitivity, 29, 31
Alternative/augmentative communication systems, 304—316; see also Communication
Alternative seating, 39, 75, 288—302; see also specific systems
Aluminum construction, 319, 323
Ambulatory clients, 98—102
American Sign Language, 310
Amigo™, 267
Amputation, 46
Amputee seating, 106
Ancient history, 331
Ankle-foot orthosis (AFO), 62, 162, 165
  head-injured patient, 230
  standing aids and, 279
Anterior pelvic tilt, 340
Antithrust block, 161
Antithrust seat, 340—341
Arm support
  elderly clients, 99—102
  high-level quadriplegics, 246
  invalid chairs, 331

juvenile seating goals, 58
muscular dystrophy, 175
spinal cord-injured, 244
trays and, 58, 69, 87, 94, 248
trunk flexion and, 344
Arthrogryposis, 46, 113, 220—224
Arthroplasty, 136
Assessment, 38—39
  cerebral palsy patient, 158—165
  communication system, 314—316
  head-injured patient, 228—229
  muscular dystrophy patient, 173—174
  for powered mobility, 264, 267—270
  pressure sore risk, 160
Asymmetrical sitting, 63, 155
  pelvic obliquity and, 132
  scoliosis and, 161
  spinal orthosis and, 72
Ataxia, 152
Athetosis, 152
Athletics, see Wheelchair sports
Automated shape assessment, 108

B

Back, sitting forces at, 66
Back height
  for spinal cord-injured, 244, 247
  sports chairs and, 250
Back support, see Trunk support
Balancing, of wheels, 320
Balloon, Rick, 284
Base, 11
  cerebral palsy patient, 160
  client assessment for, 38—39
  engineering aspects, 26—27
  high-level quadriplegics, 246
Basketball, 318—319, 324, 327
Bath chair, 332—333
Bathing, 51, 53—54, 300
Bathing, osteogenesis imperfecta children, 204, 207—208
Baxter and D'Astous criteria, 136, 138
Bead Matrix System, 364
Bead-seat system, 178
Bean bag
  alternative sitting, 290—291, 295—296
  for fixed deformity child, 80
  for self-abusive patients, 256
  stretcher, 229
Behavior modification, 256
Belts, durability of, 28—29
Bicycles, 185, 271
Biomechanics, 3—4, 188—189
Bliss Symbol Board, 13, 16, 77, 304, 310
Blistering, 327